RHETORIC OF HEALTH AND MEDICINE AS/IS

RHETORIC OF HEALTH AND MEDICINE AS/IS

THEORIES AND APPROACHES FOR THE FIELD

EDITED BY

Lisa Melançon

S. Scott Graham

Jenell Johnson

John A. Lynch

Cynthia Ryan

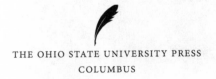

THE OHIO STATE UNIVERSITY PRESS

COLUMBUS

Library of Congress Cataloging-in-Publication Data

Names: Melançon, Lisa K., editor. | Graham, S. Scott, editor. | Johnson, Jenell M., 1978– editor. | Lynch, John (John Alexander), 1976– editor. | Ryan, Cynthia, editor.

Title: Rhetoric of health and medicine as/is : theories and approaches for the field / edited by Lisa Melançon, S. Scott Graham, Jenell Johnson, John A. Lynch, and Cynthia Ryan.

Description: Columbus : The Ohio State University Press, [2020] | Includes bibliographical references and index. | Summary: "Examines how rhetoric can be used to study the social, cultural, economic, and political aspects of health and medicine. Addresses interdisciplinary perspectives"—Provided by publisher.

Identifiers: LCCN 2020011960 | ISBN 9780814214466 (cloth) | ISBN 0814214460 (cloth) | ISBN 9780814278178 (ebook) | ISBN 0814278175 (ebook)

Subjects: LCSH: Communication in medicine. | Health. | Rhetoric.

Classification: LCC R118 .R44 2020 | DDC 610.1/4—dc23

LC record available at https://lccn.loc.gov/2020011960

Cover design by Alexa Love
Text design by Juliet Williams
Type set in Adobe Minion Pro

CONTENTS

FOREWORD

JUDY Z. SEGAL

HERE IS an exchange that I documented, in a postsurgical recovery room, at a Canadian hospital, winter 2012:

> NURSE: What's your pain like, on a 10-point scale?
> ME: About a 6.
> NURSE: I'll add some fentanyl.
> ME: No, please, don't. I'd rather be in pain than nauseated.
> NURSE: Can't let you out of recovery as long as your pain is a 6. What is it now?
> ME: 4.

And then I was given my things and discharged.

I have many such field notes. I've had more than a few medical encounters in my life, and, if I am able, whenever I am being charted by a health professional, I chart them right back: I transcribe our dialogue—as well as some overheard conversations—because what we say to each other, especially at moments of our uncertainty, is enormously important. *As* a set of dispositions and theoretical orientations, Rhetoric of Health and Medicine (RHM) *is* an assembly of procedures aimed at discovering what's going on, in contexts of health and medicine, when people act discursively on other people. As we seem in North America to be living in an age of health itself (an age when we are invited, relentlessly, to consider our diet, exercise, weight, blood pressure, bowel movements, states of mind, cholesterol level, energy level, consumption of drugs—as well as, increasingly, our personal responsibility for all of that), rhetoricians of health and medicine have important work to do. They can help us figure out how to navigate our health-world critically, and then, it might follow, sensibly. Rhetoricians can help us also enact a health citizenship that doesn't end at the boundaries of our individual bodies; they can help us sort through health ideologies, health politics and policies, health insurance, and health inequities—health power in general.

So, I've not been surprised to notice that, while my own students once were drawn to RHM in the course of their study of rhetoric more broadly, many of them now are drawn to rhetoric more broadly in the course of their study of RHM. During undergraduate and graduate courses in the field, students learn, for example, that J. Blake Scott (2003) turned critical attention to the rhetoric, ethics, and politics of HIV testing; Carol Berkenkotter (2008) illuminated the rhetoric of psychiatric case histories, tying this medical genre to its times; Lisa Keränen (2010) explored the role of rhetorical character—and trust—in a medical-research controversy; Kimberly Emmons (2010) made a case for "rhetorical care of the self" as a critical response to depression discourse; Amy Koerber (2013) composed a rhetorical history of infant feeding; Jenell Johnson (2014) composed a rhetorical history of lobotomy; Marika Seigel (2014) offered a rhetorical-usability critique of pregnancy manuals; S. Scott Graham (2015) used an expansive rhetorical theory to reconfigure problems of pain and pain medicine; Colleen Derkatch (2016) theorized the rhetorical boundary work that Western medicine does to keep Complementary and Alternative Medicine at its borders; Robin Jensen (2016) viewed "involuntary childlessness" through a rhetorical-historical lens; and Melanie Yergeau (2018) wrote about autistic identity and the "demi-rhetoricity" assigned to the "neuroqueer/ed."[1] Teachers/researchers/authors in RHM have captured adherents to their projects because the theoretical frameworks, methodologies, topics, and questions that characterize RHM are compelling, capacious, and current.

And also because of this: a hallmark of rhetorical criticism has always been, and is, increasingly, its interventionist and ameliorative mood in the face of its questions. Kenneth Burke (1973) wrote his rhetorical critique of *Mein Kampf,* and placed it before a wide audience in talks and publications: "[L]et us try to discover," he said, "what kind of 'medicine' [Hitler] concocted,

---

1. This is a list of book-length studies only, and, of course, a partial list. See http://medicalrhetoric.com/bibliography for many more titles in RHM.

that we may know, with greater accuracy, exactly what to guard against, if we are to forestall the concocting of similar medicine in America" (p. 191). (We might want to think further about Burke's project.) As one of many rhetorical critics with a similarly optimistic impulse, Barbara Warnick (1992) wrote that the "advocate critic" seeks "to persuade, to change readers' perspectives through the process of criticism" (p. 233). Intervention and amelioration are clearly desiderata of much work in RHM. In 2003, a formative year for the discipline, Scott (referring to Celeste Condit speaking of the rhetoric of science) wrote that the rhetorician "must also be a *rhetor* in the fully civic sense of that word" (p. 30).

A central question in rhetorical study is "Who is persuading whom of what, and what are the means of persuasion?"[2] As it forms and re-forms, directs and redirects, this question, RHM has composed a discipline that has a complex relation to disciplinarity. We can say that RHM is *inter*disciplinary, as it traverses several fields, both to identify partners in study (often, for example, deploying methods of the social sciences) and to isolate objects of study (medical research, health policy, and so on). Already-formed *interdisciplines,* like Health/Medical Humanities, Science and Technology Studies, and Disability Studies, include RHM, but not in a mode that is simply *multi*disciplinary—for multidisciplinarity would require demarcating fields; how might any of these inquiry-based projects map rhetoric precisely in contrast to sociology (the work, for example, of Conrad, 2007, on medicalization), or anthropology (Mol, 2008, on "the logic of care"[3]), or philosophy (Hacking, 1999, on "interactive kinds"), or literary studies (Belling, 2012, on the discursive drivers of health anxiety)? And RHM is *trans*disciplinary—to the extent that, like narrative studies, for example, it is a framework somewhat portable across many research disciplines. In considering RHM's disciplinary self and its disciplinary relations, it is useful, I think, to see it also as *poly*disciplinary: along with some core commitments (as, for example, to the suasive nature of discourse) and core values (typically, values of social justice), RHM has many expressions. It is "poly" in the way of polyamory: it is open to opportunities for alliance, and it may shape-shift a little to make each relationship work.

RHM's polydisciplinary inclinations provide one reason that it is interesting to mobilize an **as/is** framework in the first place: we can talk about RHM

---

2. This may not be every rhetorician's central question. It is the one that I learned from my mentor, Nan Johnson, and it has never failed me. Professor Johnson taught me also to ask "How do we come to believe what we believe, and what would it take to make us change our minds?"

3. It is not easy to "discipline" Mol, who is an ethnographer and philosopher; Mol has been a professor of anthropology and of political theory.

as having field coherence while it *is* a diverse set of practices and partnerships. Field identification with practical diversity characterizes this welcome volume of essays. One definition of rhetorical criticism is "criticism performed by a rhetoric critic" (Segal, 2005, p. 7). The definition is more than tautological: a rhetorical critic is, in the first instance, a person trained within a scholarly tradition on public discourse into a rhetorical subjectivity and sensitivity that suggest certain habits of mind. The "rhetorical subjectivity" of the authors in this volume binds their essays together, while their projects range widely and testify to the reach, the agility, and the usefulness, of RHM.

The foci and questions of the essays furthermore enact an essential principle of rhetoric itself: *kairos*—discursive action at the opportune moment, the fitness of that action to contingencies of time and place. *Kairos* is central to discursive performance if rhetoricians are also rhetors. The essays here both arise from and return something to exigent rhetorical situations. The essays are appropriate both internally, to their location within RHM and its associated disciplines, and externally, to their location in matters and material conditions that concern us right now.

I can specify the *kairotic* virtues of this volume by addressing, for example, the essays in its second section, on representations and online health. In 2009 Karen Kopelson and I each published an essay on internet health. My essay, doing one kind of RHM (basically, Aristotelian analysis, tilted sociologically) appeared in *Written Communication*. It argued that since people seek out information on the web in various states of mind—ranging from middle-of-the-night panicked to just health-curious—critics might invoke the *rhetorical triangle* to help sort out internet persuasions. They should, that is, consider not only the source of information (the speaker) and the information provided (the subject)—which is what most critics at the time were doing—but also the users of sites (the audience). Sources, I argued, don't have to be unreliable, or their information wrong, for an internet health search to be a negative or even harmful experience. Kopelson's essay, doing another kind of RHM (textual study, primarily, tracking the e-patient as they emerged rhetorically in medical literature) appeared in the *Journal of Advanced Composition*. Kopelson asked this question: how is medicine, including its project of gatekeeping for medical authority, responding to the emerging e-patient—and how should it? She identified six types of physician responses. She provided documentary evidence that, while some doctors reject and even vilify the patient who comes in with stacks of what are seen as time-wasting printouts, the savvy doctor works collaboratively with the e-patient, not least because that patient type is here to stay. Kopelson represented this collaborative relation in a positive light. Her worry, though, by the end of the essay, was that patients are sometimes recruited too enthusiastically to responsibility for their own care, and this is not always in their best interests.

As different as they were in their questions and their methods, our essays were both motivated by a sense that health care in the internet age could be improved. In 2009 millions of people were doing health-related internet searches, some taking printouts to their doctors; there was definitely room for improvement in integrating patient web activity into practices of health/medicine. At the time, in journals across disciplines—in medicine and bioethics and consumer health informatics—experts were writing about the internet-using patient, how they should behave (mostly, cautiously), and how doctors should behave in their presence (mostly, tolerantly). Kopelson and I had rhetorical contributions to make to that conversation. For the very reason that our essays were *of their time,* though, they invite supplementation by essays suited to conditions *of this time.* Using an *as/is* framework, three essays in this volume turn rhetorical attention to an already transformed set of contingencies with respect to health/medicine and the web.

Kessler views the web not as a source of information constituting a rhetorical problem but as a site of patient narrative and illness identity formation. Kessler studies particular websites to gain access to ways that people with autoimmune disorders negotiate boundaries of self and not-self. With one set of online posts, she introduces a person who experiences her own immune system as a kind of traitor to the self ("not me"); with another, she introduces a person who views her ostomy pouch—a prosthesis necessitated by her autoimmune disorder—as an ally ("part of me"). Kessler's study incites an ameliorative rhetorical move: Kessler mobilizes her cases to talk about health/illness identity and its rhetoric, as she works to erode the power of binaries, including the binary of what is socially constructed and what is materially imperative.

Friz and Overholt are interested in a different sort of identity issue exposed in life online. They take up the rhetoric of a smartphone application for self-tracking, training their attention on "Eve by Glow," described on its home page as an "app for your period and sex life." Friz and Overholt specify the problematics of biopower, surveillance, self-surveillance, big data, and neoliberalism, by examining the particular ways that Eve establishes a morality of self-monitoring in its users—users significantly self-monitoring not for, say, heart rate or calorie consumption but rather for reproductive fitness and control. The essay stands as a kind of rhetorical cautionary tale.

The third essay in the section, by Singer and Jack, is on rhetorical representations of chronic illness. Making a case for viewing *chronicity* as a tool for identification, Singer and Jack turn their attention to Pinterest "pins" posted by people with chronic health conditions. Singer and Jack's ameliorative purpose is to weaken the force of gender and ability norms in identifications and representations of people with chronic illness—both for people with those conditions and for health professionals. "Pins," they argue, are rhetorical opportunities to destabilize those norms by representing in a digital instant the real lives of people living in chronicity. Their ameliorative purpose extends to their address to other rhetoricians whom they urge to deploy chronicity heuristically in their own work.

I began this essay with an anecdote. It was about things that people say to each other—inescapably suasive things—that may arise out of uncertainty or anxiety, and that may be more instrumental than true. We need importantly to scrutinize the things people say in contexts of health and medicine. Locations for saying them are even now being invented. Rhetoricians of health and medicine have looked at medical journal articles, health policy documents, doctor–patient interviews, illness narratives, drug ads, instructions to patients, deathbed conversations, as some of the loci of the rhetoric of health and medicine. Now we take our rhetorical subjectivity to, for example, web texts, smartphone apps, and Pinterest. In the age of health itself, almost anywhere might become a locus of our attention. Our methods of rhetorical study are expanding too, as are the reasons to hone them. The essays in this volume are a hopeful testament to our polydisciplinarity and the usefulness of our work.

REFERENCES

Belling, C. (2012). *A Condition of Doubt: The Meanings of Hypochondria*. New York: Oxford University Press.

Berkenkotter, C. (2008). *Patient tales: Case histories and the uses of narrative in psychiatry*. Columbia, SC: University of South Carolina Press.

Burke, K. (1973). *The Philosophy of Literary Form*. Berkeley, CA: University of California Press.

Conrad, P. (2007). *The medicalization of society: On the transformation of human conditions into treatable disorders*. Baltimore, MD: Johns Hopkins University Press.

Derkatch, C. (2016). *Bounding biomedicine: Evidence and rhetoric in the science of alternative medicine*. Chicago, IL: University of Chicago Press.

Emmons, K. (2010). *Black dogs and blue words: Depression and gender in the age of self-care*. New Brunswick, NJ: Rutgers University Press.

Graham, S. S. (2015). *The politics of pain medicine: A rhetorical-ontological inquiry*. Chicago, IL: University of Chicago Press.

Hacking, I. (1999). *The social construction of what?* Cambridge, MA: Harvard University Press.

Jensen, R. E. (2016). *Infertility: Tracing the history of a transformative term*. College Park, PA: Pennsylvania State University Press.

Johnson, J. (2014). *American lobotomy: A rhetorical history*. Ann Arbor, MI: University of Michigan Press.

Keränen, L. (2010). *Scientific characters: Rhetoric, politics, and trust in breast cancer research.* Tuscaloosa, AL: University of Alabama Press.

Koerber, A. (2013). *Breast or bottle? Contemporary controversies in infant-feeding policy and practice.* Columbia, SC: University of South Carolina Press.

Kopelson, K. (2009). Writing patients' wrongs: The rhetoric and reality of information age medicine. *JAC: A Journal of Rhetoric, Culture, & Politics, 29*(1–2), 353–404.

Mol, A. (2008). *The logic of care: Health and the problem of patient choice.* London, UK: Routledge.

Scott, J. B. (2003). *Risky rhetoric: AIDS and the cultural practices of HIV testing.* Carbondale, IL: Southern Illinois University Press.

Segal, J. Z. (2005). *Health and the rhetoric of medicine.* Carbondale, IL: Southern Illinois University Press.

Segal, J. Z. (2009). Internet health and the 21st-century patient: A rhetorical view. *Written Communication, 26*(4), 351–369. https://doi.org/10.1177/0741088309342362

Seigel, M. (2014). *The rhetoric of pregnancy.* Chicago, IL: University of Chicago Press.

Warnick, B. (1992). Life in context: What is the critic's role? *Quarterly Journal of Speech, 78,* 232–237.

Yergeau, M. (2018). *Authoring Autism / On Rhetoric and Neurological Queerness.* Durham, NC: Duke University Press.

INTRODUCTION

The Rhetoric of Health and Medicine As/Is

LISA MELONÇON, S. SCOTT GRAHAM,

JENELL JOHNSON, AND JOHN LYNCH

THE RHETORIC of health and medicine (RHM) is a growing and vibrant field and incorporates scholars from, most notably, communication, composition, rhetoric, linguistics, and technical and professional communication. To ask questions about the role of rhetoric—both as analytic and productive frameworks—in health and medicine is to engage with broader theoretical and ethical concerns about health-care systems and the many participants in those systems. Scholars studying RHM argue that the field is concerned not only with the discursive aspects of health and medicine as a set of discrete practices but also with how health-care and medical issues circulate in all the social, cultural, economic, and political aspects of our world. Indeed, the rhetoric of health and medicine is principally concerned with gaining a better understanding of the conceptualization and representation of health and the complex ways in which culture (broadly construed) influences the delivery and consumption of health care.

The rhetoric of health and medicine draws from numerous sources. The rhetoric of science is one wellspring. Rhetoricians, in the wake of Thomas Kuhn, Michel Foucault, and others, contributed to the cross-disciplinary dismantling of science's objectivist pretensions (Simons, 1990) and offered an emphasis on argumentation as a commonplace across disciplines despite the appearance of fragmentation and discontinuity (Nelson, Megill, & McCloskey, 1987). Further work complicated and enriched these beginning assumptions (e.g., Gross & Keith, 1997). That work also extended the reach of the rhetoric of science into areas with medical implications, like abortion, genetics, HIV/AIDS, and psychiatry (Berkenkotter, 2008; Condit, 1999; Scott, 2003). From here, the conceptual move to a focus on health and medicine was inevitable. Segal's (2005) oft-cited *Health and the Rhetoric of Medicine* inaugurated the field. Another wellspring is methodological, as rhetoricians of health and medicine turned to historical research, archives, and qualitative social science methods like ethnography, focus groups, and interviews (Melonçon & Scott, 2018). Such a move has been valuable, but it also raises challenges about the core identity of RHM (Scott, Segal, & Keränen, 2013) and tensions as scholars negotiate the commonalities and differences in rhetoric's scholarly practices and those of critical/qualitative health communication (Lynch & Zoller, 2015).

The history of RHM and its relationships to its antecedent fields and its objects of study complicate naming and understanding it. Answers to "what is RHM?" are, as should be obvious to most scholars, fraught with ideological and disciplinary power. Is RHM a *subdiscipline* of rhetoric or even the rhetoric of science? Is it interdisciplinary because of its methodological pluralism? Is it transdisciplinary in its object of study, melioristic bias, and overlap with the broader transdiscipline of health humanities? Like Scott and Melonçon (2018), "We are confident in identifying RHM as an emerged movement, [but] we are not as comfortable calling it a disciplinary one, instead preferring to call it a field of inquiry guided by rhetoric but shaped by and drawing upon a range of disciplinary and interdisciplinary bodies of scholarship" (p. 3). Similarly, Judy Segal (foreword) offers *polydisciplinarity* as a term to capture the diverse modalities within which the movement we name here "RHM" operates.

The range of scholarship that shapes RHM into a field or polydiscipline calls for a comprehensive account of the critical apparatus—the theoretical and methodological foundations—necessary to serve a wider range of scholars within and outside the field that can set the stage for RHM's continued evolution. Our goal here is to simultaneously ground and orient the field in a way that invokes discussions and that also challenges both the grounding and the orienting. While the field seems to be coalescing, particularly in its methodological pluralism and theory building, our experience putting together this volume points to the challenges and opportunities for grounding a new field's identity. In so doing, this volume explores how scholars use rhetoric in theoretical and practical ways to examine the discourses of health and medicine and how those discourses create meaning within a wide variety of scientific, technical, practical, and political sites.

To capture those concepts and their deployment within RHM, as well as the continued evolution of the ideas and the field, we offer the distinction of "as/is."[1] First, RHM can be seen **as** a theoretical construct that guides research and thinking in the field. Additionally, the concepts can be explored in the **is** stance as a way to define the boundaries of the field. Both orientations are necessary to any scholarly field or discipline. Both offer a conceptual and methodological core that provides coherence and continuity, and both allow for a diversity of approaches that ensure flexibility and growth. For example, let's take the concept that is part of the field's name: *rhetoric*. For many years, scholars have argued that rhetoric is way of analyzing existing discourse and of providing a framework for creating it. *As* provides us an entryway into thinking about different rhetorical concepts as theoretical underpinnings. *Is* provides us an entryway into thinking about how rhetorical theories can potentially be applied in practice.

The goal of this framing is twofold. First, we want to reflect on the diversity of concepts grounding RHM and guiding the critical scholarship produced under that name. Second, we want to nudge—and even push—scholars in the rhetoric of health and medicine to appraise what it is exactly that we do and what sets RHM apart from other related fields, such as medical sociology, narrative medicine, and health communication. This endeavor means taking a critical stance to determine what is at stake when we say that we are *rhetoricians* of health and medicine. Such an approach seemed fitting to us in this moment. RHM's conceptual and methodological diversity calls for such a contemplation at this moment in order to compel us as a field of inquiry to consider the entailments of our conceptual identifications and what are made by those concepts and their integration into rhetorical criticism of health and medicine. That contemplation will, of course, reflect the diversity of extant practices and likely spur others to invent additional concepts and applications of both old and new concepts to health and medicine.

Each of the chapters reflects on this dual approach and comes to a different conclusion about what it means, but all seek in some way to answer the question of just what we mean when we say "rhetoric of health and medicine." The chapters offer examples of where to look for rhetorically rich artifacts in the domains of health, illness, disease, and medicine; they push our thinking about which rhetorical theories, concepts, terminology, and methodologies are effective in understanding those artifacts; and they challenge RHM scholars to think critically not only about *what* we do, and *how*, but also *why* and *for whom*. While the as/is framework seeks to draw the chapters together

---

1. This idea was in part inspired by the collection by Shepherd, St. John, and Striphas (2010), who gathered together scholars in communication who identified key theoretical terms—*communication as*. The emphasis on theory building and its connection to practice are key components of RHM's identity.

with a unified objective, they do not speak with a unified voice. Instead, the volume seeks to offer a robust conversation, a dialogue, a multiplicity of perspectives on the question of where this emergent movement—at this critical moment in its development—has been and where it is going. Further, we invited responses from established RHM scholars (Lyne, Scott, and Keränen) to frame each section and then provide future directions for others to consider. In doing so, the responses push on the framework by putting the idea of As/Is into practice. This move, as expected, raises more questions than it may answer, but it provides space for future work to enter while still providing an orientation to establish an identity. The incorporation of responses also make the volume one that can be integrated into the growing number of RHM courses because the sections make ready-made units (http://tek-ritr.com/rhm-as-is/) while still being a rich source for researchers.

OVERVIEW OF THE CHAPTERS

The sections that we have devised represent important scholarly areas within RHM. They overlap in many ways, a feature that reveals the complexity of the field and the intersections between approaches to examining discourses of health and medicine. The sections described here were chosen because of their importance in providing a foundation of RHM as a unique scholarly endeavor that is different from, yet related to, rhetorical studies in general.

The sections move in a direction that also underscores the ideas of As/Is by starting with the complexity of the field and then moving to more specific concerns such as the physical/corporeal body that is the focal point/site of health care and medicine; self-identity and community that stems from this material (and nonmaterial) state; and attention to other-, social-, institutional-representations of identities, practices, and communities. Finally, each section concludes with an essay written by an expert respondent, an individual from RHM who responds to the common themes and concepts in the chapters and then simultaneously challenges and advances the field's understanding and application of the concepts. The respondent's role, then, is to suggest ways that the concepts could and potentially should evolve in the next stages of research.

Interdisciplinary Perspectives

By its very nature, research in health and medicine is cross-, inter-, and trans-disciplinary. As RHM begins to establish itself as an emerging field, scholars require an understanding of the relationship between this field and those that are already established and that are closely related. Thus, the call for papers for this collection specifically asked for scholars to discuss the relationship of RHM with other scholarly areas. The three essays in this section engage conversations with the most closely related disciplines/fields: the rhetoric of science, disability studies, and health/medical humanities. Focusing on the relationship between RHM and interdisciplinary perspectives allows readers the opportunity to situate their own work within several areas, making both useful and necessary connections between their work and that of other scholars.

Derkatch and Spoel provide an account of our research on food, public health, and health citizenship to show one way that rhetoric of health and medicine widens the scope of the health humanities as an interdisciplinary field from the realm of health research and practice to a broader sphere of human life. From the health and medical humanities to disability studies, the next chapter, by Holladay and Price, focuses on the intersections between disability studies and RHM and illuminates common theoretical commitments and fruitful paths for future scholarship, while also highlighting the distinctions of each field. The final chapter in this section, by Winderman and Landau, focuses on the rhetoric and science and the concept of *rehumanization* as a rhetorical process of pathos that affectively modulates public emotion and can intervene in a dehumanizing rhetorical ecology to return distinctly human attributes to patients. All three areas are complementary and overlapping and, yet, separate from RHM. The section closes with a response by Lyne that helps to situate the necessity of understanding the relationships among and between different fields of inquiry.

Representations and Online Health

From the early days of RHM, scholars have been concerned with how health and illness are represented, both in the biomedical literature and in public spaces (Scott, 2003; Segal, 2005; Emmons, 2010). The rhetorical modes used to portray health and illness can have powerful effects on patient and stakeholder communities. Perhaps nowhere is this clearer than in the evolving representational spaces where issues like sexuality and disability intersect with notions of health and illness. Concomitant with RHM's exploration of these issues, a great deal of attention has been paid to online spaces that have proved very fertile ground for developing patient and disease advocacy communities. Indeed, the affordances of the web in terms of reach beyond biomedical audiences and supporting interactivity have allowed for the development of powerful communities devoted to alternative representations of health and illness.

While our methodologies have become more nuanced and innovative over the last several years, RHM scholarship still endeavors to assist a variety of stakeholders in understanding a continuum of representations of health and illness. It is crucial that scholars in RHM continue to pursue a fuller understanding of the complexity of these representations if we are to maintain this key facet of our identity. Accordingly, this section engages different modes of re/presenting health and illness specifically in online environments. The diverse approaches, however, bring into sharp focus the continued necessity of critical work that examines how health and illness is represented, particularly digital spaces that have become an important part of monitoring, assessing, and representing health and illness.

Molly Kessler invokes Barad's theory of intra-activity to investigate how social media advocacy related to invisible illness states different modes of living with autoimmune conditions. In so doing, she challenges rhetoricians of health and medicine to move beyond primarily linguistic approaches to representation toward accounts that better address patients' lived experiences. Additionally, Amanda Friz and Stacey Overholt unpack the biopolitical imperatives directing citizen-consumers to buy and use technologies that quantify, measure, and track health and habits. In so doing, they explore the ovulation-monitoring app Eve and its ramifications for contemporary notions of self-surveillance in the age of wearable technologies and big data. Finally, Sarah Ann Singer and Jordynn Jack explore different representations of chronic illness on the social media platform Pinterest. In so doing, they showcase how rhetoricians can use the notion of "chronicity" to explore the rhetorical processes of identification and disidentification as a part of online discourses of chronic illness. This section ends with Scott's essay, which argues that representations "also make, configure, and instantiate." This stance of making matters because RHM scholarship attends to both RHM *as* and RHM *is* in its representations of materiality and language that are "about careful, precise, and embedded attention to emergent, mutual conditioning and co-configuring processes."

Health Citizenship and Advocacy

RHM work in health citizenship and advocacy is grounded in the theoretical framework of health activism (Zoller, 2005), an approach that challenges existing structures including power, race, gender, and economics. With an increasing emphasis in field methods (McKinnon, Asen, Chavez, & Howard, 2016) and participatory methods (Middleton, Hess, Endres, & Senda-Cook, 2015), RHM scholars can contribute to important conversations in and around public health. Essays in this section intervene in conversations about the importance of combining a rhetorical perspective with critical approaches to challenge, and to offer solutions to, public health problems.

As Keränen notes in her response to this section, all authors "implicitly take up [the] Isocratean tradition of *synercheste*, the practice of using discourse to arrive at knowledge and determine action" (p. 227, this volume). Each of the chapters in Health Citizenship and Advocacy examines specific sites that bring together members of communities and representatives of health-care discourse (e.g., programs, educators, translators) seeking to negotiate more egalitarian, context-appropriate constellations of power, gender, race, and economics. In chapter 7, Kuehl, Drury, and Anderson address the deliberative processes through which two groups grappling with complex, notably diverse, health issues—breastfeeding and substance abuse—arrive at understandings about the nuances of these issues and associated health behaviors through participation in conversations about the unique definitions and challenges posed. Maher's chapter takes on the disparities between minority and Caucasian mortality rates from sudden infant death syndrome (SIDS) nationwide and in the Baltimore, Maryland, area specifically. Situating their case study in a widely distributed public health campaign SLEEP SAFE created for Baltimore residents, Maher examines how parents affected by the loss of an infant from SIDS play an integral role in efforts to reach African American populations less effectively addressed by the better-known, mainstream Back to Sleep campaign. Hickman's chapter on reaching out to Latin@ health consumers through enlisting the support of experienced *promotoras* to address health risks to the population furthers the emphasis on using discourse to develop knowledge and strategize context-specific action plans for improved dietary choices. Drawing on Chicano feminist/*mujeris* pedagogies, Hickman discusses a participatory approach that rebalances power and incentives for effective health changes. This section as a whole demonstrates that exploring the rhetoric of health and medicine *as/is* proves a necessary step in identifying the crucial role that discourses play in creating knowledge about and responses to health and medical issues in a multifaceted society.

While each section highlights an important area of scholarship in RHM, theoretical and methodological innovations are also present that cut across each of these areas. As Scott and Melonçon (2018) argue, some of the most innovative research methodologies in rhetorical studies can be found in RHM. The standard practices of rhetorical criticism, which have focused on a range of critical objects from single texts to visual images to broader social movement campaigns, can be found in this volume (e.g., Derkatch & Spoel; Maher; Winderman & Landau). Others extend familiar rhetorical methods to social media (Friz & Overholt; Singer & Jack). Many of these methods are invigorated by incorporation of new theoretical insights. For example, Holladay and Price's rhetorical criticism is enriched by an engagement with disability studies, and Kessler turns to new materialisms to reframe rhetorical criticism as the examination of practices rather than representation. Other scholars illustrate for us the benefits of incorporating rhetorical sensibilities with social science research methods. Many essays in this collection combine focus groups or interviews and participant-observation with rhetorical insight (Kuehl, Drury, & Anderson; Hickman). Overall, readers will find the richness and innovation in RHM's research methods on display here.

This volume, while not wholly theoretical, is attempting to make the same moves specific to RHM. The emphasis on theory and practice provides scholars (and students) the opportunity to see new ways of approaching this emerging field and to gain a foundational understanding of the capacious boundaries that RHM scholars are already setting. The emphasis on RHM *As/Is* encourages scholars to consistently imagine what RHM could do as theory and practice. As individual arguments, the chapters show the diversity and range of RHM scholarship. As sections, the chapters and responses become vital arguments that highlight an area of RHM scholarship that grounds the field now and likely will in the future. As a volume, the authors show the strength of rhetorical scholarship as the rhetoric of health and medicine and the breadth of what is the rhetoric of health and medicine.[2]

REFERENCES

Berkenkotter, C. (2008). *Patient tales: Case histories and the uses of narrative in psychiatry.* Columbia, SC: University of South Carolina Press.

Condit, C. (1999). *The meanings of the gene: Public debates about human heredity.* Madison, WI: University of Wisconsin Press.

Emmons, K. (2010). *Black dogs and blue words: Depression and gender in the age of self-care.* New Brunswick, NJ: Rutgers University Press.

Gross, A., & Keith, W. M. (Eds.). (1997). *Rhetorical hermeneutics: Invention and interpretation in the age of science.* Albany, NY: State University of New York Press.

Lynch, J. A., & Zoller, H. (2015). Recognizing differences and commonalities: The rhetoric of health and medicine and critical-interpretive health communication. *Communication Quarterly, 63*(5), 498–503. https://doi.org/10.1080/01463373.2015.1103592

---

2. The editors gratefully acknowledge the financial support of the University of South Florida, Department of English, who helped to make this book possible.

McKinnon, S. L., Asen, R., Chavez, K., & Howard, R. G. (Eds.). (2016). *text+field: Innovation in rhetorical method*. University Park, PA: The Pennsylvania State University Press.

Melonçon, L., & Scott, J. B. (Eds.). (2018). *Methodologies for the rhetoric of health and medicine*. New York, NY: Routledge.

Middleton, M. K., Hess, A., Endres, D., & Senda-Cook, S. (2015). *Participatory critical rhetoric: Theoretical and methodological foundations for studying rhetoric in situ*. Lanham, MD: Lexington.

Nelson, J. S., Megill, A., & McCloskey, D. N. (Eds.). (1987). *The rhetoric of the human sciences language and argument in scholarship and public affairs*. Madison, WI: University of Wisconsin Press.

Scott, J. B. (2003). *Risky rhetoric: AIDS and the cultural practices of HIV testing*. Carbondale, IL: Southern Illinois University Press.

Scott, J. B., & Melonçon, L. (2018). Manifesting methodologies for the rhetoric of health and medicine. In L. Melonçon & J. B. Scott (Eds.), *Methodologies for the rhetoric of health and medicine* (pp. 1–23). New York, NY: Routledge.

Scott, J. B., Segal, J. Z., & Keränen, L. (2013). Commentary: The rhetorics of health and medicine: inventional possibilities for scholarship and engaged practice. *Poroi, 9*(1), Article 17.

Segal, J. Z. (2005). *Health and the rhetoric of medicine*. Carbondale, IL: Southern Illinois University Press.

Shepherd, G. J., St. John, J., & Striphas, T. (Eds.). (2010). *Communication as . . . Perspectives on theory*. Thousand Oaks, CA: Sage.

Simons, H. W. (Ed.). (1990). *The rhetorical turn: Invention and persuasion in the conduct of inquiry*. Chicago, IL: University of Chicago Press.

Zoller, H. M. (2005). Health activism: Communication theory and action for social change. *Communication Theory, 15*(4), 341–364.

SECTION 1

INTERDISCIPLINARY PERSPECTIVES

CHAPTER 1

Health Humanities as an Interdisciplinary Intervention

Constitutive Rhetoric, Genre, and Health Citizenship

COLLEEN DERKATCH AND PHILIPPA SPOEL

WHAT CAN RHETORIC of health and medicine (RHM) contribute to a wider health humanities research agenda? In this chapter, we provide one answer to this question by drawing on our ongoing collaborative research on public discourse about "local" food and food sustainability (Derkatch & Spoel, 2017; Spoel & Derkatch, 2016, 2020). In this research, we have examined the rhetorical formation of health citizenship in materials produced by public health units and activist organizations about food production, distribution, and consumption. None of the materials we examine are explicitly "medical," nor are they directly about health: they do not refer to diagnoses or disease, doctors or treatments, nor are they meant to guide health-care policy or practice. The documents do not seek to reduce health-care costs or to speed up wait times. Further, while they may guide consumers toward making healthy choices, they do not explain or illustrate what health is, or how to get and maintain it. And yet, what the documents do show is that "health" is constituted rhetorically even in materials that are not directly about either medicine or health. Public discourse about local and sustainable food simultaneously enacts values about individual and community health by modeling how to be a "good" health citizen. In this chapter, we provide an account of our research on food, public health, and health citizenship to show one way that RHM widens the scope of the health humanities as an interdisciplinary field from the realm of health research and practice to a broader sphere of human life.

Health humanities emerged out of, and in response to, the medical humanities (Chambers, 2009; Jones, Blackie, Garden, & Wear, 2017; Jones, Wear, & Friedman, 2014; Shapiro, Coulehan, Wear, & Montello, 2009). Definitions of these overlapping fields are multivalent but typically invoke the "humanizing" potential of humanities instruction within the health professions as a means of expanding practitioners' capacities for empathy and care, and for understanding patients' unique "lifeworlds" through artistic expression, literary study, and narrative analysis (see, e.g., Brody, 2011; Charon, 2001; Frank, 2014; Whitehead & Kuper, 2015).[1] One of the central arguments for health humanities over medical humanities is that the term *medical* situates lived bodily experience in too narrow a frame, one of illness and active pursuit of care, whereas *health* situates it within a broader frame of living by encompassing all the factors that affect health (Crawford, Brown, Baker, Tischler, & Abrams, 2015; Crawford, Brown, Tischler, & Baker, 2010; Jones et al., 2014; Jones et al., 2017). Advocates of health humanities over medical humanities rightly emphasize, as Goldberg does, that within this wider frame, the field "must not have as its central goal the advance[ment] of the practice and science of medicine" but a broader consideration of the intersections between health and human life (as cited in Jones et al., 2014, p. 7). These are laudable goals for the health humanities, and yet, despite these and other efforts to enrich the health part of "health humanities," there has been surprisingly little consideration of what is signified by the humanities part of "health humanities." In what follows, we argue that a broader perspective on what the humanities are and do—that they constitute a rich range of research disciplines in their own right—offers a more compelling and robust means of opening to inquiry complex questions and challenging issues in health and medicine.

We begin by situating RHM *as* (in this collection's "as/is" formulation) an exemplar of a health humanities field rooted in a set of vibrant and rigorous research disciplines with their own generative theoretical frameworks and methodologies. These disciplines, which include history, philosophy, literary and language studies, and rhetoric (among others), are not artful antidotes to technoscientific medicine but instead produce robust knowledge about health, medicine, and human life. Neither are these disciplines "humane." Indeed, their power often resides in their ability to pose incisive questions and to probe, through close analysis and critique, for answers that lay bare institutional, disciplinary, and ideological agendas that may not otherwise come into view. Research in RHM is therefore not ancillary to other methods of health research,

---

1. *Lifeworld* is a term from Elliott Mishler (1984) to describe "patients' multi-faceted, contextualised and meaningful accounts" of illness (Barry, Stevenson, Britten, Barber, & Bradley, 2001, p. 487).

examining the "softer" side of medicine, but makes possible distinctive lines of inquiry for producing knowledge about health and health care by investigating the symbolic means through which individuals and groups are induced, through methods both conscious and unconscious, toward certain beliefs and actions and away from others. We illustrate through the example of rhetoric that humanities-based research on health produces knowledge in its own right, even—and, for us, especially—outside the walls of hospitals and clinics.

To demonstrate the richness and rigor of RHM within a wider health humanities research agenda, we then articulate one version of what RHM *is* by describing how we position and mobilize rhetorical theory and analysis in our research on emerging intersections in North America between public health discourse and food activism. Specifically, we show how a rhetorical perspective expands and complicates current knowledge about changing norms and values of neoliberal health citizenship within contemporary Western culture. The conceptual-methodological resources of constitutive rhetoric and rhetorical genre theory, in particular, allow us to trace the situated symbolic means through which the "good" health citizen is increasingly interpellated as someone who not only takes responsibility for her personal health but, through the consumption and support of local/sustainable food, also accepts and fulfills her responsibilities to care for the local economy, the community's well-being, and the natural environment. Drawing on the findings of our collaborative project, we outline in this chapter some ways that rhetorical research enriches and refines the focus of humanities scholarship on questions of ideology in health (care)—questions that may not be even asked, let alone answered, by scholars within the professional fields of health and medicine.

RHM AS AN EXEMPLAR OF HEALTH HUMANITIES

To situate RHM vis-à-vis health humanities, we begin by outlining different valences of "health humanities" and its cognate (and antecedent) field, medical humanities. As we discuss below, there are some key distinctions between the two fields, but, importantly, they share gaps in their ability to anticipate the full range of potential contributions of the humanities to health and medicine—gaps that, we argue, scholarship in RHM is particularly well poised to fill. While health professions curricula often incorporate "arts" such as literary study and creative writing or philosophical exercises to prompt reflection in student practitioners, rhetoric is not so easily applied as a program of self-development. Because rhetoric resists the standard invocation of the humanities as a guide to ethical or professional development within health and medical programs, RHM can exemplify how the constellation of disciplines that compose the humanities do more than serve an instrumental role in health professions education. Our own research on food-activist rhetoric, for example, may not apply directly to health-care education or practice, but it indirectly informs both by illuminating how "health" is constituted in public discourse more widely. The language and values of "health" are taken up and reconfigured within contemporary culture by multiple actors for multiple purposes and with multiple effects—which only partially align with the language and values of "health" in professional-institutional contexts. Understanding the wider meanings and rhetorical functions of "health" matters because they are central to what we value and how we live our lives, particularly as physical health increasingly becomes a proxy for personal and moral health.

In this section, we extend arguments by our colleagues in rhetoric, Gouge (2016) and Segal (2013), both of whom illustrate the extent to which the "humanities" as envisioned in medical/health humanities programs are typically premised on a model of humanist education that has been long outmoded in the humanities' traditional disciplinary homes in departments of English, history, philosophy, and so on. Gouge considers how posthumanist scholarship can "interrogate some of the basic assumptions about agency and knowledge" in research on practitioner-patient communication (p. 2), whereas Segal (2013) maintains that medical humanities might best be taught in medical schools not as separate (often elective) courses but as an integrative model of "Humanities across the Curriculum" (p. 232), embedded within and essential to physician training rather than merely an optional add-on.

We extend Gouge's and Segal's arguments in two ways. First, we expand on their argument (especially Segal's) that an ideal health humanities curriculum would be less inward-facing, focused on student-physician study of primary materials from the "arts" (e.g., novels, poems, visual art), and more outward-facing, incorporating into medical teaching and practice research on health *from* the humanities (e.g., in scholarly critical-secondary articles and books). Second, we continue their work in shifting the focus of medical/health humanities beyond investigation of the (clinical) health professions. We take up both threads of our argument simultaneously, beginning with an account of the medical humanities as it is most commonly instantiated.

The Humanities in Medicine

In their typical delivery, most medical humanities programs consist primarily of exposing medical students to art, history, literature, and philosophy (Atkinson, Evans, Woods, & Kearns, 2015; Gillis, 2008; Macneill, 2011; Polianski &

Fangerau, 2012; Saffran, 2014; Tsevat, Sinha, Gutierrez, & DasGupta, 2015). The very idea of medical humanities (and health humanities, for that matter) is premised to some extent on Snow's postulation of the "two cultures" of science and the humanities (Polianski & Fangerau, 2012; Segal, 2013), that medicine is both a science and an art (Solomon, 2015). For instance, Viney, Callard, and Woods (2015) cited "two common narratives" of medical humanities, both of which are grounded firmly in the two-cultures perspective: "First, there is a service or utilitarian model" in medical education and practice wherein the humanities are responsible for "humanising the objectivity of biomedicine" (p. 2); and second, where "the medical humanities is presented as a counter-balance to the restrictive and restricted views of science" (p. 3). Chiapperino and Boniolo (2014) similarly described the purpose of medical humanities as both "to improve the quality of the humane relationship among doctors, clinical professionals and patients" and to foster in practitioners "a deeper understanding of what medicine is and attempts to [be]" (p. 378). In each of these examples, the first standard narrative of the medical humanities adopts an "additive" approach (Evans & Greaves, 1999), in that the humanities are added to soften medicine's seemingly "hard" bioscientific edge, whereas the second narrative is "integrative" (Evans & Greaves, 1999) because it situates medicine within a larger sociohistorical contextual framework.

Regardless of which of these narratives is adopted, the humanities themselves are seldom figured as more than ancillary to medicine, as instruments for improving medical education (Atkinson et al., 2015; Belling, 2006; Brody, 2011; Shapiro et al., 2009) and practice (Brody, 2011; Chiapperino & Boniolo, 2014; Polianski & Fangerau, 2012). Recently, however, an undercurrent of critique of this instrumental model has begun to develop as scholars have increasingly recognized the importance of the humanities within medicine for introducing a space for ambiguity about and questioning of medicine's fundamental assumptions. Rather than "benign and servile" (Macneill, 2011), the humanities within medicine may, for instance, inadvertently serve as a tool of governance (Atkinson et al., 2015; Bleakley, Marshall, & Brömer, 2006; Petersen, Bleakley, Brömer, & Marshall, 2008; Viney et al., 2015). Engaging medical students and doctors in reflective exercises such as literary analysis and personal writing may, for example, "individualise systemic failures [of medicine], compensating structurally-induced overwork and poor management with the arts" (Petersen et al., 2008, p. 2). Similarly, in the practice of narrative medicine—a model of narrative practice premised on listening to and honoring patients' individual stories of illness (Charon, 2001)—trust and empathy could become mechanisms of ensuring patient compliance (Bishop, 2008). To wit: if the ideal of narrative medicine is for physicians to identify with their patients to care more effectively for them, then the pragmatic end of that "empathic engagement" (Charon, 2001, p. 1898) may simply be to persuade patients to follow doctor's orders (Gouge, 2016).

Further, as numerous critiques of medical humanities have illustrated, calls for more "humane" and "patient-centered" practitioners (Petersen et al., 2008, p. 2) occurred alongside the rise of neoliberal-consumerist models of health and health care centered on patient choice. In this perspective, medical humanities both rose out of and symptomizes larger systemic problems within medicine. Atkinson et al. (2015) phrased the problem succinctly:

> While the medical humanities has done a lot to challenge dominant medical perspectives, it seldom if ever ventures beyond a neoliberal, humanist notion of the individual body-subject and associated conceptualizations of responsibility, rights, and risk management to really explore alternative "collective" and "relational" approaches to "flourishing." (p. 77)

The focus in medical humanities is generally so squarely on making better doctors (Segal, 2013) that other, often-structural problems within health and health care become harder to see. But what if the medical humanities' most significant contribution to medicine will be to produce not better doctors but better patients? Or better health consumers? Or better policymakers, city planners, or cultural critics? We return below to questions such as these, and to how RHM is well poised to answer them, but first we turn our attention to health humanities as a response to medical humanities.

Over the past decade, there has been a major push to reconceive the field of medical humanities by widening its scope beyond medical education and practice to encompass health more broadly (e.g., Crawford et al., 2010; Segal & Richardson, 2006; Squier, 2007; Tsevat et al., 2015). In most cases, the broadening of the field from "medical" to "health" refers to extending the application of the humanities to a wider range of health professions, including nursing, mental health, occupational therapy, physiotherapy, and mental health (Crawford et al., 2010; Jones et al., 2017; Tsevat et al., 2015). Although Atkinson et al. (2015) rejected the label of "health humanities" in favor of "critical medical humanities" (p. 78), their core arguments resonate with those for the emergent field of health humanities as an interdiscipline that employs the humanities to improve health education and practice.

Some scholars who advocate for health humanities as a more comprehensive version of medical humanities do attend to health itself as a construct (including rhetoricians such as Gouge, 2016, and Segal, 2013), but, overall, the new field remains inward-looking, focused on health professions education and practice. One irony of the health humanities, then, is that it replicates some of the same gaps it was intended to fill within the field it superseded: by adopting a narrow perspective on health—in this case, health in the context of professional education and care—health humanities in general does not sufficiently conceptualize health as it is produced outside of institutional contexts, thereby limiting its potential reach as a field of academic research and teaching. Of course, the emphasis on education and practice in health humanities is understandable: although scholars of the humanities and health can be found at universities across departments and faculties, core programs for research and teaching in both fields are typically housed in and funded by faculties of medicine or health sciences (and so, the logic goes, should be of primary benefit to the practitioners educated within them). For this very reason, however, we believe that a broader conception of the field is necessary: by housing medical/health humanities programs under the same disciplinary umbrella as the communities they research (e.g., studying medicine from within a school of medicine), researchers are necessarily constrained by the terms of their objects of study.[2]

Rhetorician Kenneth Burke (1966) would describe the present institutional-structural constraints of medical/health humanities as a problem of terministic screens. That is, medicine's terministic screen—its governing perspective, language, and logic—affects what can be seen, and said, in much of the medical and health humanities. We might think of this problem as one of directional perspective: by viewing the humanities through the lens of medicine instead of the reverse, viewing medicine through the lens of the humanities, scholarship in the field is restricted to a certain range of views that are consonant with a medical worldview. We do not believe that this restricted perspective undermines the health humanities as much as it simply limits it. So, part of a wider conception of health humanities would be to turn its inward-facing gaze at least partly outward.

Rhetoric as a "Hard" Humanities Discipline

If one limitation of both medical and health humanities is that their interpretation of "health" is restricted to the realm of health-care practice, a more

---

2. On Twitter, for example, bioethicist Carl Elliott (2016) pointed out that one potential intellectual consequence of housing medical/health humanities programs within medical schools is the potential stifling of critical perspectives on medical education and practice: "There is a difference between studying a subject and putting him on your promotion and tenure committee." In the interests of disclosure, one of us (Derkatch) participated in this Twitter conversation.

significant limitation of both fields is that their interpretation of "humanities" is narrower still. As Belling (2006) and Polianski and Fangerau (2012) argued, the humanities are typically figured in both fields as "soft" disciplines vis-à-vis medicine, where their value is seen, problematically, to lie in "softening the [hard] edges of science" through narrative interpretation, personal reflection, and elicitation of feeling (Belling, 2006, p. 3). Even though Crawford and colleagues (2010) described the humanities "as disciplines in their own right" (p. 6) in their initial call for the more inclusive term *health humanities,* they constitute those disciplines primarily as expressive arts (e.g., visual art, dance, drama, and poetry) rather than as research disciplines.

Most strikingly, the humanities continue to be characterized as instruments for individual practitioner development (see, e.g., Bleakley, 2019; Bleakley et al., 2006; Chiapperino & Boniolo, 2014; Chiavaroli, 2017; Gillis, 2008; Kumagi, 2017; Petersen et al., 2008; Polianski & Fangerau, 2012; Tsevat et al., 2015; Wear, 2009). In focusing on producing better practitioners, many commentators unwittingly interpret *humanities* as synonymous with *humanism.* Even the more nuanced accounts of medical/health humanities remain concerned primarily with aesthetics, ethics, and physician identity/self-development through self-expression. For instance, although Bleakley et al. (2006) drew on scholars whose intellectual commitments resist humanist application (such as Deleuze and Guattari, Derrida, Foucault, and Latour), ultimately, they maintained that the goal of humanities learning in medical settings is to engage student medical practitioners in a process of "aesthetic and ethical identity formation" (p. 197). They argued that their position is guided by an interest in producing "humane" medicine, rather than "humanistic" or "humanitarian" medicine (p. 203), but their end goal remains the personal development of practitioners within a humanistic framework. Similarly, other progressive accounts of the humanities' potential contributions to health and health care nevertheless figure the humanities as pedagogical rather than epistemological instruments (e.g., Klugman, 2017; Lam, 2019)—that is, as tools exclusively for teaching rather than also for producing knowledge.

In our view of rhetoric as an exemplar research discipline within the health humanities, we share Segal's (2013) admonishment of humanistic justifications of the field:

Medical school . . . is not a project of human improvement. Humanism is a philosophy, focusing on individuals, their potential, their will, and their power; and most scholars working now in the humanities are not humanists. Humanities scholars think about human beings not, in the first instance, as individuals, with individual potential for greatness, but as actors in social and cultural contexts, living within systems, using language, under constraints. Medical humanities should use the resources of the humanities, the work that humanities scholars actually do. (p. 231)

Similarly, Catherine Belling (2006), an English-department-trained literature scholar working in a medical school, asked: "Is my role as a humanities scholar to teach humaneness by example? I hope I do that anyway; but is it my job more than it is the job of a biochemistry professor?" (p. 5). In her bracing critique of the "softness" of the humanities as taken up in medical programs, Belling called for "exacting standards and precision" in the analysis of primary literary texts within medical settings (p. 3), rather than viewing such texts as vehicles of content that mirror the actual conditions of medicine and teach desirable character traits. She tasked medical (and health) humanities scholars with the project of reckoning with how their teaching and research relate to the "wider, perhaps harder, academic humanities" (p. 4).[3]

The conception of the humanities as humanizing and identity-forming disciplines is thus rooted in a too-instrumental understanding of what humanities research is and does. We therefore agree with Belling (2006), Gouge (2016), Polianski and Fangerau (2012), and Segal (2013) that the medical/health humanities require "a more solid methodological and theoretical basis" (Polianski & Fangerau, 2012, p. 122), and we believe that RHM can provide a blueprint for establishing that basis. For one, the texts that rhetorical scholars study in the context of health and medicine (whether those texts are written, spoken, or visual) are generally not "great works" of literature, philosophy, or history. The texts that rhetorical scholars analyze are typically unglamorous—antidepressant advertisements (Emmons, 2008), anatomy laboratories (Fountain, 2014), infant-feeding policy (Koerber, 2013), pregnancy manuals (Seigel, 2014)—and do not promise to reveal a "soul" or "heart" of medicine.

Certainly, not all researchers in other humanities disciplines study materials of high culture, but we would argue that this is a fortiori true in RHM, and that the topics and texts of our research generally resist canonization as exemplars of the human condition. Further, as a matter of disciplinary orientation, rhetorical research generally foregrounds agency as distributed, knowledge

---

3. It is worth noting that Belling could, herself, have made more of the place of humanities *scholarship* in her essay, rather than focusing solely on the teaching of primary texts to health science students, although this oversight seems to be largely a factor of context and audience—her editorial-style article is published in *Atrium*, an academic magazine published by the Center for Bioethics and Medical Humanities at the Northwestern University Feinberg School of Medicine. Certainly, Belling's scholarly research demonstrates no such oversight.

and meaning as contingent, and discourse as always embedded in and mediated by context. In their typical subject-matter and approach, rhetorical studies of health and medicine thus resist a standard humanistic interpretation and open space for other ways of viewing how the humanities can contribute to health research, education, and practice.

One of the main spaces that rhetorical research on health opens up is that it can ask questions that are conceptually prior to questions usually asked by other health researchers (Segal, 2009). The answers to these "prior questions"—answers often unattainable through more conventional health research methods—can provide important insight into matters that affect health. To draw examples from our own research, for instance, while other health researchers might ask whether locally produced food is healthier than food produced at a distance, or why some people eat healthily while others do not, we are able to ask how public discourse about food and food activism instantiates values about what it means to be a good health citizen. As we argue below, models of health citizenship are not limited to the specific contexts within which they are formed. Rather, they characterize individuals' health beliefs and behaviors generally, across contexts. For example, if someone learns from public health materials that being a good health citizen in the realm of food means being a smart consumer (Derkatch & Spoel, 2017), that model of being a smart consumer may well inform how that person makes decisions in other areas of health as well, such as which health products to acquire (pharmaceuticals or supplements, say), which practitioners to see (doctors or naturopaths, say), and which precautionary health measures to take or not (vaccinations, say). If we, as health citizens, define who we are partly by the values we hold and the choices we make, then a rhetorical approach to health and medicine can intervene at a higher point of access than a more instrumental application of the humanities in medicine such as narrative medicine because it offers insight not only into individual beliefs and behaviors in the clinic but also into the social-ideological frameworks within which patients and practitioners are primed for those beliefs and behaviors.

In the remainder of this chapter, we address how public discourse about food sustainability and local food functions as a contextual framework, located beyond the clinic, for priming contemporary values and actions of health citizenship. To demonstrate the distinctive contributions of rhetorical theory and analysis to investigating this dimension of health and health care, we unpack how two conceptual-methodological perspectives from rhetorical studies, constitutive rhetoric and genre theory, have facilitated our own research on prior questions in the formation of health citizenship in public discourse about food sustainability and local food.

RHM IS A MODE OF CRITICAL INQUIRY

Our motivation to enter into conversation with scholars in food studies and critical public health has necessitated careful reflection on how our rhetorical approach contributes worthwhile insights that are not available in those fields through other forms of research, including other humanities-based approaches. A significant part of our contribution to those conversations lies simply in how, as rhetoricians, we proceed with our research. As a mode of inquiry, rhetoric constitutes "both a critical-hermeneutic and an empirical practice that centers on persuasion, on all of the ways in which we act on each other (and ourselves) by influence, through methods both conscious and unconscious, through various communicative means" (Derkatch, 2016, p. 13). Accordingly, to answer prior questions about local food and food sustainability, such as those we identify above, we have undertaken rigorous textual and contextual analysis of "situated uses and effects of language (or symbolic action)" in public health and community-based discourse (Spoel & Den Hoed, 2014, p. 272). Our goal has been to bring our specific, humanities-based approach of fine-grained attention to language to bear on the texts we examine as a means of understanding how they work and what rhetorical action they perform in the world. Examining rhetorical action within and across texts and text-types (or genres) in food-related discourse focuses attention on the mediating effects of language and communicative forms in the constitution of individual and community identities and values, as well as overlapping, and possibly conflicting, types of health citizenship.

Within critical health studies, the concept of health citizenship has been identified as a key component of contemporary neoliberal approaches to health care and health promotion. It refers to the set of civic rights and obligations that "public health systems and policies both presume and encourage" as responsibility for health and well-being is increasingly transferred from state-level public agencies to individuals as consumers within a market economy (Spoel, 2014, p. 565; see also Brown, 2019; Henderson & Petersen, 2002; Petersen, Davis, Fraser, & Lindsay, 2010; Porter, 2011). In contrast to earlier approaches to health citizenship and care based on social entitlement and the welfare state, the "New Public Health" (Petersen & Lupton, 1996) characterizes the "good citizen" as an individual who performs their civic duty of taking responsibility for their own well-being by actively becoming informed about and practicing a healthy lifestyle (Spoel, 2014).[4]

---

4. Health citizenship is similar to the broader, more amorphous concept of "biological citizenship" (Majdik, 2014; Rose & Novas, 2004) in that it reconstitutes citizen identities in terms other than (though not necessarily disconnected from) the traditional criterion of

Drawing on the concepts of constitutive rhetoric and rhetorical genre theory, our research has illuminated the discursive formation of "good" health citizens in public health and food-activist documents as individuals who take responsibility for their own health as well as the health of the community, the environment, and the economy by supporting and consuming local and sustainable food. In the sections below, we outline two specific contributions of our research to broader scholarship in the health humanities: first, we show how public health promotion of local foods reproduces market-based ideologies that could potentially undermine the very aims of public health; and, second, we show how the emergent genre of the food charter may constrain the effectiveness and reach of the social-discursive action that the genre itself is intended to perform.

Our ultimate aim in this section is to illustrate how RHM produces rigorous and substantive knowledge about health. In our own case, for example, rather than supporting the development of more "humane" health-care practitioners or exemplifying the artistic-expressive value of the humanities, our research seeks to deepen understanding of the complex and evolving ways in which rhetorics of health simultaneously reveal and shape the social-ideological frameworks that undergird contemporary health citizenship and individual health beliefs and behaviors. The power of rhetoric as a mode of inquiry for the fields with which our research intersects, such as critical public health and food studies, is that its close attention to language use in context allows us to map within our research site of public discourse about local and sustainable food "the constellation of symbolic and material rhetorics that influence daily life and public meanings and practice" (Scott, Segal, & Keränen, 2013, n.p.).

Constitutive Rhetoric and the Formation of the Neoliberal Health Citizen

Our first inquiry into the rhetorical formation of health citizenship vis-à-vis food-activist discourse employed Maurice Charland's (1993) well-known theory of constitutive rhetoric to investigate promotion of "local" food in Canadian regional public health units (Derkatch & Spoel, 2017). Constitutive rhetoric extends Louis Althusser's (1968/1971) concept of interpellation,

---

nationality. Although these concepts are sometimes used interchangeably, the literature on health citizenship emphasizes more specifically the rights and obligations of individuals to contribute to the common good by maintaining their own health primarily through personal lifestyle and behavior (Porter, 2011).

or "hailing," to describe the process through which subjects are constituted by the very discourses with which they are addressed.[5] Charland (1993) argued that the *peuple québécois* was rhetorically constituted in the early 1980s as a sovereignty-seeking collective by the publication of a provincial policy document that characterized Québec citizens as "oppressed" by the Canadian national government (p. 216). This study illustrated how individuals and groups are constructed as subjects discursively, who then reaffirm that subjectivity as they engage in action in the social world. The discursive constitution of identity is a dynamic process that can occur in any context to transform addressees of discourse into subjects of that same discourse. In RHM, the framework of constitutive rhetoric has been employed to illuminate the discursive construction of, for example, headache patients in clinical practice (Segal, 2005) and boundaries between mainstream and alternative medicine in medical journals (Derkatch, 2016).

In our research (Derkatch & Spoel, 2017), we found that public health materials that promote local foods discursively constitute four overlapping and partly contradictory forms of health citizenship that call forth civic imperatives to maintain or enhance individual health, environmental health, regional economic health, and community health through the consumption and support of local food. Each of these four facets of health citizenship (individual, economic, community, and environmental) carries its own, overlapping sets of obligations and expectations for what and how we should eat. Despite their emphasis on environmental sustainability and community well-being, however, the dominant ideal of health citizenship advanced in these materials is one of economic prosperity, whereby informed consumers support the interests of the neoliberal state through individualized lifestyle behaviors, particularly by consuming goods produced and distributed through private enterprise. By exhorting individuals to "buy local," public health discourse therefore frames responsible health citizenship principally in consumerist terms that constrain the range of available options for citizens to engage in meaningful action vis-à-vis their food systems.

With respect to our contributions as humanities-based researchers to knowledge about health, one core finding of this project is that, despite efforts within the public health materials we examined to broaden contemporary

_____

5. Althusser (1968/1971) explained that "interpellation or hailing . . . can be imagined along the lines of the most commonplace everyday police (or other) hailing: 'Hey, you there!'" Upon hearing this call, Althusser argued, "the hailed individual will turn round. By this mere one-hundred-and-eighty-degree physical conversion, he becomes a subject. Why? Because he has recognized that the hail was 'really' addressed to him, and that 'it was really him who was hailed' (and not someone else)" (p. 174).

understandings of "health" to include responsibility for the community and for the environment, the dominant characterization of the ideal health citizen continues to be that of an informed individual who has the desire and knowledge (and necessary resources) to accept responsibility for personal or family health by consuming goods produced and distributed through private enterprise. Accordingly, our rhetorical perspective has allowed us to show that in their promotion of local food, public health agencies may in some cases be inadvertently advancing private, market interests over those of public health. Examining how different forms of health citizenship are called forth and prioritized in public health discourse can therefore shed important light on where health practitioners and scholars might intervene more effectively against the potentially harmful effects of the "responsibilization" of health (Guthman, 2008, p. 1173)—the downloading of responsibility for health from the state onto individuals—that may jeopardize the very goals of public health to support health across populations.

Genre Theory and the Social Action of Health Citizenship

Following our initial study of the rhetorical constitution of health citizenship in public health discourse about local food, we sought to better understand the ideological tensions between public welfare and neoliberal values such as individual prosperity and self-reliance in the constitution of contemporary health citizenship. Accordingly, the next phase of our research (Spoel & Derkatch, 2016, 2020) focused on the rhetorical forms and functions of the "food charter" as a key emergent genre within the broader landscape of public health discourse about local food, food sustainability, and community food security. Food charters are nonbinding visioning documents that articulate core value statements about what their authors hope to achieve for their food system, most notably with respect to food security and food sustainability within the community. By 2019 at least fifty Canadian communities and regions across four provinces and one territory have adopted or are developing their own food charter, the majority of which have been produced by community groups under the auspices of public agencies such as public health units. Current scholarship on this new genre focuses on its purposes, content, and best practices for development without querying the genre's own significance or effects. As humanities-based scholars of rhetoric, we contribute to this conversation an ability to track how food charters enact situated, contingent visions of community food sustainability and food security, allowing us to address prior questions about the values instantiated by the genre of the food charter itself, as well as its impact on the situations, purposes, and communities it serves.

Drawing on Keränen's (2008) characterization of genre as a valuable "meso-level" concept for RHM, we employed genre as a lens for revealing how each regional health agency's rhetorical actions at once reflect and reconfigure broader ideological tensions about health citizenship within current public health discourse about food. As Hyland (2002) maintained, the ability of rhetorical research to unpack the complex relations between texts and contexts helps "reveal the social, cultural, ideological, and political foundations of texts; the ways they evolve and change in response to their contexts; and how this also works to reshape those contexts" (p. 124). Paré's (2002) similar theorization of genre as a key site of ideological and institutional struggle led us to investigate how the textual-contextual forms and functions of the community food charter may inadvertently advance private, market interests over those of public health and food security. We found in our analysis, for example, that one key action performed by current Ontario food charters is the advancement of community values and identities that principally address certain sorts of citizens, such as farmers, food workers, and consumers, over others, such as those who are poor, elderly, or living with disabilities or illness.

More significantly, we found that the terminologies and argumentative structures characteristic of the food charter genre may actually impede the very action the genre is intended to perform: namely, to produce meaningful social-structural change within regional food systems to support the health and welfare of all citizens in ecologically and economically sustainable ways. Although food charter proponents view the genre as a form of deliberative rhetoric, oriented to facilitating future action, our analysis reveals it instead to be primarily epideictic, instantiating present-day values about community identity, social justice, and sustainability. On closer scrutiny, we found that the values espoused in food charters contain ideological and logical incongruences, concealed within the genre itself, that may prevent charters from achieving their intended goals. For a valorized genre such as the food charter, reconsideration of what the genre is and what it does can therefore reveal potential sites of amelioration for the communities who value and use the genre. In the studies we have outlined above, by drawing on constitutive rhetoric and rhetorical genre theory, we have sought to produce rigorous, textured knowledge about health citizenship and public health discourse that is distinct from but complementary to knowledge about health produced by researchers in other disciplines.

CONCLUSION

While much important work in RHM produces knowledge that may be applied more or less directly to improving the communicative dimensions of health-care practices, our ongoing collaborative research on public health discourse about local food, food sustainability, and food security is concerned primarily with deciphering the constitutive functions of these rhetorical practices rather than improving their instrumental effectiveness. (On constitutive versus instrumental rhetorics, see Cox & Pezzullo, 2016, p. 16.) Thus, our main objective has been to produce knowledge that enriches our understanding of the complex, situated ways that public health discourse intersects with other prominent, ideologically inflected discourses circulating in contemporary North American culture. This approach concerns itself first and foremost with generating critical insights about the rhetorical conditions that prime our values, attitudes, and actions as health citizens in contexts beyond institutional or clinical health-care settings. Although we hope that the results of our research will interest policymakers and practitioners in public health and food activism, we, along with Segal (2005), resist the idea that humanities research on health, and rhetorical research in particular, must be applied in order to be useful. Here, we differ from some of our colleagues in RHM, who distinguish rhetorical contributions to health and medicine from other humanities-based research on health precisely because they see RHM as more oriented to application (e.g., Angeli & Johnson-Sheehan, 2018), but we do not see this difference of perspectives as problematic: RHM has a long history of embeddedness within health education and practice, so it is no surprise, and is indeed an asset, that much of the work of the field faces inward, toward the health professions. Our point remains that expanding the health (and medical) humanities more generally to encompass broader and yet sharper conceptions of the humanities as a suite of research disciplines will enrich the possibilities for what humanities-based research on health can do epistemologically as well as pedagogically.

In our reflection on the constitutive and generic effects of public health discourse about food, we have tried to illustrate the place and significance of RHM within the larger realm of the health humanities. Rhetoric furnishes a rich set of theoretical-conceptual resources for investigating matters of health and medicine that may have instrumental value for researchers seeking their direct application in health-care settings. But we believe that as RHM comes of age—and the launch in 2018 of its first dedicated journal, *Rhetoric of Health and Medicine,* is one indication of the field's maturity—it is equally important to articulate with conviction and precision its place as a scholarly field that produces significant knowledge about health unavailable through other means, and that this knowledge has value in its own right, rather than principally or exclusively in relation to health-care professions and practices. Knowledge produced through research in RHM advances critical understanding of how our values, beliefs, and behaviors as health citizens are constituted through prevalent and ideologically inflected discourses of health and well-being.

REFERENCES

Althusser, L. (1968/1971). *Lenin and philosophy, and other essays* (B. Brewster, Trans.). London, UK: New Left Books.

Angeli, E., & Johnson-Sheehan, R. (2018). Introduction to the special issue: Medical humanities and/or the rhetoric of health and medicine. *Technical Communication Quarterly, 27*(1), 1–6.

Atkinson, S., Evans, B., Woods, A., & Kearns, R. (2015). "The medical" and "health" in a critical medical humanities. *Journal of Medical Humanities, 36*(1), 71–81.

Barry, C. A., Stevenson, F. A., Britten, N., Barber, N., & Bradley, C. P. (2001). Giving voice to the lifeworld: More humane, more effective medical care? A qualitative study of doctor-patient communication in general practice. *Social Science & Medicine, 53*(4), 487–505.

Belling, C. (2006). Toward a harder humanities in medicine. *Atrium, 3*, 1–5.

Bishop, J. P. (2008). Rejecting medical humanism: Medical humanities and the metaphysics of medicine. *Journal of Medical Humanities, 29*(1), 15–25.

Bleakley, A. (2019). Invoking the medical humanities to develop a #MedicineWeCanTrust. *Academic Medicine.* Advance online publication. https://journals.lww.com/academicmedicine/toc/2019/10000

Bleakley, A., Marshall, R., & Brömer, R. (2006). Toward an aesthetic medicine: Developing a core medical humanities undergraduate curriculum. *Journal of Medical Humanities, 27*(4), 197–213.

Brody, H. (2011). Defining the medical humanities: Three conceptions and three narratives. *Journal of Medical Humanities, 32*(1), 1–7.

Brown, M. M. (2019). Don't be the "Fifth Guy": Risk, responsibility, and the rhetoric of hand-washing campaigns. *Journal of Medical Humanities, 40*(2), 211–224.

Burke, K. (1966). *Language as symbolic action: Essays on life, literature and method.* Berkeley, CA: University of California Press.

Chambers, T. (2009). Manifesto for medicine studies. *Atrium, 7,* 4–5.

Charland, M. (1993). Constitutive rhetoric: The case of the peuple québécois. In T. W. Benson (Ed.), *Landmark essays in rhetorical criticism* (pp. 213–234). Davis, CA: Hermagoras.

Charon, R. (2001). Narrative medicine: A model for empathy reflection, profession, and trust. *Journal of the American Medical Association, 286*(15), 1897–1902.

Chiapperino, L., & Boniolo, G. (2014). Rethinking medical humanities. *Journal of Medical Humanities, 35*(4), 377–387.

Chiavaroli, N. (2017). Knowing how we know: An epistemological rationale for the medical humanities. *Medical Education, 51*, 13–21.

Cox, R., & Pezzullo, P. C. (2016). *Environmental communication and the public sphere* (4th ed.). London, UK: SAGE.

Crawford, P., Brown, B., Baker, C., Tischler, V., & Abrams, B. (2015). *Health humanities*. London, UK: Palgrave Macmillan.

Crawford, P., Brown, B., Tischler, V., & Baker, C. (2010). Health humanities: The future of medical humanities? *Mental Health Review Journal, 15*(3), 4–10.

Derkatch, C. (2016). *Bounding biomedicine: Evidence and rhetoric in the new science of alternative medicine*. Chicago, IL: University of Chicago Press.

Derkatch, C., & Spoel, P. (2017). Public health promotion of "local food": Constituting the self-governing citizen-consumer. *Health: An Interdisciplinary Journal for the Social Study of Health, Illness and Medicine, 21*(2), 1–17. https://doi.org/10.1177/1363459315590247

Elliott, C. [FearLoathingBTX]. (2016, May 10). @prof_goldberg @ColleenDerkatch There is a difference between studying a subject and putting him on your promotion and tenure committee. Retrieved from https://twitter.com/FearLoathingBTX/status/730058219175862272

Emmons, K. (2008). Narrating the emotional woman: Uptake and gender in discourses on depression. In H. Clark (Ed.), *Depression and narrative: Telling the dark* (pp. 111–126). Albany, NY: State University of New York Press.

Evans, M., & Greaves, D. (1999). Exploring the medical humanities. *British Medical Journal, 319*(7219), 1216.

Fountain, T. K. (2014). *Rhetoric in the flesh: Trained vision, technical expertise, and the gross anatomy lab*. New York, NY: Routledge.

Frank, A. (2014). Being a good story: The humanities as therapeutic practice. In T. Jones, D. Wear, & L. D. Friedman (Eds.), *Health humanities reader* (pp. 13–25). New Brunswick, NJ: Rutgers University Press.

Gillis, C. M. (2008). Medicine and humanities: Voicing connections. *Journal of Medical Humanities, 29*(1), 5–14.

Gouge, C. (2016). "Getting the knowledge right": Patient communication, agency, and knowledge. *Journal of Medical Humanities, 37*(1), 1–17.

Guthman, J. (2008). Neoliberalism and the making of food politics in California. *Geoforum, 39*, 1171–1183.

Henderson, S., & Petersen, A. (2002). Introduction: Consumerism in healthcare. In S. Henderson & A. Petersen (Eds.), *Consuming health: The commodification of health care* (pp. 1–10). New York, NY: Routledge.

Hyland, K. (2002). Genre: Language, context, and literacy. *Annual Review of Applied Linguistics, 22*, 113–135.

Jones, T., Blackie, M., Garden, R., & Wear, D. (2017). The almost right word: The move from *medical* to *health* humanities. *Academic Medicine, 92*(7), 932–935.

Jones, T., Wear, D., & Lester D. Friedman. (2014). Introduction. In T. Jones, D. Wear, & L. D. Friedman (Eds.), *Health humanities reader* (1–9). New Brunswick, NJ: Rutgers University Press.

Keränen, L. (2008). *Rhetorics of health and medicine*. Roundtable presentation at the meeting of the Rhetoric Society of America Conference, Seattle, WA.

Klugman, C. (2017). How health humanities will save the life of the humanities. *Journal of Medical Humanities, 38*, 419–430.

Koerber, A. (2013). *Breast or bottle? Contemporary controversies in infant-feeding policy and practice*. Columbia, SC: University of South Carolina Press.

Kumagi, A. (2017). Beyond "Dr. Feel-Good": A role for the humanities in medical education. *Academic Medicine, 92*, 1659–1660.

Lam, A. (2019). To dwell at the border. *Tendon, 1*. Retrieved from https://hopkinsmedicalhumanities.org/tendon-magazine/issue-1-borders/to-dwell-at-the-border/

Macneill, P. U. (2011). The arts and medicine: A challenging relationship. *Medical Humanities, 37*(2), 85–90.

Majdik, Z. (2014). Biological citizenship. In T. Thompson (Ed.), *Encyclopedia of health communication* (pp. 105–106). Thousand Oaks, CA: SAGE.

Mishler, E. G. (1984). *The discourse of medicine: Dialectics of medical interviews.* Norwood, NJ: Ablex.

Paré, A. (2002). Genre and identity: Individuals, institutions, and ideology. In R. Coe, L. Lingard, & T. Teslenko (Eds.), *The rhetoric and ideology of genre* (pp. 57–71). Cresskill, NJ: Hampton.

Petersen, A., Bleakley, A., Brömer, R., & Marshall, R. (2008). The medical humanities today: Humane health care or tool of governance? *Journal of Medical Humanities, 29*(1), 1–4.

Petersen, A., Davis, M., Fraser, S., & Lindsay, J. (2010) Healthy living and citizenship: An overview. *Critical Public Health, 20*(4), 391–400.

Petersen, A., & Lupton, D. (1996). *The new public health: Health and self in the age of risk.* London, UK: SAGE.

Polianski, I. J., & Fangerau, H. (2012). Toward "harder" medical humanities: Moving beyond the "two cultures" dichotomy. *Academic Medicine, 87*(1), 121–126.

Porter, D. (2011). *Health citizenship: Essays in social medicine and biomedical politics.* Berkeley, CA: University of California Medical Humanities Press.

Rose, N., & Novas, C. (2004). Biological citizenship. In A. Ong & S. J. Collier (Eds.), *Global assemblages: Technology, politics, and ethics as anthropological problems* (pp. 439–463). Oxford, UK: Blackwell.

Saffran, L. (2014). "Only connect": The case for public health humanities. *Medical Humanities, 40*(2), 105–110.

Schryer, C. F., & Spoel, P. (2005). Genre theory, healthcare discourse, and professional identity formation. *Journal of Business and Technical Communication (Special Issue on Medical Rhetoric), 19*(3), 249–278.

Scott, B., Segal, J. Z., & Keränen, L. (2013). Rhetorics of health and medicine: Inventional possibilities for scholarship and engaged practice. *POROI, 9*(1). Retrieved from http://ir.uiowa.edu/cgi/viewcontent.cgi?article=1157&context=poroi

Segal, J. Z. (2005). *Health and the rhetoric of medicine.* Carbondale, IL: Southern Illinois University Press.

Segal, J. Z. (2009). Rhetoric of health and medicine. In A. A. Lunsford, K. H. Wilson, & R. A. Eberly (Eds.), *The SAGE handbook of rhetorical studies* (pp. 227–246). Los Angeles, CA: SAGE.

Segal, J. Z. (2013). Suffering and the rhetoric of care. In M. J. Hyde & J. A. Herrick (Eds.), *After the genome: A language for our biotechnological future* (pp. 219–233). Waco, TX: Baylor University Press.

Segal, J. Z., & Richardson, A. (Co-organizers). (2006, October). *Health Humanities Conference.* Conference convened at Green College, University of British Columbia, Vancouver, BC.

Seigel, M. (2014). *The rhetoric of pregnancy.* Chicago, IL: University of Chicago Press.

Shapiro, J., Coulehan, J., Wear, D., & Montello, M. (2009). Medical humanities and their discontents: Definitions, critiques, and implications. *Academic Medicine, 84*(2), 192–198.

Solomon, M. (2015). *Making medical knowledge.* Oxford, UK: Oxford University Press.

Spoel, P. (2014). Health citizenship. In T. L. Thompson (Ed.), *Encyclopedia of health communication* (Vol. 2, pp. 565–567). London, UK: SAGE.

Spoel, P., & Den Hoed, R. C. (2014). Places and people: Rhetorical constructions of "community" in a Canadian environmental risk assessment. *Environmental Communication: A Journal of Nature and Culture, 8*(3), 267–285.

Spoel, P., & Derkatch, C. (2020). Resilience and self-reliance in Canadian food charter discourse. *Poroi 15*(1), Article 8.

Spoel, P., & Derkatch, C. (2016). Constituting community through food charters: A rhetorical-genre analysis. *Canadian Food Studies, 3*(1), 46–70.

Squier, S. M. (2007). Beyond nescience: The intersectional insights of health humanities. *Perspectives in Biology and Medicine, 50*(3), 334–347.

Tsevat, R. K., Sinha, A. A., Gutierrez, K. J., & DasGupta, S. (2015). Bringing home the health humanities: Narrative humility, structural competency, and engaged pedagogy. *Academic Medicine, 90*(11), 1462–1465.

Viney, W., Callard, F., & Woods, A. (2015). Critical medical humanities: Embracing entanglement, taking risks. *Medical Humanities, 41*(1), 2–7.

Wear, D. (2009). The medical humanities: Toward a renewed praxis. *Journal of Medical Humanities, 30*(4), 209–220.

Whitehead, C., & Kuper, A. (2015). A false dichotomy. *Canadian Medical Association Journal, 187*(9), 683–684.

CHAPTER 2

Mediating Minds

Disability Studies and the Rhetoric of Mental Health

DREW HOLLADAY AND MARGARET PRICE

BUILDING AND MAINTAINING connections to related fields must be a central component of defining the rhetoric of health and medicine (RHM) and of distinguishing its intellectual contributions from other scholarship that takes up similar topics. The field of disability studies (DS) shares not only topics with RHM but also a critical stance toward ideologies of health and illness and a focus on the vital role of discourse in identifying and challenging those ideologies. Supported by the recent development of scholarship at their intersection, we believe that RHM and DS will continue to illuminate common theoretical commitments and fruitful paths for future scholarship; at the same time, the juxtaposition of these two fields highlights the distinct types of knowledge and critique offered by rhetorical theory.

In this chapter, we demonstrate the utility of combining disability- and rhetoric-oriented approaches to yield valuable insights into the cultural construction of mental health and disorder, with implications for scholarship, advocacy, and public action. As a critical apparatus, RHM allows scholars to investigate the many ways that minds are mediated through culture, institutions, individuals, and our own conceptions of self. Further, DS's commitment to centering the perspective of disabled and ill subjects can productively combine with medical rhetoric scholarship, which often focuses on the production and negotiation of knowledge within expert communities. Together, the two fields open avenues for investigating the creation, circulation, and evolution of persuasive arguments related to mental health and mental disability.

We begin with an overview of DS and its theoretical orientation toward topics and sites commonly taken up in RHM. From this overview we highlight three central theoretical concepts employed frequently in DS, *the social model of disability, normality,* and *ableism,* and demonstrate their usefulness in analyzing how bodily and mental difference are defined and then deployed in discussions related to health and medicine. Next, we review existing scholarship that combines DS with rhetorical theory and situate these pieces in relation to the academic identity of RHM. Finally, we describe implications for the more specialized study in RHM. To illustrate, we discuss a few central themes related to mental health and disorder that make fertile avenues for our emerging field: circulating constructions of mental health, mental health and medical technology, and translation potential in research from psychiatry and neuroscience.

OVERVIEW OF DS

DS is itself a relatively new field, having cohered in the 1980s following the growth of the modern disability rights movement in previous decades (Charlton, 2000; Shakespeare, 2006; Shapiro, 1993). Like other critical academic fields, DS mobilized the political conviction of the rights movement to critique the academic and professional establishments that perpetuated inequality. Those working in DS sought to change the cultural conversations surrounding disability (and its commonplace counterpart, normalcy), identifying the ways that people with disabilities were vilified and feared, pitied and infantilized, segregated and ignored (Brueggemann, 1999; Davis, 1995; Erevelles, 2000; Linton, 1998; Longmore, 2003; Mitchell & Snyder, 2001; Wendell, 1996; Wilson & Lewiecki-Wilson, 2001). DS has incorporated methods from a range of disciplines, including philosophy, cultural studies, literary criticism, sociology, anthropology, and rhetorical theory.

While DS scholars recognized the role of popular discourses, they also paid attention to medical institutions that closely governed the identities and opportunities afforded people with various disabilities. Most importantly, medical institutions created and legitimized a deficit view of disability, constructing disability as brokenness, a lack, an abnormality, and a problem to be rectified. Medical discourse, in what would become known as the *medical model* or *individual model,* tends to assume that disability reflects an underlying disease or disorder in an individual; accordingly, interventions focus on physical aids or pharmaceuticals that will correct or ameliorate the "problem" and return the individual to a normal state. In the medical model, social and political circumstances surrounding disability are, at best, secondary to the physical or biological disorder, and in many cases considered irrelevant to planning disability interventions.

In contrast to the medical model, the disability rights movement—and DS scholars thereafter—offered the *social model of disability*, which asserts that disability is a social, not an individual, phenomenon: "it is society which disables physically impaired people. Disability is something imposed on top of our impairments, by the way we are unnecessarily isolated and excluded from full participation in society" (Union of the Physically Impaired Against Segregation, 1976, p. 3). As such, the social conditions that produce disability—policies, prejudices, environments—should be changed to accept with equity people with impairments. While traditional conceptions of disability may focus on the individual body limited by an impairment, Lennard J. Davis (1995) reminded us that "the disabled body is not a discrete object but rather a set of social relations . . . The body . . . has been conceptualized as a simple object when it is in fact a complex focus for competing power structures" (p. 11). Further, Davis argued that "the object of DS" is not the individual body or mind but rather "the set of social, historical, economic and cultural processes that regulate and control the way we thought about and think through the body" (p. 2). From this perspective, the cultural and political settings in which bodies and minds emerge become an essential site for investigation and critique, and changes to those settings are central to the protection and expansion of disability rights. Consequently, the work of DS scholarship often focuses on explicating how institutions and other social groups construct disability as an issue of individual limitation or tragedy, signifying deviance and needing to be pitied and/or "overcome." In response to these circulating cultural narratives of disability, DS scholars have proposed new ways of conceptualizing both individual and society in relation to disability, including revised definitions of health, independence/interdependence, care, disease/illness, and disability itself. Organizations devoted to disability rights have used the power of these reconceptualizations to petition for more equitable access and representation in society.

The social model of disability has been thoroughly debated and repeatedly critiqued within the field of DS (see Clare, 1999; Crow, 1996; Shakespeare, 2006, 2013). An important overview of these critiques comes from Kafer's (2013) *Feminist Queer Crip*, which explained the complexity (and heterogeneity) of DS approaches to medicine, culture, and politics. As Kafer noted, DS scholars do not reject medical approaches out of hand, nor do they rely exclusively on the ideal of the "barrier-free utopia" (Shakespeare, 2013) that the conventional social model suggests. Pointing out the sexist and racist roots of the development of the social model, as well as its lack of attention to materiality, Kafer drew on materialist feminist DS theory to propose a *political-relational* approach, which recognizes that "*both* impairment and disability are social" and that "disability is experienced in and through relationships" (pp. 7–8). Although Kafer is one of the best-known proponents of this materialist feminist DS model, her work draws upon scholars of feminist materialism both within and outside DS. These include Rosemarie Garland-Thomson (2011), who has argued that disability inheres neither in individual bodies nor in the environment, but rather in the emergent fit/misfit between the two; and Nirmala Erevelles (2011), who argues that the "becoming" of disability is inseparable from the material histories of race, global politics, and colonialism.

One important concept for scholars who expose and explain the cultural construction of disability has been *normality*. Influenced by the writing of Michel Foucault, many DS scholars write about the norm as the primary mechanism by which the disabled are marked as deviant. Reflecting on his methods, for example, Davis (1995) wrote that he "[directs] the spotlight not so much on disability . . . as on the notion of normalcy that makes the idea of disability (as well as the ideas of race, class, and gender) possible" (p. 158). Building on the work of Judith Butler and Rosi Braidotti, DS scholar Dan Goodley (2013) connected this theoretical orientation back to the body, which he described as "a field where intersecting material and symbolic forces converge; a surface where multiple codes of sex, class, age, race, and so forth, are inscribed" (p. 636). In this arrangement, the norm cannot remain a "natural," status-quo ideal against which any deviance is measured; instead, even the most "normal" bodies and minds are subject to the forces of normativity.

> The normative body is understood as being fashioned and materialized through cultural, political and social conditions ranging from surgery to self-help. The non-normative body—a body that appears as an object of fear and curiosity—is therefore considered an opportunity to think through values, ethics and politics that congregate around such bodies. (Goodley, 2013, p. 636)

By investigating normality as a social process rather than an objective fact, scholars in DS simultaneously identify disability as an "open" category without assumed negative valence and also disrupt the authority of biomedical views of disability based upon normative ideas of ab/normality and dis/ability.

Prevailing mainstream attitudes, however, continue to consider the disabled body and mind as Other—physically, visually, psychologically, behaviorally, and politically. According to DS, ableism appears not only through discrimination and violence but also through the social governing of normality across groups of people, both disabled and nondisabled. In *Contours of Ableism*, Fiona Kumari Campbell (2009) wrote that, while definitions of ableism are varied, "a chief feature of an ableist viewpoint is a belief that impairment or disability (irrespective of 'type') is inherently negative and should the opportunity present itself, be ameliorated, cured or indeed eliminated" (p. 5). In DS ableism represents the forces that oppress people with disabilities while also demanding conformity to a cultural ideal or stereotype. As Goodley (2013) wrote, ableism is always active: "the dominant ableist self is ready and willing to bring disabled people back into the norm (re/habilitate, educate) or banish them (cure, segregate) from its ghostly centre" (p. 640). While physical separation or lack of access may be its most obvious forms, ableism also functions in subtle ways to discipline nonnormative bodies and minds. Mitchell and Snyder (2001) described how disability may be "prostheticize[d]," brought back into "a regime of tolerable deviance" (pp. 6–7): "If disability falls too far from an acceptable norm, a prosthetic intervention seeks to accomplish an erasure of difference all together [*sic*]; yet, failing that, as is always the case with prosthesis, the minimal goal is to return one to an acceptable degree of difference" (p. 7). The normative body is the ideal and measure of all other bodies; ableism is the cultural force that disciplines individuals into more normative states and appearances. As Campbell (2009) argues, ableism may stem in part from unease with "bodies that ooze or are leaky, especially those that are fat, distressed, sick, dying, addicted and appear impermanent" (32).

Rhetoric and DS

Rhetorical scholars have made significant connections to DS in the past three decades, and much of this scholarship gave rise to methods and topics we now associate with RHM. In 1995 Brenda Jo Brueggemann published an article in *Rhetoric Review* on Deaf culture and American Sign Language, followed in 1997 with a resonant personal account of "'(almost) passing" and then "'coming out' as a deaf person" and its relation to her teaching of writing in *College English*. Brueggemann's (1999) book *Lend Me Your Ear* treated these and other related topics in much greater depth. In one chapter on "the audiologist's authority," she rooted the field of audiology in the designation of all hearing loss as pathology and rhetorically analyzed the interpretation of hearing test reports. Also in 1999 Brueggemann and James Fredal's essay "Studying Disability Rhetorically" posited rhetoric as a tool to help "explain, question, critique, and theorize disability" (p. 129) and showed the relevance of key terms from rhetorical theory for studies of disability (pp. 132ff). In 2001 the collection *Embodied Rhetorics: Disability in Language and Culture*, edited by Wilson and Lewiecki-Wilson, brought together a large group of rhetorical scholars to make an array of explicit connections with the field of DS, including Catherine Prendergast's reflections on medical, academic, and cultural representations of schizophrenia. This period also saw the publication of a number of articles and book chapters connecting rhetoric and DS (Barton, 2001; Brueggemann, Cheu, Dunn, Heifferon, & White, 2001; Dunn & De Mers, 2002; Feldmeier White, 2002; Lewiecki-Wilson, 2001, 2003; Lindgren, 2004; McRuer, 2004; Morse, 2003; Mossman, 2002).

From the mid-2000s, many scholars combining rhetoric and DS began to pursue more specialized topics and rhetorical contexts. Many scholars have made direct connections between RHM and DS (Jack, 2014; Price, 2011; Walters, 2014; among many others). Other texts have drawn broader connections between the disciplines, including Duffy and Yergeau's (2011) co-edited special issue of *DS Quarterly* on Disability and Rhetoric and Dolmage's (2013) wide-ranging volume *Disability Rhetoric*. DS scholars have also examined methodology closely, asking both what methodologies are used in DS and also what the unique affordances and constraints of DS methodology might be (see Minich, 2016; Ostrove & Rinaldi, 2013; Price, 2012).

POTENTIAL DIRECTIONS FOR RHM AND MENTAL HEALTH

Building on the record of current scholarship on rhetoric and DS, we propose a few potential directions of research in RHM, focused on mental health, in which DS approaches may be especially useful. As our field already understands, the concepts from DS we reviewed earlier—the political-relational model of disability, normativity, and ableism—can only be sustained through rhetorical uptake and circulation in public and private discourse. Combined with existing theoretical analyses of RHM, these concepts help maintain a focus on the cultural effects of medical discourse, the perspective of patients and users, and the political context of appeals to health. Each of the following sections points to relevant concepts and studies currently used in RHM and the unique contribution of the rhetorical perspective.

Circulating Constructions of Mental Health

Perhaps the most direct way that DS concepts can inform RHM research is in the analysis of cultural artifacts related to health. DS has a deep archive of such work in many disciplines and methodologies, including empirical research, cultural studies, ethnography, critical discourse analysis, media studies, and autobiography. While a majority of this work is directed toward physical and sensory disabilities, the concepts outlined earlier can be readily applied to mental disabilities as well. Accordingly, rhetoricians can use a DS frame to analyze different definitions of "mental health" and their circulation in expert and lay discourses.

Scholarship in rhetorical studies has investigated the ontology of mental health (Reynolds, 2008; Segal, 2011), "neurorhetorics" (Jack, 2010), diagnostic categories in psychiatry (Berkenkotter, 2008; Berkenkotter & Ravotas, 1997; McCarthy & Gerring, 1994; Price, 2010), identities and qualities attributed to mental health conditions (Heilker & King, 2010; Heilker & Yergeau, 2011; Jack, 2014 Johnson, 2010; Price, 2011; Yergeau, 2015, 2018), feminist studies of psychiatry (Donaldson, 2011; Nicki, 2001), and brain science (J. Johnson, 2010, 2014; D. Johnson, 2008; D. Johnson Thornton, 2011). By orienting research toward disability and illness as well as health, rhetoricians can investigate the ideals of the normative mind alongside the "deviant" minds that bring the norm into relief. Rhetorical scholars can examine how problems are ascribed to individuals with mental disabilities rather than the contexts in which they do not have support or access. In one common refrain in public discourse, children with mental disabilities are constructed as a burden to public education; in arguments for the segregation of these students, attention is often drawn to a particular diagnosis (such as attention-deficit hyperactive disorder or autism spectrum disorder) and the onus placed on the individual to conform to the educational environment. Moreover, sex and race play central roles in the diagnoses that schoolchildren receive; for example, Black boys are more likely to receive diagnostic labels that identify them as defiant or aggressive (Adams & Erevelles, 2016; Erevelles, 2000). The persuasiveness of the separation argument is dependent on individualizing the disability and seeing that disability as a justification for inequitable treatment and access—views that can be described as ableist. In contrast, some educational advocacy groups call for changes in the school environment and increases in instructional support to accommodate the needs of different students, including those with mental disabilities. Similar arguments can be seen in debates around the treatment of the homeless, justification for high rates of incarceration, denials of workplace accommodation, and critiques of the welfare state.

A DS critique of normality includes a critique of the phrase *mental health* itself (Price, 2010), thus making space for other discursive possibilities, including *c/s/x* or *neurodiversity*. These other possibilities, quickly glossed in this paragraph, overlap in some cases but are not identical. The consumer/survivor/ex-patient (c/s/x) movement emerged in the late 1960s, and its current proponents argue for a model of mental health that empha-sizes acceptance, and peer support over medication and institutionalization (see Morrison, 2005). The c/s/x movement, like the overlapping Mad Pride movement, emphasizes mental disability as a minority identity and the need to question standard conceptions of mental health; for instance, as the mission statement of the Icarus Project ("Mission, Vision, & Principles," n.d.) asserts, "We envision a new culture that allows the space and freedom for exploring different states of being, and recognizes that breakdown can be the entrance to breakthrough." The neurodiversity movement, which began with autism self-advocacy in the 1990s, argues that autism should be viewed as part of human diversity rather than as a medical disorder. Activists in these various movements engage directly with scientific and medical ideologies in order to offer alternative views of mental health. For example, Bradley Lewis's (2006) *Moving Beyond Prozac* is a critique of the psychiatric profession but also a call to action for psychiatrists, offering detailed suggestions for ways that psychi-atric practices might be reformed.

Rhetoricians are uniquely equipped to study the creation and circula-tion of such public arguments. As Miller (2010) noted about classical texts in rhetoric, "the ancients were astute observers of the workings of rhetorical power, particularly in the public realm" (p. 19); and in the past two centuries rhetoric has continued to be considered "the art of public discourse" (p. 31). Foundational scholars of the New Rhetoric, like Kenneth Burke, Chaim Perel-man, and Lucie Olbrechts-Tyteca, frequently focused on public discourse and political argumentation. In relation to RHM, Segal (1997) studied metaphors in public policy, where "biomedicine supplies the terms in which the health policy debate takes place" (p. 218). More recently, Keränen edited a special issue of the *Journal of Medical Humanities* focused on rhetoric and publics; as Keränen (2014) argued, "a rhetorical model of publics presents an inclusive vision of health and medicine as networked, public exchange and encourages us to see participants in health and medical processes as more than consum-ers, clients, and patients" (p. 103).

With this history of engagement with public issues, RHM scholars are well placed to analyze activist discourse that seeks to, in addition to resist-ing biomedical language, *reframe* it in more equitable terms. Autistic blogger Cohen-Rottenberg (2009) exemplified this rhetorical strategy in her article "If I Could Rewrite the DSM-IV Criteria for Autism." After stating that the inclusion of autism in the DSM[1] is "deeply offensive" to her, Cohen-Rottenberg

---

1. The *Diagnostic and Statistical Manual of Mental Disorders,* American psychiatry's handbook for the description of mental disorders and their symptoms.

reflected on why she wanted to create a new version: "I thought it might be fun to rewrite the diagnostic criteria, line by line, so that the text describes us as something more than walking collections of mysterious pathologies" (para. 2). In this brief example, she replaces language of abnormality and devaluation with a statement of understanding:

2. ~~apparently inflexible adherence to specific, nonfunctional routines or rituals~~
2. An innate capacity for self-care that manifests itself in the creation of comforting routines and a fascination with patterns of all kinds.

Cohen-Rottenberg reframed the psychiatric description, which identifies atypical childhood behaviors as manifestations of dysfunction, in new, positive terms like *self-care* and used the affirming language of *creativity* and *fascination*. Combining RHM and DS perspectives to this text, one can describe how Cohen-Rottenberg is using epideictic appeals to discredit psychiatric observation and elevate autistic self-knowledge, adapting a medical genre to influence its purpose and connotation, and openly resisting medicalization of behavior—all with the political (and rhetorical) aim of shifting popular conceptions of autism. Rhetoricians can also work to include c/s/x and neurodiverse (also termed neurodivergent/neuroqueer) perspectives like Cohen-Rottenberg's in academic discourse (Jones & Brown, 2012) as well as advocating for their inclusion in public debates around issues like health care.

In addition to political and scientific discourses, rhetoricians can also use this approach to analyze the work of formal mental health advocacy organizations, like Autism Speaks and the National Alliance on Mental Illness (NAMI), building on previous scholarship on medical advocacy (Keränen, 2014; Koerber, 2013; Kopelson, 2013; Pezzullo, 2003; Segal, 2007). Mental health, like other disability and illness categories, is culturally suspended between ideologies of science, medicine, morality, and personhood; advocacy groups must navigate a complicated rhetorical terrain to voice their positions. Autism Speaks, for instance, has repeatedly taken up the tropes of epidemic and cure as the impetus for its work, and NAMI foregrounds biological descriptions of schizophrenia to demonstrate the "reality" of the condition and the need for treatment; both of these rhetorical strategies reinforce medicalized views of mental disability and can, as Angela K. Thachuk (2011) argued, actually *increase* stigma attached to these conditions. Further, the issue of rhetorical agency in representation is especially fraught for mental health advocacy groups since the interests of people with mental disabilities are more likely to be communicated by others, whether family, caretakers, or medical professionals. In the case of autism or other common childhood diagnoses like ADD/ADHD, eating disorders, and (increasingly) bipolar disorder, parents stand in as agents for the person with a diagnosis that carries *kakoethos* (Johnson, 2010) and the status of "demi-rhetor" (Yergeau, 2015). Finally, some advocacy groups, such as the Autistic Self-Advocacy Network, have taken a disability rights approach to their work, offering rhetoricians sites to not only study the application and circulation of DS-related concepts but also to work as allies to increase self-representation and social justice.

Another area ripe for study is the concept of *mental health literacy* (see Jorm, 2012; White & Pike, 2013), which indicates that mental health knowledge requires translation in another sense: to the public, and to consumers themselves. Rhetoricians should investigate the implications of *literacy* in this context, given that the phrase is used (as other deployments of *literacy* often are) to measure compliance with cultural norms rather than knowledge or fluency in a particular discourse. The routinely valorized concept of literacy here describes how fully patients accept their doctor's opinions of their diagnoses and appropriate treatments. Building on DS analyses of medical intervention, RHM scholars can trace the way that mental health treatments are described and justified in ableist (and also racist, sexist, and classist) terms. Although mental health literacy work does pay some attention to issues of cultural difference or patients' difficulty trusting health-care professionals, the consistent conclusion is simply that patients need to be better educated (rather than, for example, that perhaps medical practices might need to change). For instance, Jorm (2012; drawing upon Lee et al., 2010) stated that "some languages lack words to adequately describe concepts such as depression" (p. 231). This statement—which is situated within a very brief three-paragraph section subtitled "Mental Health Literacy and Cultural Diversity"—seems to ignore the possibility that "some" languages might enable concepts that Western health-care practitioners do not understand.

MENTAL HEALTH AND MEDICAL TECHNOLOGY

In DS, medical technology has been scrutinized for its connection with "compulsory able-bodiedness" (McRuer, 2006a) and the government of normality as well as their individualizing effects. Technology plays a pivotal role in the persuasiveness of descriptions of mental abnormality and, in tandem, the cultural acceptance of treatments that focus on the individual. As we describe below, the tools of DS and RHM can be usefully applied to discussions of medical imaging and surveillance technology.

Medical Imaging. As medical imaging technology becomes more refined, the visual representation of disease increases in prominence both within expert communities and in the popular imagination. While images of cancerous cells or skeletal X-rays are common in writing on science and medicine, none is more ubiquitous than the brain scan. While these scans are far from transparent and require expert interpretation, they often function as evidence with given authority in popular reports that, for example, tie different brain states to mental disorders; as Fitzpatrick (2012) wrote, "like the tabloid pictures, once brain scans are in the public domain, the brightly colored images are also freed from the controlled experimental context during which they were obtained" (p. 193). While Fitzpatrick cautioned that "we cannot draw conclusions from looking at functional brain images without the full scientific context" (194), she acknowledged the power and "allure" that they have gained in popular accounts of the brain and behavior (see also Beaulieu, 2002; Weisberg, Keil, Goodstein, Rawson, & Gray, 2008; Weisberg, Taylor, & Hopkins, 2015).

Rhetorical scholars have interrogated the use of medical imaging (Dolmage, 2015; D. Johnson, 2008; Jack & Appelbaum, 2010; Teston, 2012); however, the lens of DS helps maintain a focus on consequences for people with mental disabilities when brain imaging affects the broader discourse of mental health. For instance, imaging is sometimes used as part of the apparatus that justifies moves such as confinement in institutions, and brain scans have been offered in court proceedings as evidence of legal insanity or mitigated responsibility (Erickson, 2010; Rembis, 2014; Rushing, 2014); this is part of the medical-carceral apparatus on which DS has focused (Ben-Moshe, Chapman, & Carey, 2014). In a recent *New York Times* article, one neuroscientist explained that "neurological immaturity may contribute to criminal behavior" and that brain scans should be used as evidence in sentencing of juveniles, while another argued that "brain scan data" demonstrates that "young adults are just as capable of restraint as older adults" (Requarth, 2017). Brain imaging also appears in popular discourse as a confirmation of biomedical constructions of mental disability, where colorful representations of electrical activity and neurochemistry act as proof for the sole relevance of medical interventions. In an observation that mirrors DS arguments regarding representation, S. Scott Graham (2015) wrote that the authority of neuroimaging in establishing the existence of pain, even when it seems to hold some benefit for the individual patient, can "still [be] an act of epistemic violence," since "patient subjective report is still not trusted, and these patients still are not authorized to speak and be heard" (p. 144). By connecting Graham's argument to work in DS—for example, Alyson Patsavas (2014) on chronic pain, or

Ellen Samuels (2014) on "biocertification"—RHM scholars can demonstrate that such epistemic violence is rooted in ableist ideology that discredits the voice of people with disabilities more broadly, and thus "fibromyalgics and migraineurs" (Graham, 2015, p. 144) have political interests in common with anyone whose credibility, health, or rationality is subject to the confirmation of brain imaging technologies.

Technologies of Surveillance and Control. Historically, designations of mental illness mark individuals for increased suspicion, scrutiny, and surveillance. The rapid growth of technology related to health and medicine has significant ramifications for people with mental disabilities: while many medical technologies monitor physical signs of illness, those related to mental health also monitor the subject and her behavior. Rhetoricians of health and medicine can contribute to critiques of mental health technology by recognizing the topoi used to inspire that technology's development, justify its use, and defend its effects—topoi that often derive from negative stereotypes, like the violent and incoherent schizophrenic or the emotionless child with autism. Again, the DS stance encourages a focus on the ways in which the disability, and the disabled person, are constructed by a culture that assumes a stable "norm" rather than the deliberations of expert communities that create and apply the technology. For example, the Koenigs Lab at the University of Wisconsin–Madison uses the threat of criminal deviance to justify its study of "psychopathic prison inmates." A primary source of data for the researchers here is "multimodal brain imaging to identify structural and functional abnormalities in the psychopaths' brains," and its conclusions "could have profound implications for the clinical and legal management of psychopathic criminals" ("Koenigs Lab"). Some proponents of biological criminology believe that genetic studies and medical imaging can be used to identify a risk of, and perhaps even predict, criminal behavior. Adrian Raine, author of *The Anatomy of Violence: The Biological Roots of Crime,* argued that "parole boards are making . . . predictive decisions every day" and that "biological measures . . . could only improve the prediction" (qtd. in T. Adams, 2013). As with Graham's discussion of pain sufferers above, in this situation biomedical and genetic tests testify in place of the individual, with direct consequences for the length and nature of their incarceration.

By taking a DS stance and emphasizing the perspective of the *user* (or *subject*), rhetoricians can demonstrate how technologies related to mental health are predicated on a return to the norm and encourage the monitoring of difference. In her analysis of mHealth technologies, Teston (2016) "challenges narratives of scientific and medical progress that often accompany the emergence of wearable technologies" (p. 253) and shows that the pursuit of a "culture of health" can leave untouched health disparities in populations without access. Like Teston's (2016) use of the concept of precarity to illustrate rhetorical disconnects, work in RHM can take up DS critiques of medical technology to "[help] identify systemic inequities hiding out in a host of material-discursive forces" (p. 266). DS critiques often focus on the goal of normality—as rehabilitation or prosthesis—in medical interventions; mental health treatments, while not always visible, have similar aims. Pharmaceuticals are nearly ubiquitous in psychiatric treatment, most of which seek to rehabilitate abnormal brain states and return the user to normative behavior (see Segal, 2011, for a detailed explanation of these goals in pharmaceutical advertisements). In line with similar DS arguments toward medicine, some mental health advocates have criticized psychiatry's focus on compliance with pharmaceutical treatment without sufficient personal and community support. How, then, might RHM scholars respond to the development of compliance-tracking technologies? One recent report in the *Journal of Clinical Psychiatry* described how ingestible sensors in pills that communicate with wearable devices and smartphones will help doctors keep track of when patients are taking their medications (Profit et al., 2016). Developers pitch this "digital medicine system" as a way to help patients take control of their own health, yet they fail to address the implications of such surveillance power in the hands of doctors (and, inevitably, institutions that oversee health insurance, government assistance, and criminal justice).

Developers attach different purposes to wearable technologies for children such as Reveal, a bracelet designed to be worn by children with autism to monitor physiological signs of stress and send data to a parent's or caregiver's smartphone. Like many medical devices, the bracelet's description uses the language of empowerment prominently and notes its ability to be "a tool for self-regulation," presumably for older users ("Reveal," para. 2). Other stated purposes, though, implicate a desire to anticipate and control nonnormative behavior: the bracelet's smartphone app allows the user to "track observed behavior" with notes and will "notify you of an oncoming meltdown" ("Reveal"). Since the bracelet itself simply transmits the wearer's heart rate, the app cannot use the data produced to distinguish between anxiety and other emotional states like excitement. The user, however, makes notes to accompany the rise and fall of the wearer's pulse, notes that might include (as shown in the app's illustration) the duration of an "episode," the current activity ("getting dressed"), or nonnormative behaviors ("arm flapping"). One can imagine a seamless integration between such tracking and the dominant form of therapy for autism, applied behavioral analysis, whose practices have been condemned by autism self-advocates and DS scholars (Broderick, 2011;

Ne'eman, 2010; Yergeau, 2018). Rhetoricians can analyze the gaps between such devices' stated purposes and the interests of disability self-advocates, as well as the discourse surrounding the devices in medical, professional, and governmental contexts. For example, with regard to the Reveal bracelet, rhetorical scholars can recognize the division of normal/acceptable and abnormal/unacceptable behaviors in the device's description, as well as its primary audience of parents and caretakers rather than people with mental disabilities themselves; a DS stance might relate that division of behavior to normative, ableist assumptions and the primary audience to a history of discrimination in which others are given authority over people with disabilities. By combining RHM and DS in this instance, the mechanisms of logic and persuasion may be connected to historical inequities as well as the political project to address them.

CONCLUSION

The late DS scholar Tobin Siebers (2008) wrote of disability's powerful, but often hidden, influence in the cultural imagination: disability "represents a diacritical marker of difference that secures inferior, marginal, or minority status, while not having its presence as a marker acknowledged in the process" (p. 7). The silent effects of disability—and ableism—hold particularly strong influence in RHM, where treatments bring individuals back into bodily and mental normality and health is often synonymous with ability. While critical theories of health and disease are endemic to RHM, we believe that DS has much to offer through its rich research tradition, methodologies, and emphasis on the knowledge produced by marginalized subjects. Voices advocating intersectionality in DS can support RHM as it dialogues with feminist, queer, racial, and transnational perspectives on health discourse and communication (Goodley, 2013; Kafer, 2013; McRuer, 2006b). Most concretely, rhetoricians can contribute to activist discourses that work toward equity and justice.

REFERENCES

Adams, D. L., & Erevelles, N. (2016). Shadow play: DisCrit, dis/respectability, and carceral logics. In D. J. Connor, B. A. Ferri, & S. A. Annamma (Eds.), *DisCrit: Disability studies and critical race theory in education* (pp. 131–144). New York, NY: Teachers College Press.

Adams, T. (2013). How to spot a murderer's brain. *The Guardian*, May 11. Retrieved from https://www.theguardian.com/science/2013/may/12/how-to-spot-a-murderers-brain

American Psychiatric Association. (2013). *Diagnostic and statistical manual of mental disorders* (5th ed.). Arlington, VA: Author.

Barton, E. (1996). Negotiating expertise in discourses of disability. *TEXT, 16,* 299–322.

Barton, E. (2001). Discourses of disability in the *Digest. JAC: A Journal of Composition Theory, 21*(3), 555–581.

Beaulieu, A. (2002). Images are not the (only) truth: Brain mapping, visual knowledge, and iconoclasm. *Science, Technology, & Human Values, 27*(1), 53–86.

Ben-Moshe, L., Chapman, C., & Carey, A. C. (Eds.). (2014). *Disability incarcerated: Imprisonment and disability in the United States and Canada.* New York, NY: Palgrave Macmillan.

Berkenkotter, C. (2008). *Patient tales: Case histories and the uses of narrative in psychiatry.* Columbia, SC: University of South Carolina Press.

Berkenkotter, C., & Ravotas, D. (1997). Genre as tool in the transmission of practice over time and across professional boundaries. *Mind, Culture, and Activity, 4*(4), 256–274.

Broderick, A. (2011). Autism as rhetoric: Exploring watershed rhetorical moments in Applied Behavior Analysis discourse. *Disability Studies Quarterly, 31*(3). Retrieved from http://dsq-sds.org/article/view/1674/1597

Brueggemann, B. J. (1995). The coming out of Deaf culture and American Sign Language: An exploration into visual rhetoric and literacy. *Rhetoric Review, 13*(2), 409–420.

Brueggemann, B. J. (1997). On (almost) passing. *College English, 59*(6), 647–660.

Brueggemann, B. J. (1999). *Lend me your ear: Rhetorical constructions of deafness.* Washington, DC: Gallaudet University Press.

Brueggemann, B. J. (2005). Delivering disability, willing speech. In C. Sandahl & P. Auslander (Eds.), *Bodies in commotion: Disability and performance* (pp. 17–29). Ann Arbor, MI: University of Michigan Press.

Brueggemann, B. J., Cheu, J., Dunn, P., Heifferon, B., & White, L. (2001). Becoming visible: Lessons in disability. *College Composition and Communication, 52*(3), 368–398.

Brueggemann, B. J., & Fredal, J. A. (1999). Studying disability rhetorically. In M. Corker & S. French (Eds.), *Disability discourse* (pp. 129–135). Philadelphia, PA: Open University Press.

Campbell, F. K. (2009). *Contours of ableism: The production of disability and abledness.* New York, NY: Palgrave Macmillan.

Charlton, J. I. (2000). *Nothing about us without us: Disability oppression and empowerment.* Berkeley, CA: University of California Press.

Clare, E. (1999). *Exile and pride: Disability, queerness, and liberation.* Cambridge, MA: SouthEnd.

Cohen-Rottenberg, R. (2009). If I could rewrite the DSM-IV criteria for autism. Retrieved from http://www.journeyswithautism.com/2009/12/20/if-i-could-rewrite-the-dsm-iv-criteria-for-autism/

Crow, L. (1996). Including all of our lives: Renewing the social model of disability. In C. Barnes & G. Mercer (Eds.), *Disability & illness: Exploring the divide* (pp. 55–72). Leeds, UK: Disability.

Davis, L. J. (1995). *Enforcing normalcy: Disability, deafness, and the body.* London, UK: Verso.

Dolmage, J. (2005). Between the valley and the field: Metaphor and disability. *Prose Studies, 27*(1), 108–119.

Dolmage, J. (2006). Breathe upon us an even flame: Hephaestus, history and the body of rhetoric. *Rhetoric Review, 25*(2), 119–140.

Dolmage, J. (2013). *Disability rhetoric.* Syracuse, NY: Syracuse University Press.

Donaldson, E. J. (2011). Revisiting the corpus of the madwoman: Further notes toward a feminist disability studies theory of mental illness. In K. Q. Hall (Ed.), *Feminist disability studies* (pp. 91–113). Bloomington, IN: Indiana University Press.

Duffy, J., & Yergeau, M. (Eds.). (2011). Disability and rhetoric [Special Issue]. *Disability Studies Quarterly, 31*(3). Retrieved from http://dsq-sds.org/issue/view/84

Dunn, P. A., & De Mers, K. D. (2002). Reversing notions of disability and accommodation: Embracing universal design in writing pedagogy and web space. *Kairos, 7*(1). Retrieved from http://kairos.technorhetoric.net/7.1/coverweb/dunn_demers/

Erevelles, N. (2000). Educating unruly bodies: Critical pedagogy, disability studies, and the politics of schooling. *Educational Theory, 50*(1), 25–47.

Erevelles, N. (2011). *Disability and difference in global contexts.* New York, NY: Palgrave Macmillan.

Erickson, S. K. (2010). Blaming the brain. *Minnesota Journal of Law, Science & Technology, 11,* 27–77.

Fahnestock, J. (1986). Accommodating science: The rhetorical life of scientific facts. *Written Communication, 3*(3), 275–296.

Feldmeier White, L. (2002). Learning disability, pedagogies, and public discourse. *College Composition and Communication, 53*(4), 705–738.

Fitzpatrick, S. M. (2012). Functional brain imaging: Neuro-turn or wrong turn? In M. M. Littlefield & J. M. Johnson (Eds.), *The neuroscientific turn: Transdisciplinarity in the age of the brain* (pp. 180–198). Ann Arbor, MI: University of Michigan Press.

Garland-Thomson, R. (2002). Integrating disability, transforming feminist theory. *NWSA Journal, 14*(3), 1–32.

Garland-Thomson, R. (2011). Misfits: A feminist materialist disability concept. *Hypatia, 26*(3), 591–609.

Goodley, D. (2013). Dis/entangling critical disability studies. *Disability & Society, 28*(5), 631–644.

Graham, S. S. (2015). *The politics of pain medicine: A rhetorical-ontological inquiry.* Chicago, IL: University of Chicago Press.

Heilker, P., & King, J. (2010). The rhetorics of online autism advocacy: A case for rhetorical listening. In S. A. Selber (Ed.), *Rhetorics and technologies: New directions in writing and communication* (pp. 113–133). Columbia, SC: University of South Carolina Press.

Heilker, P., & Yergeau, M. (2011). Autism and rhetoric. *College English, 73*(5), 485–497.

Jack, J. (Ed.). (2010). Neurorhetorics [Special Issue]. *Rhetoric Society Quarterly, 40*(5).

Jack, J. (2014). *Autism and gender: From refrigerator mothers to computer geeks.* Urbana-Champaign, IL: University of Illinois Press.

Jack, J., & Appelbaum, L. G. (2010). "This is your brain on rhetoric": Research directions for neurorhetorics. *Rhetoric Society Quarterly, 40*(5), 411–437.

Johnson, D. (2008). "How do you know unless you look?" Brain imaging, biopower and practical neuroscience. *Journal of Medical Humanities, 29,* 147–161.

Johnson, J. (2010). The skeleton on the couch: The Eagleton affair, rhetorical disability, and the stigma of mental illness. *Rhetoric Society Quarterly, 40*(5), 459–478.

Johnson, J. (2014). *American lobotomy: A rhetorical history.* Ann Arbor, MI: University of Michigan Press.

Johnson Thornton, D. (2011). Neuroscience, affect, and the entrepreneurialization of motherhood. *Communication and Critical/Cultural Studies, 8*(4), 399–424.

Jones, N., & Brown, R. L. (2012). The absence of psychiatric c/s/x perspectives in academic discourse: Consequences and implications. *Disability Studies Quarterly, 33*(1). Retrieved from http://dsq-sds.org/article/view/3433/3198

Jorm, A. F. (2012). Mental health literacy: Empowering the community to take action for better mental health. *American Psychologist, 67*(3), 231–243.

Kafer, A. (2013). *Feminist, Queer, Crip.* Bloomington, IN: Indiana University Press.

Keränen, L. (2014). Public engagements with health and medicine. *Journal of Medical Humanities, 35*(2), 103–109.

Koenigs Lab. (n.d.). Retrieved from http://koenigslab.psychiatry.wisc.edu/

Koerber, A. (2013). *Breast or bottle? Contemporary controversies in infant feeding policy and practice.* Columbia, SC: University of South Carolina Press.

Kopelson, K. (2013). Risky appeals: Recruiting to the environmental breast cancer movement in the age of "pink fatigue." *Rhetoric Society Quarterly, 43*(2), 107–133.

Lewiecki-Wilson, C. (2001). "Doing the right thing" vs. disability rights: A response to Ellen Barton. *JAC, 21*(4), 870–881.

Lewiecki-Wilson, C. (2003). Rethinking rhetoric through mental disabilities. *Rhetoric Review, 22*(2), 156–167.

Lewis, B. (2006). *Moving beyond Prozac, DSM, and the new psychiatry: The birth of postpsychiatry.* Ann Arbor, MI: University of Michigan Press.

Lindblom, K., & Dunn, P. A. (2003). The roles of rhetoric in constructions and reconstructions of disability. *Rhetoric Review, 22*(2), 167–174.

Lindgren, K. (2004). Bodies in trouble: Identity, embodiment, and disability. In B. G. Smith & B. Hutchison (Eds.), *Gendering disability* (pp. 145–165). New Brunswick, NJ: Rutgers.

Linton, S. (1998). *Claiming disability: Knowledge and identity.* New York, NY: New York University Press.

Longmore, P. K. (2003). *Why I burned my book and other essays on disability.* Philadelphia, PA: Temple University Press.

Lunsford, S. (2005). Seeking a rhetoric of the rhetoric of dis/abilities. *Rhetoric Review, 24*(4), 330–333.

McCarthy, L. P., & Gerring, J. P. (1994). Revising psychiatry's charter document: DSM-IV. *Written Communication, 11*(2), 147–192.

McRuer, R. (2004). Composing bodies; or, De-composition: queer theory, disability studies, and alternative corporealities. *JAC, 24*(1), 47–78.

McRuer, R. (2006a). Compulsory able-bodiedness and queer/disabled existence. In L. J. Davis (Ed.), *The disability studies reader* (2nd ed., pp. 88–99). New York, NY: Routledge.

McRuer, R. (2006b). *Crip theory: Cultural signs of queerness and disability.* New York, NY: New York University Press.

Mission, vision, & principles. (n.d.). Retrieved from http://theicarusproject.net/mission-vision-principles

Miller, C. R. (2010). Should we name the tools? Concealing and revealing the art of rhetoric. In D. Coogan & J. Ackerman (Eds.), *The public work of rhetoric: Citizen-scholars and civic engagement* (pp. 19–38). Columbia, SC: University of South Carolina Press.

Minich, J. A. (2016). Enabling whom? Critical disability studies now. *Lateral, 5*(1).

Mitchell, D. T., & Snyder, S. L. (2001). *Narrative prosthesis: Disability and the dependencies of discourse.* Ann Arbor, MI: University of Michigan Press.

Morrison, L. J. (2005). *Talking back to psychiatry: The psychiatric consumer/survivor/ex-patient movement.* New York, NY: Routledge.

Morse, T. A. (Ed.). (2003). Symposium: Representing disability rhetorically. *Rhetoric Review, 22*(2), 154–202.

Mossman, M. (2002). Visible disability in the college classroom. *College English, 64*(6), 645–659.

Ne'eman, A. (2010). The future (and the past) of autism advocacy, or why the ASA's magazine, *The Advocate,* wouldn't publish this piece. *Disability Studies Quarterly, 30*(1). Retrieved from http://dsq-sds.org/article/view/1059/1244

Nicki, A. (2001). The abused mind: Feminist theory, psychiatric disability, and trauma. *Hypatia, 16*(3), 80–104.

Ostrove, J. & J. Rinaldi. (2013). Introduction to special issue: Self-reflection as scholarly praxis. *Disability Studies Quarterly, 33*(2).

Patsavas, A. (2014). Recovering a cripistemology of pain: Leaky bodies, connective tissue, and feeling discourse. *Journal of Literary and Cultural Disability Studies, 8*(2), 203–218.

Pezzullo, P. (2003). Resisting "National Breast Cancer Awareness Month": The rhetoric of counter-publics and their cultural performances. *Quarterly Journal of Speech, 89*(4), 345–365.

Prendergrast, C. (2001). On the rhetorics of mental disability. In J. C. Wilson & C. Lewiecki-Wilson (Eds.), *Embodied rhetorics: Disability in language and culture* (pp. 45–60). Carbondale, IL: Southern Illinois University Press.

Price, M. (2011). *Mad at school: Rhetorics of mental disability and academic life.* Ann Arbor, MI: University of Michigan Press.

Price, M. (2012). Disability studies methodology: Explaining ourselves to ourselves. In K. M. Powell & P. Takayoshi (Ed.), *Practicing research in writing studies: Reflexive and ethically responsible research* (pp. 159–186). New York, NY: Hampton Press.

Profit, D., Rohatagi, S., Zhao, C., Hatch, A., Docherty, J. P., & Peters-Strickland, T. S. (2016). Developing a digital medicine system in psychiatry: Ingestion detection rate and latency period. *Journal of Clinical Psychiatry, 77*(9), e1095–e1100.

Raine, A. (2013). *The anatomy of violence: The biological roots of crime.* New York, NY: Vintage.

Rembis, M. (2014). The new asylums: Madness and mass incarceration in the neoliberal era. In L. Ben-Moshe, C. Chapman, & A. C. Carey (Eds.), *Disability incarcerated: Imprisonment and disability in the United States and Canada* (pp. 139–159). New York, NY: Palgrave Macmillan.

Requarth, T. (2017). A California court for young adults calls on science. *New York Times,* April 17. Retrieved from https://www.nytimes.com/2017/04/17/health/young-adult-court-san-francisco-california-neuroscience.html

Reveal: Empowered care for autism. (2016). Retrieved from https://www.indiegogo.com/projects/reveal-empowered-care-for-autism--2#/

Reynolds, J. F. (2008). The rhetoric of mental health care. In B. Heifferon & S. C. Brown (Eds.), *Rhetoric of healthcare: Essays toward a new disciplinary inquiry* (pp. 149–159). New York, NY: Hampton.

Rösler, F. (2012). Some unsettled problems in behavioral neuroscience research. *Psychological Research: An International Journal of Perception, Attention, Memory, and Action, 76*(2), 131–144.

Rushing, S. E. (2014). The admissibility of brain scans in criminal trials: The case of Positron Emission Tomography. *Court Review, 50*(2), 62–69.

Samuels, E. (2014). *Fantasies of identification: Disability, gender, race.* New York: NYU Press.

Scutti, S. (2016). Scientists confirm genetics of schizophrenia. *Cable News Network,* October 19. Retrieved from https://www.cnn.com/2016/10/19/health/schizophrenia-genome-study/index.html

Segal, J. Z. (1997). Public discourse and public policy: Some ways that metaphor constrains health (care). *Journal of Medical Humanities, 18*(4), 217–231.

Segal, J. Z. (2007). Illness as argumentation: A prolegomenon to the rhetorical study of contestable complaints. *Health, 11*(2), 227–244.

Segal, J. Z. (2011). What, in addition to drugs, do pharmaceutical ads sell? The rhetoric of pleasure in direct-to-consumer advertising for prescription pharmaceuticals. In D. Dysart-Gale & J. Leach (Eds.), *Rhetorical questions of health and medicine* (pp. 9–32). Lanham, MD: Lexington.

Shakespeare, T. (2006). *Disability rights and wrongs*. London, UK: Routledge.

Shakespeare, T. (2013). *Disability rights and wrongs revisited* (2nd ed.). London, UK: Routledge.

Shapiro, J. P. (1993). *No pity: People with disabilities forging a new civil rights movement*. New York, NY: Times Books.

Siebers, T. (2008). *Disability theory*. Ann Arbor, MI: University of Michigan Press.

Teston, C. (2012). Moving from artifact to action: A grounded investigation of visual displays of evidence during medical deliberations. *Technical Communication Quarterly, 21*(3), 187–209.

Teston, C. (2016). Rhetoric, precarity, and mHealth technologies. *Rhetoric Society Quarterly, 46*(3), 251–268.

Thachuk, A. K. (2011). Stigma and the politics of biomedical models of mental illness. *International Journal of Feminist Approaches to Bioethics, 4*(1), 140–163.

Union of the Physically Impaired Against Segregation. (1976). *Fundamental principles of disability*. London, UK: Author.

Walters, S. (2014). *Rhetorical touch: Disability, identification, haptics*. Columbia, SC: University of South Carolina Press.

Weisberg, D. S., Keil, F. C., Goodstein, J., Rawson, E., & Gray, J. R. (2008). The seductive allure of neuroscience explanations. *Journal of Cognitive Neuroscience, 20*(3), 470–477.

Weisberg, D. S., Taylor, J. C. V., & Hopkins, E. J. (2015). Deconstructing the seductive allure of neuroscience explanations. *Judgment & Decision Making, 10*(5), 429–441.

Wendell, S. (1996). *The rejected body: Feminist philosophical reflections on disability*. New York, NY: Routledge.

White, K. & Pike, R. (2008). The making and marketing of mental health literacy in Canada. In B.A. LeFrançois, R. Menzies & G. Reaume (Eds.), *Mad matters: A critical reader in Canadian Mad studies* (pp. 239–252). Toronto: Canadian Scholars' Press.

Wilson, J. C., & Lewiecki-Wilson, C. (Eds.). (2001). *Embodied rhetorics: Disability in language and culture*. Carbondale, IL: Southern Illinois University Press.

Won, H., de la Torre-Ubieta, L., Stein, J. L., Parikshak, N. N., Huang, J., Opland, C. K., . . . Geschwind, D. H. (2016). Chromosome conformation elucidates regulatory relationships in developing human brain. *Nature, 538*(7626), 523–527.

Yergeau, M. (2015). *Autism and demi-rhetorical subjects*. Paper presented at Feminism(s) & Rhetoric(s), Tempe, AZ, October.

Yergeau, M. (2018). *Authoring autism: On rhetoric and neurological queerness*. Durham, NC: Duke University Press.

CHAPTER 3

From HeLa Cells to Henrietta Lacks

Rehumanization and Pathos as Interventions for the Rhetoric of Health and Medicine

EMILY WINDERMAN AND JAMIE LANDAU

AS A FOREMOTHER of the rhetoric of science, Martha Solomon brought rhetorical theory to bear on public health injustices. In 1985 she published an analysis of progress reports from the forty-year United States Public Health Service Study of Untreated Syphilis in the Negro Male in Macon County, Alabama, 1932–1972—colloquially known as the Tuskegee Syphilis Study.[1] Solomon argued that the progress reports, published in major medical journals from 1936 to 1973, functioned as "rhetoric of dehumanization" that allowed the study to evade ethical outcry despite the fact that a therapeutic dose of penicillin could have been administered to those affected as early as 1945 (p. 231). Partly because the published reports "avoided emotionally connotative language," researchers and readers could passively observe and dissociate themselves from the afflicted men and their families, deflecting attention from structural racism, human suffering, and the possibility of intervention (pp. 237–238, 244). While Solomon condemned the dehumanizing characteristics of this particular prose, she also lamented dehumanization as a more general feature of scientific writing writ large (p. 241). Although Solomon's critique of the reports appeared decades before the rhetoric of health and medi-

---

1. The naming of this study is deeply tethered to public memory efforts. Originally titled "The United States Study of Untreated Syphilis in the Negro Male," Tuskegee University's Legacy Museum renamed the study and we engage that title. For an analysis of the memory-work implications of this naming, see Lynch (2019).

cine (RHM) emerged as a discipline, her article is often cited as foundational to this work (Jensen, 2015a; Lynch & Zoller, 2015; Segal, 2009), even among health communication scholars more oriented toward social scientific methodologies (e.g., Babrow & Mattson, 2003; Dutta & Zoller, 2008).

Solomon would likely value the recent rhetorical shift to *rehumanization,* what we claim is a newly emergent function and feature of pathos-laden popular science writing today. In the passage that closed her essay, Solomon (1985) rehabilitated emotion as central to a humane pursuit of scientific knowledge:

> While all of us appreciate the importance of reason in human affairs, we also recognize the value of human emotion in tempering our behavior. Insistence on objectivity and detachment is a great asset in the pursuit of knowledge, but that stance reflects only one aspect of a broad spectrum of human concerns . . . If allegiance to objectivity and detachment blinds us to other values, it produces neither human behavior nor sound science. (p. 245)

Following calls to consider the role of pathos in health discourse (Condit, 2013; Waddell, 1990; Winderman & Condit, 2015) and to create progressive public health messages (Gronnvoll & Landau, 2010), we suggest that the scholarly fields of the rhetoric of science, health, and medicine are uniquely suited to theorizing the possibilities and perils of rehumanizing rhetoric—when people who have experienced structural dehumanization are recentered as human. Unlike the progress reports, a growing number of contemporary nonfiction books about public health written by science writers and doctors are intensely emotional and foster relationships between doctors, patients, and readers.[2] Our chapter calls scholars to consider *rehumanization* as a fruitful concept for RHM. In particular, we argue that *rehumanization* is a rhetorical process of pathos that affectively modulates public emotion to intervene upon a dehumanizing rhetorical ecology and return distinctly human attributes to patients. We identify two rhetorical strategies that work affectively to rehumanize patients: personification and rebuilding familial networks of affiliation. Not only do we suggest that the rhetoric of science, health, and medicine can be understood *as* areas of scholarship that distinctively theorize *rehumanization,* but also we show how rehumanization *is* put into practice by science writer Rebecca Skloot (2010) in the award-winning bestselling book

---

2. Although we focus on Rebecca Skloot's (2010) *The Immortal Life of Henrietta Lacks* as an exemplar, we recognize as siblings other recent nonfiction, such as Siddhartha Mukherjee's best-selling book, *The Emperor of All Maladies: A Biography of Cancer* (2010), as well as earlier books by Oliver Sacks.

The Immortal Life of Henrietta Lacks.[3] Skloot weaves together more than 1,000 hours of interviews with the Lacks family and doctors, archival research, histories of medical racism, and self-reflexivity to write a nonfiction "biography" about Henrietta Lacks and HeLa cells. Henrietta Lacks was a low-income African American woman who sought treatment from cervical cancer in 1951 at Johns Hopkins Hospital. Taken without her consent or knowledge, her cells became the first to thrive independently of a human host in a laboratory and made possible major medical advancements, ranging from the polio vaccine to in-vitro fertilization. Skloot's book demonstrates that while RHM *is* rooted in earlier scholarly advances made by the rhetoric of science, it also possesses a rhetorical capacity *as* unique unto itself: the practical ability to show how popular science writing can rehumanize patients who have been dehumanized.

This chapter proceeds in three parts. First, we outline the theoretical underpinnings of *rehumanization* by reviewing literature on dehumanization, rehumanization, and the role of affect, emotion, and pathos in science, health, and medicine. Second, we demonstrate rehumanization in practice with the case study of *The Immortal Life of Henrietta Lacks.* We close with implications for teaching students, training clinicians, and the potential perils of rehumanizing rhetoric.

FROM DEHUMANIZATION TO REHUMANIZATION

This chapter holds that *rehumanization is* a worthy project for RHM scholars because structural racism in US medical research has systematically dehumanized and harmed African American communities, implicating the medical knowledge gleaned along the way. Indeed, the US government's Syphilis Study at Tuskegee University was not an unfortunate aberration in an otherwise racially just history of medicine; as Harriet A. Washington (2006) noted, "Dangerous, involuntary, and nontherapeutic experimentation upon African Americans has been practiced widely and documented extensively since at

---

3. Named by more than sixty critics as one of the best books of 2010, *The Immortal Life of Henrietta Lacks* also won countless awards, including the American Association for the Advancement of Science's Award for Excellence in Science Writing and best-book awards from the National Academy of Science, the National Academy of Engineering, and the Institute of Medicine. Additionally, the book was adopted as common reading for over 130 universities. Finally, Oprah Winfrey's Harpo Films acquired the rights to the book when it first published, and then HBO Films co-produced and aired the movie on April 22, 2017, with Winfrey starring as Deborah Lacks, Henrietta's daughter. While outside the scope of this analysis, for many reasons we do not believe that the film does rehumanizing work comparable to the book's.

least the eighteenth century" (p. 7). Whether it be J. Marion Sims perfecting his vaginal fistula surgery on nonconsenting enslaved women before he would consider treating white women, state-sponsored forced sterilizations of predominantly African American women, or nineteenth-century medical schools illegally and unethically procuring African American corpses for student anatomical dissection, to name a few, dehumanization is often the recursive rhetorical maneuver necessary to justify these practices (Washington, 2006). Furthermore, this history of medical dehumanization has shaped our medical epistemologies, limiting more socially robust conceptualizations of patients and the larger affiliative contexts in which humans experience health and illness. As Jason E. Glenn argued, "The use of [dehumanized] persons for research helped produce a dehumanized body of medical knowledge that has been detached from a greater understanding of humans as primarily social-symbolic rather than purely biological beings" (p. 115). In other words, as researchers produce knowledge with dehumanized patients, those dehumanizing assumptions shape larger conceptualizations of humanity and then re-emerge in future study design, treatment protocols, and communication.

What exactly constitutes a dehumanizing rhetoric? Dehumanization is a strategy and symptom of intergroup conflict, social fragmentation, political aggression, violence, discrimination, and oppression that happens at the institutional, social, and interpersonal levels (Haslam, 2006; Smith, 2011; Stollznow, 2008). As Cheng (2001) claimed, "Dehumanization has long been *the* tool of discrimination" (p. 26). Dehumanization is even a predictor of genocide (Waller, 2016). Dehumanization occurs when one group denies the humanity of another group, often through social practices of emotional distancing. While scholars debate the exact quality of "humanity" or "humanness" that dehumanization denies, Haslam's (2006) literature review reveals two dimensions of dehumanization pertinent to our theory and case: (1) the likening of group members to nonhumans, such as animals, machines, or other nonliving objects (e.g., comparisons of African Americans to monkeys, Nazi propaganda portrayed Jews as rats, depictions of women as pornographic objects); and (2) the denial of "uniquely human" attributes (e.g., capacities for language, morality, pain, and emotional responsiveness). Pain perception is a particularly important emotional example insofar as African American patients have historically been characterized as less capable of feeling pain, an assumption that retains cultural currency, resulting in health disparity and moral disengagement today (Trawalter, Hoffman, & Waytz, 2012; Washington, 2006). Both forms of dehumanization involve objectification and emotional distancing, suggesting that dehumanization is distinctly affective and divisive. Furthermore, dehumanization is not only a general quality of discourse but also occurs in the use of specific language strategies, such as dissociation and naming (Grohowski, 2014; Solomon, 1985).

The history of dehumanization in medicine is an ongoing accumulation of social practices that "penetrates individual and collective bodies and minds" (Bustamante et al., 2019). Importantly for RHM, scholars have found that a number of contemporary health-care practices—including science writing—often dehumanize patients. Solomon (1985) was one of the earliest rhetorical critics to make this claim when she identified dehumanization in the scientific prose of the syphilis study reports and in medical practices undergirding the experiments. "Dehumanization is endemic in medical practice," even though it does not necessarily result from malicious intent of caretakers (Haque & Waytz, 2012, pp. 176–177). That is, dehumanization also occurs because of the structural features and psychological demands intrinsic in the medical profession that objectify patients and encourage clinicians to evacuate feelings for them. One example is mechanization, the diagnostic practice of imagining patients as mechanical systems made up of parts. Another example is the standard problem-solving method of classification, which reduces people and symptoms to systems and subsystems (from organ systems to tissues to cells to molecules). Dehumanization also increases with the development and reliance on biomedical and computer technologies in health care.

Medical dehumanization is often framed as a functional coping mechanism for reducing stress among health-care professionals. For example, while seasoned doctors Kompanje, van Mol, and Nijkamp (2015) admitted that they dehumanize patients to perform their jobs, they justified their emotional distancing as necessary:

> The dulling of empathic sense is, however, essential for practicing medicine . . . disease, pain, suffering, and death are a daily part of the work in the ICU. The health care providers expect it and are not shocked or surprised to see it 24/7, 365 days a year. Through the "dehumanization" of our patients we can deal with this. (pp. 2193–2194)

When interviewing physicians who cared for dying patients, Schulman-Green (2003) similarly discovered that they dehumanized patients by classifying them by their medical status or diagnosis, and by objectifying them (e.g., using technical words and naming people as "cases"; p. 257). Shulman-Green referred to this as "language of coping" during stressful situations, suggesting that it can lessen emotional angst and helplessness felt by physicians who cannot always cure those they encounter (p. 260). However, she worried that this language allows physicians to "isolate themselves" and "withdraw" from patients, which "sets up a divide between patients and physicians" and makes collaborative health care difficult (pp. 260–262). Yet feeling for patients cannot be uncritically prescribed as a solution to dehumanization either. Trifiletti, Di Bernardo, Falvo, and Capozza (2014) found that nurses who attributed traits perceived as uniquely human to their patients and had other affective commitments to patients saw increased stress levels compared with nurses who did not. Nonetheless, narrative medicine practitioners such as Rita Charon (2006) still strongly encourage doctors to be affectively "moved by the stories of illness" and to engage in "affiliation" with patients who are otherwise treated as commodities by the modern health-care system (p. 262).

Although the multidisciplinary literature on "dehumanization" is vast and we applaud Solomon for introducing the concept to the rhetoric of science, research about "rehumanization" is less common. Anticolonial theorist Sylvia Wynter (1970) briefly addresses *rehumanization* as a cultural practice that can counter the dehumanizing forces of capital extraction and colonial violence (p. 36). We conceptualize *rehumanization* as an intervention into existing dehumanization that returns a group's humanity or humanness that was stripped from them. Similar to how language has the dehumanizing ability to exterminate a group of people through emotional distancing, we argue that rehumanizing rhetoric can authenticate people (such as patients) by restoring their "uniquely human" attributes, especially with pathos. Kelly Wilz's (2010) rhetorical analysis of the 2004 film *Jarhead* demonstrated how rehumanizing rhetoric can productively counter dehumanization practices. Wilz argued that *Jarhead* challenges ideologies of soldiers and enemies by "rehumanizing the Other as an antidote to the virulent rhetoric of war" (p. 582). In contrast to most wartime rhetoric that dehumanizes the enemy and divides people, *Jarhead* enables identification between the spectator and soldiers, regardless of whether they are American or Iraqi. The Marine protagonist in the film ultimately refuses to kill during Operation Desert Storm, and the audience shares in this rehumanization of an "enemy," which Wilz claims can lead to peace-building efforts and to "thinking peacefully about enemies even *before* they are constructed as enemies" (p. 605). Likewise, James Kimble's (2004) rhetorical criticism of peacemaking discourse in issues of the *Ladies Home Journal* magazine published just months after World War II found that rhetorical action can *rehumanize* "enemies." Kimble asserted, "Rather than enabling and encouraging the slaughter of an inhuman enemy, here is language that puts things together—healing the wounds of war by reuniting enemies with their human qualities" (p. 65). Kimble's analysis invokes an affective dimension of rehumanization when he documents how readers of the *Ladies Home Journal* familiarized themselves with human suffering and felt compassion for people living in the former Axis nations (p. 66). Amplifying Wilz (2010) and Kimble (2004) in the context of rhetoric of science, health, and medicine, we argue that rehumanizing rhetoric can return humanness to patients and that, crucially, pathos plays a part in that process.

AFFECT, EMOTION, AND PATHOS IN SCIENCE, HEALTH, AND MEDICINE

Our concern with pathos parallels recent rhetorical studies that have taken the "affective turn" along with leading scholars of rhetoric of science who recognize the value of pathos in science, health, and medicine. For example, Jensen (2015a, 2015b) drew from Jenny Edbauer's theory of affective rhetorical ecologies to take an ecological turn in rhetoric of health scholarship. Rather than conceptualizing rhetoric as a response to a rhetorical situation composed of discrete elements, Edbauer (2005) proposed "a framework of *affective ecologies* that recontexualizes rhetorics in their temporal, historical, and lived fluxes" (p. 9). She continued, "an ecological, or affective, rhetorical model is one that reads rhetoric both as a process of distributed emergence and as an ongoing circulation process," much like how a virus spreads or energy moves between bodies (pp. 13–14). While we do not trace a rhetorical ecology as our method of criticism like Jensen does when studying the medicalization of infertility, we suggest that Skloot's book *intervenes* within an affective ecology of medical dehumanization. The notion of affective rhetorical ecologies draws from scholarship that takes seriously affect, emotion, and pathos. The turn has emerged in response to the privileging of logic and the denigration of emotion in the academy and in rhetorical studies. We briefly define these terms but ultimately lean on pathos because, much like how rehumanizing rhetoric intervenes into a dehumanizing rhetorical ecology, we argue that pathos appeals are concerted interventions into affective ecologies.

Although they cannot be easily separated from one another theoretically or in application, "affect" is conceptualized in much of the literature as a visceral bodily sensation that is physiological but sociopolitical, while "emotion" is its "sociolinguistic fixing" (e.g., Landau, 2016, p. 76; Massumi, 2002). As Seigworth and Gregg (2010) explained, affect designates the "visceral forces beneath, alongside, or generally *other than* conscious knowing . . . that can drive us toward movement" (p. 1). Operating in a register distinct from signification yet always tethered to it, affect connects bodies in less-than-fully conscious and nonlogical ways that move people together toward public feeling and social action. In her 2008 review of critical affect, Rice, referencing philosopher Brennan (2004), emphasized the embodied sociality of affect: "Affect is not personal feeling, but instead the means through which bodies act in context with each other. . . . Even at the cellular level, which might be the most elemental element, my self is rooted in others" (p. 203). In contradistinction, some scholars suggest that it is "emotion" which names or fixes that social movement. For example, emotion can be captured in words, whereas affect is impossible to put into words even while it is felt and shared among people (e.g., Landau, 2016, gasped and other people similarly felt sick when looking into a bottle labeled "ectopic pregnancy"; p. 83).

While "affect" and "emotion" are receiving renewed attention across the humanities and social sciences, pathos has long-standing importance for the rhetoric of science. Centuries ago, Aristotle conceptualized pathos as an artistic proof designed to appeal to a desired emotional capacity of an audience. While Aristotle subsumed pathos to logos, Condit (2013) expanded the concept, theorizing it as "the deliberate art for the construction of shared public emotions" (p. 3). She identified how "emotions are relational" and humans are "affiliative" animals that have a predisposition toward sharing affects that calcify "we/they" boundaries (p. 7). Condit's definition comports with critical theorist Terada's (2003) claim that pathos reflects techniques of emotional perpetuation. In other words, pathos is the rhetorical means of strategically modulating affect, public emotion, and collective affiliation.

Pathos *is* operative throughout rhetorics of science, health, and medicine, even while scientists and science writing have gone to great lengths to omit it. Echoing Solomon's (1985) conclusion that emotion is needed for sound science, Waddell (1990) observed pathos as an overlooked yet indispensable element of public engagement with science: "the privileged position enjoyed by logos in Western culture has often led to the denial of any appropriate role for pathos in science-policy formation" (p. 381). In addition to its frequent denial, emotional appeals backfired in cases of scientific controversy. According to Keränen (2010), during the infamous lumpectomy controversy that publicly tarnished the reputations of several pre-eminent clinical researchers, appeals to emotion both redeemed the characters of researchers who tampered with evidence and later demonstrated their ineptitude as scientists. Keränen wrote: "The suggestion that Poisson was guided more by emotion than reason . . . supplied further ammunition to critics who could cast him as passionate and therefore non-scientific" (p. 62). As Keränen suggested, physician-scientists are expected to conform to a narrow performance of emotional range in relationship to nonscientists, as a detached affective self-presentation remains central to their maintenance of professional identity.

Dehumanizing emotional detachment *is* quite prevalent in scientific writing itself. Rhetorical scholars noted this feature even before Solomon's (1985) analysis of the progress reports. For instance, Weaver (1953) described how, in the *Phaedrus*, Lysias's speech praises the nonlover. As an allegory for passionless discourse, Weaver argued that the nonlover lacks impulsivity and possesses a "detachment with the kind of abstraction to be found in scientific notation" (p. 9). Later rhetorical work about science writing analyzed its stylistic conventions that posture impartial objectivity and passive observation (e.g., Gross, 1991; Myers, 1990; Nelson, Megill, & McCloskey, 1990). One example is how the common trend of writing in the passive voice contributes to normalizing this disembodied scientific view. Comparing the autobiography of famed biologist Lewis Thomas with his peer-reviewed scientific research reports, Gross noted (1991), "In the autobiographical fragment, the personal is in the forefront: Thomas and his co-investigators actually upstage their fellow creatures. Clearly the rabbits are seen through human eyes" (p. 936). Like Gross's observation of the differences between scientific and autobiographical prose, we contend that when science writers practice "reflexive voicing" it "locates reader and writer and calls both to account for the impossibility of distanced, wholly objective, apolitical knowledge" (Harris, 2016, p. 118). Reflexive voicing, we argue, is itself a pathos-function that can build affiliation between researchers, readers, and patients, furthering the intersectional goal of coalition building (Harris, 2016).

Pathos *is* a key concept grounded in the rhetoric of science, health, and medicine. As a theoretical framework, pathos aligns RHM with innovative research on affect but distinguishes the emergent discipline as one that can explain how science writing like *The Immortal Life of Henrietta Lacks* can strategically modulate public emotion. RHM is particularly well positioned to make pathos-driven rehumanizing interventions in medical practice. That is, *as* an ideal discipline to encourage *rehumanizing* rhetoric, RHM can *re*-tether patients to the medical advancements that their bodies have made possible. We illustrate next how Skloot engages a pathos-driven rehumanizing rhetoric to return humanness to Henrietta Lacks's cells, an effort which also positions RHM as a field that can uniquely interrogate these efforts.

In the first part of our analysis, we demonstrate how Skloot traces an affective rhetorical ecology of dehumanizing medical racism to set the stage for a rehumanizing intervention. The book highlights how Henrietta Lacks was dehumanized through structural racism, naming, as well as through the medical practices of cell harvesting and oncological care administration.[4]

---

4. Throughout this analysis, we frequently refer to Mrs. Henrietta Lacks as Henrietta for the sake of clarity, especially when referring to multiple members of the Lacks family in conversation with one another. We recognize that this naming presumes a level of familiarity and intimacy with Mrs. Lacks that implicates a much longer racial history of infantilization of African

But Henrietta is also rehumanized through the viscerally resonant strategies of personification and reanimating that the Lackses's familial affiliations ignored throughout Henrietta's dehumanization processes. While not *mapping* a rhetorical ecology like Edbauer or Jensen, we argue that the book traces and intervenes in a dehumanizing ecology as it returns humanity to Henrietta Lacks as an African American woman, mother, sister, cousin, and—crucially—a patient. In so doing, Lacks and HeLa cells become human, and in some instances, Henrietta exceeds the corporeal boundaries of her living embodiment.

FROM HENRIETTA LACKS TO HELA CELLS: CONTEXTUALIZING A DEHUMANIZING RHETORICAL ECOLOGY

The book opens by reminding twenty-first-century readers that when Henrietta sought medical care, she was doing so in 1951 as an African American woman living in poverty when Jim Crow laws ravaged the Black body politic. As Henrietta visited Johns Hopkins, she "scurried into the hospital, past the 'colored' bathroom, the only one she was allowed to use" (Skloot, 2010, p. 13). Within two pages, we learn why Henrietta and her family were referred to Hopkins, twenty miles from their home: "not because they preferred it, but because it was the only major hospital for miles that treated black patients" (p. 15). As Skloot continues: "This was the era of Jim Crow—when black people showed up at white-only hospitals, the staff was likely to send them away, even if it meant they might die in the parking lot" (p. 15). Despite its public mandate to serve the community, Johns Hopkins segregated wards, drinking fountains, and health care. Within these first pages, Skloot positions Henrietta within a larger affective ecology of Jim Crow–based medical dehumanization, allowing readers to sense the fearful orientation African American patients experience when accessing racially segregated care.

Skloot reflects upon her own position within this ecology of dehumanization as she—a white science writer—sought out the Lacks family to write this book. In particular, Skloot animates and grapples with the fallout of this ecology: a community distrust of those who might take further advantage of the Lacks family. Skloot recalls how, in 1999, she contacted Morehouse School of Medicine's professor of gynecology Dr. Roland Pattillo, for a lead on the Lacks

---

American adults. However, we follow the lead of the Legacy Museum at Tuskegee University that has curated an exhibit entitled "Henrietta Everlasting" and "identifies the discoveries and inventions made possible by HeLa cells in various areas of biology," (Lynch, 2019, p. 71).

family. Dr. Pattillo was one of George Gey's only African American students, now teaching at this Historically Black College. When Skloot shared that she was writing a book about Henrietta and asked whether he could put her in contact with the family, Dr. Pattillo replied, "I do have the ability to put you in touch with them, but you need to answer a few questions, starting with 'Why should I?'" (p. 49). As the conversation progressed, Dr. Pattillo wanted to know what Skloot knew about "African-Americans and science" because so many had previously exploited the Lacks family (p. 50). Using her response to Dr. Pattillo as an opportunity to educate readers about medical experimentation with African Americans, Skloot "told him about the Tuskegee syphilis study like I was giving an oral report in history class" (p. 50). After narrating a history aligning with Solomon's (1985) rhetorical critique, Skloot (2010) detailed the social effects and mistrust that the study engendered in African American communities: "The news spread like pox through black communities: doctors were doing research on black people, lying to them, and watching them die" (p. 50). She also addressed conspiracies within the community that the doctors intentionally injected men with syphilis. Not fully satisfied, the response was: "'What Else?' Pattillo grumbled" (p. 50). Skloot then offered the following vignette to her audience:

> I told him I'd heard about so-called Mississippi Appendectomies, unnecessary hysterectomies performed on poor black women to stop them from reproducing, and to give young doctors a chance to practice the procedure. I'd also read about the lack of funding for research into sickle-cell anemia, a disease that affected blacks almost exclusively. (p. 50)

Although abbreviated, Skloot's conversation serves at least two pathos-functions. First, it explicates Henrietta's individuated fearful orientation about visiting the doctor. When Henrietta first located her cervical lump, she did not immediately seek medical attention. Her cousin Sadie "always figured Henrietta kept it a secret because she was afraid her doctor would take her womb and make her stop having children" (p. 14). Narrating Henrietta's individuated fear frames her as an autonomous, agential, and complex human concerned about her own health and fearful for the fate of her reproductive capacity. Second, the exchange with Dr. Pattillo demonstrates how the book explicitly animates a larger ecology of dehumanization among African American patients. These visceral accounts of dehumanization enable readers and science writers like Skloot to situate Henrietta's fears as just one instance of the African American community's justifiable distrust of medical establishments. As Skloot remarks at the end of the first chapter, "It was no surprise that she hadn't come back all those times for follow-up. . . . She, *like most black patients,* only went to Hopkins when she thought she had no choice" (p. 16; emphasis added). Even though Johns Hopkins was endowed for the benefit of the poor inhabitants of the greater Baltimore area, Black oral histories have operated with a significant level of suspicion, believing that the hospital was built for the benefit of white scientists and doctors. As Skloot observes, "Today when people talk about the history of Hopkins' relationship with the black community, the story many of them hold up as the worst offense is that of Henrietta Lacks—a black woman whose body, they say, was exploited by white scientists" (p. 168). Ultimately, Skloot attends to the dehumanizing affective ecology of medical racism while centering the emotional orientation of those impacted along the way.

Henrietta's dehumanization also occurred in the mechanized biomedical research process with the naming of her cells as "HeLa." Skloot narrates the affective dimensions of those processes. In chapter 4, "The Birth of HeLa," readers meet twenty-four-year-old Mary Kubicek who, as Gey's research assistant, was tasked with the seemingly futile and laborious job of growing immortal cells. Kubicek was technically adept in the laboratory, able to pre-cisely pipe tissue samples into a cell culture. The day she grew Henrietta's cervical cancer cells, Skloot detailed Kubicek's affective burnout, that she "was tired of cell culture—tired of meticulously cutting dead tissue like gristle from a steak, tired of having cells die after hours of work" (p. 35). After sterilizing the equipment, "only then did she pick up the pieces of Henrietta's cervix—forceps in one hand, scalpel in the other—and carefully slice them into one-millimeter squares" (p. 37). She then labeled each [test tube] as she'd labeled most cultures they grew: using the first two letters of the patient's first and last names. After writing 'HeLa,' for *Henrietta* and *Lacks,* in big black letters on the side of each tube," Kubicek placed the tubes into the incubator (pp. 37–38).

As mentioned earlier, mechanization is one structural culprit of dehuman-ization in medicine (e.g., Haslam, 2006, p. 252; Haque & Waytz, 2012). Haque and Waytz (2012) noted that focusing on less than the whole human and dis-secting people into parts is useful for diagnostic and pathological localization; in turn, medical professionals commonly refer to patients in "depersonal-ized terms, using acronyms, the body part being operated on, or the name of their disease" (p. 178). Doctors severed Henrietta's cervical cells from her body without her knowledge, labeled her "a miserable specimen" in her chart (Skloot, 2010, p. 66), and then abbreviated her cells as "HeLa." By narrating the literal embodiment of mechanized dehumanization, Skloot demonstrates how Kubicek's withdrawal from Henrietta's full humanity was an affective rela-tionship between Kubicek's body "doing science" and Henrietta's tissue sample. This misnamed mechanization had far-reaching intergenerational results, however, erasing Henrietta's identity as millions of other scientists who used HeLa cells over the next sixty years were isolated from Henrietta and mis-informed about her name. Skloot emphasizes how Henrietta's photograph, which graces the cover of her book,[5] is often absent from scientific reports and medical textbooks about HeLa cells. When the photograph is present, Henrietta Lacks is frequently misidentified as "Helen Lane" or "Helen Larson" in captions (p. 1). This dehumanization negatively impacted the Lacks family for decades, as they were uninformed about Henrietta's death or the profitable research involving her cells. Indeed, the Lacks family could not afford health insurance, demonstrating the intergenerational material impacts of Henrietta's dehumanization. Henrietta's daughter Deborah put it best: "Everything always just about the cells and don't even worry about her name and was HeLa even a person" (p. 52).

FROM HELA CELLS TO HENRIETTA LACKS: REHUMANIZING RHETORIC

Crucially, *The Immortal Life of Henrietta Lacks* does not cease at document-ing and critiquing the ecology surrounding Henrietta's dehumanization. The book simultaneously intervenes with a rhetoric of rehumanization, primarily through viscerally resonant personification and rebuilding affective familial relationships between Henrietta, the Lacks family, Skloot, readers, and, ulti-mately, the doctors and scientists who dehumanized her.

The Pathos of Personification

In general, *personification* is conceptualized as a linguistic strategy by which an inanimate idea or object is endowed with personal or human qualities (Leb-owitz & Ahn, 2016). Skloot's book personifies Henrietta Lacks in at least three ways: (1) titling the book after "Henrietta," putting her picture on the cover (Figure 1) and toggling in-text between naming her "Henrietta" and "HeLa"; (2) attributing affective agency to HeLa cells; and (3) recognizing human sub-jectivity in the medical procedure of tissue collection.

---

5. One can view the image here: https://en.wikipedia.org/wiki/The_Immortal_Life_of_Henrietta_Lacks

Skloot shifts between referring to "Henrietta" and "HeLa cells," thereby crafting a hybridized human identity that comprises a woman *and* her immortal cells. This shift occurs even within a single paragraph:

> Henrietta's cells helped launch the fledgling field of virology, but that was just the beginning. In the years following Henrietta's death, using some of the first tubes of her cells, researchers around the world made several important scientific advances in quick succession. First, a group of researchers used HeLa to develop methods for freezing cells without harming or changing them. (p. 98)

This doubled move of endowing personhood yet complicating the human boundary is notable considering the uniqueness of HeLa cells. We must remember that HeLa cells grew from Henrietta's cervical *cancer*—a type and stage of cell growth that many people wish to dissociate from their bodies based on common metaphors for cancer as enemies, invaders, alien mutations, and monsters (e.g., Mukherjee, 2010, pp. 38–39, 45, 68). Moreover, HeLa cells are unlike most malignancies because they keep growing outside of a human. By naming "Henrietta Lacks" and associating a smiling face and full body image with her name on the book's cover, Skloot rehumanizes Henrietta as a person rather than as the faceless and bodiless HeLa. At the same time, "HeLa" retains a material trace of the dehumanizing ecology that reduces "humanness" to existence at the cellular level. This is indeed a twofold biography: a biography of Henrietta and also a "biography" of HeLa cells and their rhetorical uptake.

Personification also occurs distinctly as a pathos when Henrietta's voice, emotional responsiveness, and moral outrage are agentially attributed to HeLa cells. In other words, while HeLa cells technically possess an agential quality in their capacity to grow and contaminate other cell cultures, some people interviewed in the book go further to endow HeLa cells with the "uniquely human" qualities that are often denied through dehumanization (Haslam, 2006). Perhaps the most compelling case is when Skloot and Deborah Lacks (Henrietta's daughter) visit Christoph Lengauer's lab at Johns Hopkins to view HeLa cells. After they tour the lab, Lengauer takes them to a special room set aside for HeLa cells to prevent contamination. Lengauer muses that it was "poetic justice" that HeLa contamination caused millions of dollars in damage. Deborah's reply attributes to Henrietta an emotional capacity acting vis-à-vis HeLa cells: "My mother was just getting back at scientists for keepin all them secrets from the family . . . You don't mess with Henrietta, she'll sic HeLa on your ass!" (Skloot, 2010, p. 262). Deborah personifies her mother by attributing anger and moral outrage to the contamination, explaining Henrietta's reasoning for destroying research and laboratory property. There are several other instances of the agential attribution of Henrietta's emotional capacity, including when one of the book's editors implored Skloot to remove mention of the Lacks family: "When an editor who insisted I take the Lacks family out of the book was injured in a mysterious accident, *Deborah said that's what happens when you piss Henrietta off*" (p. 7; emphasis added). Crucially, the book narrates the wide range and complexity of Henrietta's feelings and avoids reductive emotional stereotypes. To illustrate, Henrietta's children describe her as working through HeLa cells because of her deep care for those with whom she met. Sonny, who was even too young at the time of his mother's death to remember her, said, "She liked takin care of people, so it make sense what she did with them cells. I mean, people always say she was really just hospitality, you know, fixing everything up nice, making a good place, get up, cook breakfast for everybody, even if it's twenty of them" (Skloot, 2010, p. 159). In line with Washington's (2006) observation that the African medical tradition "involved physiological as well as spiritual approaches to healing," Henrietta's family believed her spirit acted through her cells (Skloot, 2010, p. 49). This attribution of a complex repertoire of agential emotions is a pathos that calibrates the dimensions of humanity that were robbed in the Henrietta to HeLa mechanization process.

Finally, personification of Henrietta Lacks is relationally constituted during her autopsy as Kubicek recognizes Henrietta's full humanity. After she passed away, Gey sent Kubicek to the morgue to collect tissue samples in case they could grow her other cells. Skloot (2010) narrates Kubicek as deeply uncomfortable in the morgue and looking in any direction to avoid Henrietta's eyes: "Then Mary's gaze fell on Henrietta's feet, and she gasped: Henrietta's toenails were covered in chipped bright red polish" (p. 90). Kubicek later confided that she had "nearly fainted" when she saw Henrietta's toenails, thinking "*Oh, Jeez, she's a real person*" (p. 91; author's emphasis). Kubicek continued, "I started imagining her sitting in her bathroom painting those toenails, and it hit me that those cells we'd been working with all this time and sending all over the world, they came from a live woman. I'd never thought of it that way" (p. 91). Since medical dehumanization often desensitizes and distances medical practitioners from patients and their pain, Kubicek's experience was an affective rupture in scientific protocol. This moment of recognition, detailed by Kubicek's visceral "gasp," indexed the work of pathos: an embodied reorientation within this dehumanizing ecology. The red nail polish returns later to capture her family's feelings about Henrietta's passing. Henrietta's cousin Sadie was perhaps more distraught about Henrietta's chipped polish than about her lifeless body, noting that for her to let her nails look that bad meant that "Hennie must a hurt somethin worse than death" (p. 92). Beyond the personification of Henrietta Lacks, rehumanization embedded her within an extended kinship network of other humans affected by her life, death, and cellular immortality. The book's arrangement of social and familial relationships intimately binds the Lacks family together along with Skloot, readers, doctors, and researchers.

The Intervening Pathos of Familial and Social Affiliations

The Immortal Life of Henrietta Lacks crafts an extended network of affiliation by narrating Henrietta's life through her relationships with Lacks family members across generations and framing her story as affecting the family. From the first chapter, where she walks into Johns Hopkins, Skloot notes that her husband "was parked under a towering oak tree outside . . . with three of his children—two still in diapers—waiting for their mother, Henrietta" (p. 1). The stark juxtaposition of Henrietta entering a medical complex while her family awaited her return outside focuses the book on her family, rather than on the individuated patient-subject. Importantly, extended kinship ties are written in their original vernacular, rather than in scientific prose. Skloot offers "A Few Words About This Book" where she notes that she invented neither characters nor events for the sake of reader intrigue. The second paragraph clarifies that she carefully narrated individuals so that "dialogue appears in native dialects; passages from diaries and other personal writings are quoted exactly as written" (p. xiii). Quoting a Lacks relative, she did so because "If you pretty up how people spoke and change the things they said, that's dishonest" (p. viii). This writing style honors the voices of the Lacks family. Yet a few pages later, in the prologue, Skloot offers a brief history lesson about how HeLa cells "have become the standard laboratory workhorse," such as aiding research on genes that cause cancer, helping the development of drugs for treating major diseases like hemophilia, polio, and Parkinson disease, and advancing the study of other health and medical issues, ranging from appendicitis to human longevity (p. 4). While this second storyline seems to circumvent emphasis on the Lackses' storyline, we argue that it emotionally moves millions of other people into their family circle or "family album."

Connecting Henrietta Lacks to her family and an extended social network means that Henrietta and HeLa cells live through generations. Rehumanizing Henrietta is more than reanimating one woman; it is about affiliating others with her cellular and familial legacy, encouraging readers to feel the racial history of a dehumanizing rhetorical ecology and how they have personally benefited from Henrietta and her cells. The six-page photo insert in the middle of the book functions as an extended "family album" that invites new patterns of social affiliation. It opens with a stained and scratched black-and-white photo of Henrietta and her husband, David, dressed up and youthful-looking while school portraits of their daughters appear beneath. The next page displays scenes that were part of Henrietta's childhood, including the Virginia log cabin former slave quarters where Henrietta was born, her mother's tombstone, and scenes from a downtown tobacco auction. Turn the pages again and Gey, Kubicek, other doctors, and lab technicians appear alongside Henrietta's death certificate and an image of her cousin, Sadie, visually blending the distinction between medicine and family. The last three pages display the Tuskegee Institute's HeLa mass production line and HeLa cells under a microscope followed by snapshots of Deborah and other Lacks family members. The caption for the largest and final picture says it was taken in 2009 and names thirteen people in the photograph and their familial relationship to Henrietta (e.g., "Henrietta's youngest son, Zakariyya"). Much like Henrietta's photo on the book's cover, this multiphoto insert authenticates and renders the Lacks family visible. Since slave owners prevented the creation and exchange of photographs and there are not representative images of Black communities in mass media, Willis (1999) argued, photographs of Black families can potentially transform racist stereotypes of community and family decay (pp. 113–116). Importantly, this insert is a larger collection of family photos—an "extended family album"—that features people who are not biologically Henrietta's family. Even doctors who distanced themselves from Henrietta through dehumanizing medical practices are included in this family album. Subsequently, we suggest that this photo album builds familial affiliations with medical professionals, as well as between black and white people in the past and present. It reassures familial unity and solidarity even through there has been (racial) discord and division, a convention of many family albums (e.g., Holland, 1991). Scholars of family photographs emphasize how they are not documentary in aim or attitude (Slater, 1995, p. 134). Rather, family photos are deeply affective and can trigger feeling and collective affiliation: "These emotions are released in us whenever we see any family photographs, even if it is of strangers, or of persons to whom we are otherwise indifferent" (Hirsch, 1981, pp. 119–120). Taken together, the family photo album rehumanizes Henrietta Lacks by crafting these expansive affiliations with doctors and whites while obscuring dehumanizing visual rhetoric.

Finally, Skloot connects her role as a science writer to the Lacks family by reflexively voicing the relational complexities of her friendship with Deborah.

Rebecca reflexively narrates frequent conversations when Deborah wavered between trusting and rejecting her and the book. Deborah held an understandable distrust of persons who previously tried to procure information about HeLa cells without an interest in Henrietta's humanity. In one of many conversations with Deborah, Rebecca narrated the events that transpired when she believed Deborah was ready to share her mother's medical records. After reaching for the records, Deborah screamed "No! . . . leaping up and diving onto the folder like it was a fumbled football, hugging it to her chest, curling her body around it" (p. 239). Although Rebecca and Deborah spent days together "laughing, elbowing, and consoling," she felt shocked that Deborah "was now running from me like I was out to get her" (p. 240). While Deborah and Rebecca mended the next day, she would often field frantic calls from Deborah during the middle of the night as she had questions about HeLa myths and scientific advances. Frequently, Deborah became anxious, accusing Rebecca of being funded by Johns Hopkins. Skloot had to continually remind her that she was financing the book's research with credit cards and loans (p. 283). When Deborah finally permitted Rebecca to view Henrietta's medical records, she remained protective of her mother's most personal information; only allowing notetaking rather than photocopying. Rebecca acknowledges this friendship to be a complicated affective attachment, reflecting the larger complicated relationship between all patients and the racial history of the HeLa cells.

CONCLUSION

Solomon (1985) closed her landmark critique with warnings about the emotionless dehumanization of the progress reports: they reinforced racial prejudice, encouraged insensitivity, polarized the relationship between "subjects" and medical investigators, and divorced scientists from human concerns (p. 245). As a result, we believe Solomon would value *The Immortal Life of Henrietta Lacks* for its rehumanization of patients. *Rehumanization is* a productive concept for scholars of RHM because it serves *as* a tool for theory development, criticism, and creation. It connects us to the discipline's theoretical and analytical foundations, demonstrating how rhetoricians of science like Solomon have long been concerned with these issues. Importantly, rehumanization might perform reparative work, encouraging science writers and medical practitioners to adjust their discourses and affiliate with patients, especially those whose vulnerability is deeply rooted in systemic (medical) racism. Specifically, we argued that Skloot's book intervened in a rhetorical ecology of dehumanization by employing strategies of pathos to personify HeLa cells as Henrietta and to build relationships between the Lacks family, Skloot, readers, doctors, and researchers.

Moreover, we suggest RHM might further develop rehumanizing strategies *as* practical recommendations for training health-care professionals. We cautiously make this claim because rehumanization has been a critical strategy to justify eliminating women's reproductive rights. On the one hand, we're hopeful that the book is already being used to teach future scientists, evidenced by its inclusion in introductory biology courses (Resendes, 2015). Landau found the book nested next to technical nursing manuals in her college's library. As a pedagogical resource, the book assists in teaching medical racism to undergraduates. While Winderman used the book in a "Rhetoric of Health and Medicine" course as an end-of-semester narrative to tie concepts together, Landau assigned the book in her "Health Communication and Rhetoric of Cancer" class at a predominantly white institution, where she found that it set off a fission of feelings for Henrietta and race-based medical injustices (Landau & Thornton, 2015, p. 513). Just as Haraway (1998) famously advocated for a situated embodiment of science rather than an impartial view from nowhere, our students affectively connected to Henrietta and African American patients.

There are perils to the rhetorical uptake of *rehumanization,* of which critics must remain on guard. Reproductive advocates have long been aware of the dangerous rhetoric of "fetal personhood" deployed by anti-abortion groups and politicians (Condit, 1990). When a fetus is constituted as human complete with feelings and enabling affiliations for the political purpose of preventing rights to an abortion, then the more difficult task for the RHM is to distinguish between progressive rehumanization that works in service of gender and racial justice and regressive rehumanizing rhetoric that limits reproductive autonomy. Yet, as Wilz (2010) reminded us, "we must look for modes of rehumanization where they appear even impartial and imperfect in form" (p. 591). Despite the potential for regressive uptake, rehumanization has promise for advancing other issues discussed by RHM scholars, ranging from informed consent, patient privacy, and doctor–patient communication to philosophical inquiries into what Hyde (1986) once titled his review of five books—"treating the patient as a person" (p. 456). Indeed, rhetoricians of health and medicine should seriously consider rehumanization as an intervention into a dehumanizing ecology. In this chapter, we have only just begun to document the ways in which rehumanization and pathos move our bodies and discipline in new directions.

REFERENCES

Babrow, A. S., & Mattson, M. (2003). Theorizing about health communication. In T. L. Thompson, A. Dorsey, & K. I. Miller (Eds.), *Handbook of health communication* (pp. 35–61). Mahwah, NJ: Lawrence Erlbaum.

Bustamante, P., Jashnani, G, & Stoudt, B.G. (2019). Theorizing cumulative dehumanization: An embodied praxis of "becoming" and resisting state-sanctioned violence. *Social and Personality Psychology Compass, 13*(1), e12429.

Charon, R. (2006). *Narrative medicine: Honoring the stories of illness.* New York, NY: Oxford University Press.

Cheng, A. (2001). *The melancholy of race: Psychoanalysis, assimilation, and hidden grief.* New York, NY: Oxford University Press.

Condit, C. M. (1990). *Decoding abortion rhetoric: Communicating social change.* Urbana, IL: University of Illinois Press.

Condit, C. M. (2013). Pathos in criticism: Edwin Black's communism-as-cancer metaphor. *Quarterly Journal of Speech, 99*(1), 1–26.

Dutta, M. J., & Zoller, H. M. (Eds.). (2008). *Emerging perspectives in health communication: Meaning, culture, and power.* New York, NY: Routledge.

Edbauer, J. (2005). Unframing models of public distribution: From rhetorical situation to rhetorical ecologies. *Rhetoric Society Quarterly, 35*(4), 5–24.

Glenn, J.E. (2015). Dehhumanization, the *symbolic gaze,* and the production of biomedical knowledge. In J.R. Ambrose & S. Broeck (Eds.), *Black knowledges/Black struggles: Essays in critical epistemology* (pp. 112–144). Liverpool, UK: Liverpool University Press.

Grohowski, M. (2014). Moving words/words that move: Language practices plaguing U.S. servicewomen. *Women & Language, 37*(1), 121–130.

Gronnvoll, M., & Landau, J. (2010). From viruses to Russian roulette to dance: A rhetorical critique and creation of genetic metaphors. *Rhetoric Society Quarterly, 40*(1), 46–70.

Gross, A. G. (1991). Does rhetoric of science matter? The case of the floppy-eared rabbits. *College English, 53*(8), 933–943.

Haque, O. S., & Waytz, A. (2012). Dehumanization in medicine: Causes, solutions, and functions. *Perspective on Psychological Science, 7*(2), 176–186.

Haraway, D. (1998). Situated knowledges: The science question in feminism and the privilege of partial perspective. *Feminist Studies, 14*(3), 575–599.

Harris, K. L. (2016). Reflexive voicing: A communicative approach to intersectional writing. *Qualitative Research, 16*(1), 111–127.

Haslam, N. (2006). Dehumanization: An integrative review. *Personality and Social Psychology Review, 10*(3), 252–264.

Hirsch, J. (1981). *Family photography: Context, meaning, and effect.* New York, NY: Oxford University Press.

Holland, P. (1991). Introduction: History, memory, and the family album. In J. Spence & P. Holland (Eds.), *Family snaps: The meanings of domestic photography* (pp. 1–14). London, UK: Virago.

Hyde, M. (1986). Treating the patient as person: Book review. *Quarterly Journal of Speech, 72*(4), 456–500.

Jensen, R. E. (2015a). An ecological turn in rhetorical of health scholarship: Attending to the historical flow and percolation of ideas, assumptions, and arguments. *Communication Quarterly, 63*(5), 522–526.

Jensen, R. E. (2015b). Improving upon nature: The rhetorical ecology of chemical language, reproductive endocrinology, and the medicalization of infertility. *Quarterly Journal of Speech, 101*(2), 329–353.

Keränen, L. (2010). *Scientific characters: Rhetoric, politics, and trust in breast cancer research.* Tuscaloosa, AL: University of Alabama Press.

Kimble, J. (2004). Feminine style and the rehumanization of the enemy: Peacemaking discourse in *Ladies Home Journal, 1945–1946. Women and Language, 27*(2), 65–70.

Kompanje, E. J. O., van Mol, M. M., & Nijkamp, M. D. (2015). "I just have admitted an interesting sepsis." Do we dehumanize our patients? *Intensive Care Medicine, 41*(12), 2193–2194.

Landau, J. (2016). Feeling rhetorical critics: Another affective-emotional field method for rhetorical studies. In S. L. McKinnon, R. Asen, K. R. Chávez, & R. G. Howard (Eds.), *text + field: Innovations in rhetorical method* (pp. 72–85). University Park, PA: Pennsylvania State University Press.

Landau, J., & Thornton, D. (2015). Teaching rhetoric of health and medicine to undergraduates: Citizens, interdisciplinarity, and affect. *Communication Quarterly, 63*(5), 527–532.

Lebowitz, M. S., & Ahn, W. (2016). Using personification and agency reorientation to reduce mental health clinicians' stigmatizing attitudes towards patients. *Stigma and Health, 1*(3), 176–184.

Lynch, J. A. (2019). *The origins of bioethics: Remembering when medicine went wrong.* Lansing, MI: Michigan State University Press.

Lynch, J. A., & Zoller, H. (2015). Recognizing differences and commonalities: The rhetoric of health and medicine and critical-interpretive health communication. *Communication Quarterly, 63*(5), 498–503.

Massumi, B. (2002). *Parables for the virtual: Movement, affect, and sensation.* Durham, NC: Duke University Press.

Mukherjee, S. (2010). *The emperor of all maladies: A biography of cancer.* New York, NY: Scribner.

Myers, G. (1990). *Writing biology: Texts in the construction of social knowledge.* Madison, WI: University of Wisconsin Press.

Nelson, J. S., Megill, A., & McCloskey, D. N. (Eds.). (1990). *The rhetoric of the human sciences: Language and argument in scholarship and public affairs.* Madison, WI: University of Wisconsin Press.

Resendes, K. R. (2015). Using HeLa cell stress response to introduce first year students to the scientific method, laboratory techniques, primary literature, and scientific writing. *Biochemistry and Molecular Biology Education, 43*(2), 110–120.

Rice, J. E. (2008). The new "new": Making a case for critical affect studies. *Quarterly Journal of Speech, 94*(2), 200–2012.

Schulman-Green, D. (2003). Coping mechanisms of physicians who routinely work with dying patients. *OMEGA: Journal of Death & Dying, 47*(3), 253–264.

Segal, J. Z. (2009). Rhetoric of health and medicine. In A. A. Lunsford, K. Wilson, & R. A. Eberly (Eds.), *The SAGE handbook of rhetorical studies* (pp. 227–245). Thousand Oaks, CA: SAGE.

Seigworth, G., & Gregg, M. (Eds.). (2010). *The affect theory reader.* Durham, NC: Duke University Press.

Skloot, R. (2010). *The immortal life of Henrietta Lacks.* New York, NY: Broadway Books.

Slater, D. (1995). Domestic photography and digital culture. In M. Lister (Ed.), *The photographic image in digital culture* (pp. 129–146). London, UK: Routledge.

Smith, D. L. (2011). *Less than human: Why we demean, enslave, and exterminate others.* New York, NY: St. Martin's.

Solomon, M. (1985). The rhetoric of dehumanization: An analysis of the medical reports of the Tuskeegee syphilis project. *Western Journal of Communication, 49*, 233–247.

Stollznow, K. (2008). Dehumanisation in language and thought. *Journal of Language and Politics, 7*(2), 177–200.

Trawalter, S., Hoffman, K. M., & Waytz, A. (2012). Racial bias in perceptions of others' pain. *PLoS ONE 7*(11), e48546.

Terada, R. (2003). *Feeling in theory: Emotion after the "death of the subject."* Cambridge, MA: Harvard University Press.

Trifiletti, E., Di Bernardo, G. A., Falvo, R., & Capozza, D. (2014). Patients are not fully human: A nurse's coping response to stress. *Journal of Applied Social Psychology, 44*(12), 768–777.

Waddell, C. (1990). The role of pathos in the decision-making process: A study in the rhetoric of science policy. *Quarterly Journal of Speech, 76*(4), 381–400.

Waller, J. (2016). *Confronting evil: Engaging our responsibility to prevent genocide.* New York, NY: Oxford University Press.

Washington, H. A. (2006). *Medical apartheid: The dark history of medical experimentation on Black Americans from colonial times to the present.* New York, NY: Doubleday.

Weaver, R. (1953). *The ethics of rhetoric.* Chicago, IL: Regnery.

Willis, D. (1999). A search for self: The photograph and black family life. In M. Hirsch (Ed.), *The familial gaze* (pp. 107–123). Hanover, NH: University Press of New England.

Wilz, K. (2010). Rehumanization through reflective oscillation in *Jarhead. Rhetoric & Public Affairs, 13*(4), 581–610.

Winderman, E., & Condit, C. M. (2015). From trope to pathos in health scholarship: Sharing disgust in the Kermit Gosnell case. *Communication Quarterly, 63*(5), 516–521.

Wynter, S. (1970). Jonkonnu in Jamaica: Towards the Interpretation of Folk Dance as a Cultural Process. *Jamaica Journal, 4*(2), 34–48.

TO INTERDISCIPLINARY PERSPECTIVES

Mapping the Healthscape

Onto, Eco, *and* Otherwise

JOHN LYNE

FOR THOSE new to the field of rhetoric of health and medicine (RHM), it may be useful to first connect the essays in this volume to a broader lineage, which begins with the theory and practice of rhetoric and the purposes of those who study it. The definition of terms is variable, reflecting differences in theories, so I am putting my cards on the table. *Rhetoricians,* under the description here, share a concern with how language and other signifiers guide perception and yield influence. *Rhetoricians of science* share a concern with how science is articulated and applied, and with how this may shape knowledge and influence or impact participants, audiences, and stakeholders. Common points of focus are persuasion, patterns of language, paths of invention and discovery, pathos, genres, configurations, audiences, affect, and boundary crossings, along with the specific tropes and methods of the various sciences. *Rhetoricians of health and medicine* extend the repertoire and methods of rhetoric of science and turn attention to the various articulations of health and medicine within the expansive frameworks of scientific and cultural practices at every level from the local to the general. By pushing beyond the confines of institutional medicine and a narrowly construed definition of health, studies in RHM refresh the question of what comes next in expanding our understanding of these vital concerns.

Thinking of RHM as a field of investigation brings to mind the way Ludwig Wittgenstein came to see the workings of language as a serviceable weave within the patterns of life. Wittgenstein (1973) used the metaphor of a city that grows, not just by antecedently mandated structures but by the historical accretions that respond to usage patterns and create evolving formations. Drawing upon a similar metaphor to characterize the way that RHM engages a *healthscape,* one could say that it moves forward by retracing, reforming, and in some ways departing from previous studies and boundary practices. The healthscape hosts different neighborhoods, with various patterns of access and opportunity. The metaphor seems apt for a moment when the field is taking stock of its methodologies (Melonçon & Scott, 2018) and tapping into its locational resources as it anticipates its future opportunities. The essays in this volume suggest something of the range of opportunity. At the same time, they highlight the challenge of finding *composite formations* to which the research methods may contribute, and more generally, of tending to the general ecology that shapes what and how we study.

To take the Wittgensteinian metaphor a bit further, navigating a cityscape requires reliance on some directionality and mapping. Given the pervasive tension between the known and the unknown, sticking close to what is known produces reliability, but in a trade-off with the possibility of finding new paths. Academic navigation perpetually struggles with this tension. Thinking of the healthscape in this way, the questions to be addressed would include the following: (1) What is known and what can be known about the conditions and practices that bear upon health? (2) What do the practices and instrumentalities of rhetoric do, and what can they do, within and beyond those conditions? (3) What affordances might the *actual* yield toward the *possible,* that is to say, toward what might be otherwise? and (4) What are the types and features of agency within and beyond the relevant frameworks? Each of these questions presumes that certain decisions will be made about contextualization, and this becomes especially pertinent within the frame of multidisciplinarity, where contexts are notably nested within other contexts, within and beyond the framings of a particular discipline.

The "as/is" distinction with which this volume is introduced might at its broadest level be construed as calling attention, first, to the basic categories that undergird the inquiry in this field, prior to the work that we expect them to do: How should we conceptualize health? What defines the field of medicine? Indeed, in what light should we see rhetoric? These might be considered *ontological* questions, not in the metaphysical sense of that term but in the sense of specifying a set of concepts and categories that define the subject domain. The *ontological* gives way to the *ecological* as the interplay of the fundamental concepts produces its own interactive and relational space. One might think of the preceding essays as charting routes of connection in that relational space of what *is*. Along with the other essays in this volume, they reflect the breadth of possibility for studies in RHM, and hint at how a rapidly expanding medical and health landscape might be configured *otherwise*.

One emerging task of RHM is to seek a more fleshed-out ecological account of local and culturally broad elements of the healthscape. The task is energized but also complicated by an extensive interdisciplinarity and a variety of foci, as demonstrated in this section's essays. An issue that Derkatch and Spoel bring to our attention is the relative disciplinary trade-off involved in focusing on local conditions and practices as distinguished from those that are more culturally broad. The authors interrogate the formation of health citizenship, arguing that the approach that rhetoricians take to this cannot be confined to medical and health-care practices. Rather, they argue, it requires a broader framing of the way that health is defined, as well as an expansion of the way that rhetorical contexts are typically conceived. Still, the conception of rhetoric they advocate is quite recognizable as "the symbolic means through which individuals and groups are induced, through methods both conscious and unconscious, toward certain beliefs and actions and away from others" (p. 15). While taking an expansive view of "symbolic means," they draw upon theories of *genre* and *constitutive rhetoric* to shed light on cultural and ideological influences that do not always enter discourses about health. Their focus turns away from medical care and toward one of the main determinates of health—the multipatterned availability of food.

Derkatch and Spoel make the case that research focused mainly on local producers and consumers at food markets can leave in the shadows the ways in which public health requires more than individuals taking on relevant responsibilities. Criticisms such as these push the field toward a reflective assessment of its goals, and one such goal that comes under their critique is that of hitching academic scholarship to a goal of influencing medical practices—something these authors believe may be constrictive to larger theoretical objectives. For medical humanities, they argue, the typical locational commitments to medical institutions mean that whatever version of the humanities is pursued in such settings, the humanities are viewed through the lens of medical programs, rather than the reverse. Thus they advocate a broadening of the scope of concern from medical institutions to the wider determinants of health.

The essay also touches on another issue of general interest to those working in the field of RHM in that the authors advocate a conception of a rhetoric of health that is "hard," precise, and rigorous, and therefore not to be confused with something intended to soften our understanding of medical and health practices and technologies. And this puts focus on a relevant issue for advocates of RHM—the question of whether tightly disciplined methods are the only, or even necessarily the best way to define the field. In this matter some would suggest that we tread with caution, having seen other academic fields play out as one hardened set of methods against another. In some pertinent ways, one might argue, it is the very fluidity of methods and approaches that keeps studies of rhetoric from being rigidified by their internal mandates. While it can be a clarifying strategy to advocate an "as" that is conceptually distinguished from other perspectives, time will tell how fully a quest for methodological uniqueness in approaching an inherently interdisciplinary project can be realized.

One question that might be posed for Derkatch and Spoel, and for studies of this kind, is to ask what processes mutually engage state and nonstate agents. I think the authors might agree that attention to nonlocal levels of discourse need not necessarily require giving up attention to the local, and that delineating system-wide agency need not come at the expense of a better understanding of local agency. The local framing of the food co-ops might be expected to reveal what would not be visible at the more general ideological level, and vice versa. The field of RHM comprises investigations of both culturally broad and more locally concrete processes, and thinking ecologically carries further implications for the framing of the various inquiries. One of these is that the different niches of the ecology can directly or indirectly affect one another. Another is that any niche is a context that will be nested within broader contexts. This suggests that flexibility in *scope* as well as methodological interdisciplinarity will have general relevance in navigating the healthscape.

The case for an interdisciplinary alliance between RHM and disability studies (DS) is taken up by Holladay and Price, who provide a useful overview and analysis of research in DS that anticipates an increasingly productive relationship between the two fields. Themes highlighted in DS include the construction and maintenance of the normal and the need for a more robust account of the social/discursive shaping of those processes—one that is not predicated on a deficit model of disability. This suggests that there is a need for rhetorical strategies that challenge prevailing configurations and boost the conversation between RHM and DS scholars. Holladay and Price move toward an aspirational vocabulary that might speak beyond the limitations of often stigmatizing terms such as *mental health,* favoring a broader range of implicit motivational appeals, including terms such as *equity* and *rights,* which in turn suggest sites of dialogical and persuasive engagement with an expanded terrain of health. The authors invoke Kafer's argument for "a *political-relational* approach, which recognizes that *both* impairment and disability are social and that disability is experienced in and through relationships" (pp. 7–8, as cited by Holladay and Price, p. 36).

If the deficit model is to be surmounted by embracing a political-relational approach, there should a role for rhetorical critique and invention. When *ability* serves as the unmarked term in relation to the marked term *disability*, it deflects scrutiny of the environmental conditions that allow "abilities" to function. If taken-for-granted assumptions about enablement, such as the assumption that ability resides simply in the properties of the enabled person, it occludes awareness of the relational and systemic interactions between humans and their environments. Rhetorical engagement with DS may help in articulating alternative conceptions of access. A challenge to the assumption that "abilities" are an innate set of pre-given capacities might begin with the observation, well understood in DS, that disabling conditions invite development of alternative capacities and perspectives. What can we learn from the fact that blindness activates other ways of seeing, paralysis generates other ways of moving, and speechlessness leads to different ways of giving voice? History gives us an abundance of examples of artists, philosophers, and political leaders whose disabilities led to such enablements. Of course, this is not to underestimate the challenges that disabilities pose, nor to suggest that there is a simplistic symmetry between disabilities and abilities. Rather, it is an example of how scholars might rhetorically align with DS in exploring the possibilities for articulating dis/abilities—and perhaps in reconfiguring the aspirational landscape so that disability becomes understood as an opening to alternate possibilities.

It is worth noting here that the evolving possibilities for medical or quasi-medical enhancement make "good health" a receding goalpost, and this is something that deserves attention in RHM. There is an increasingly apparent issue with respect to how we gauge disability in a culture of enhancement. The ability/disability dyad has been based on the unexamined premise that "ability" is the high-water mark—a condition that might be lost or restored to a presumed state of optimal functioning. But it is increasingly complicated to determine the meaning of optimal functioning in a time when medical knowledge and health technologies increasingly call attention to the demand for enhancement, or, to use Carl Elliott's (2003) phrase, to be "better than well." If cosmetic surgery or pharmaceuticals are used in pursuit of social success or better mental performance, analogous to the way that diet and exercise regimes or gym culture can expand some abilities, then there is always the possibility that any existing condition, cast as a lack, can come to be seen as disabling. The new normal in the culture of enhancement has largely become a consumer-based model, with increasing evidence that the dialogical pair of ability/disability is being transformed accordingly. For this and other reasons, the pairing of RHM with DS is timely.

An important issue for RHM studies is the way that agency is conceptualized and articulated, and the extent to which narratives of agency should be focused on individual human capacities. Winderman and Landau examine a rhetorical strategy that personifies and locates agency within an account that might otherwise lack narrative coherence. They turn attention to how dehumanization can be reversed by rehumanizing strategies. The case of Henrietta Lacks, as narrated by Rebecca Skloot, shows the possibility of movement in either direction. First, Lacks was disconnected from the cellular lineage that she introduced, and was by that disconnection rendered invisible in the medical context. By an institutionally induced intervention, her cancerous cells were marked by only the faintest traces of the lurking metonymy that emerged from the extended narrative. "HeLa" cells had lost nearly all traces of their human genesis. The rehumanization emerging from Skloot's eye-opening narrative was a double achievement, in that it brought the original donor to the foreground and also personified her biological heritage—a rhetorical engagement by which the identity of the two was merged.

A topic of significance in rhetorical studies, the role of *pathos* in influencing both identification and motivation, should likewise be recognized as a topic brimming with possibilities for RHM. Winderman and Landau employ Edbauer's (2005) conception of affective ecologies to put the spotlight on *pathos,* and this gives us an interesting counterpoint to the rhetoric of the posthuman. This move to personifying strategies takes us to the brink of a conceptual challenge. What does it mean to humanize or dehumanize within a theoretical environment that, as Derkatch and Spoel note, beckons us *away* from the "human"? The recovery of Henrietta Lacks's agency as a point of origin for the medical uses of her cancer cells has been heralded as the correction of an injustice—the injustice of making agency and identity invisible. Might not this emphasis on human agency and identity be accounted as going against the grain of a posthuman academic frame? Granted, the rehumanization in this case recovers a broadened agency, yet it assimilates it to Lacks's identity. But what does it mean to speak of humanizing or dehumanizing if we have become suspicious of "the human"? And what does it mean to use a term such as *uniquely human* in this narrative? Does the language of "the human" not function within our multilayered "forms of life" (Wittgenstein, 1973)? Could it be that this historical episode underscores the continuing relevance of "the human" as a formation so deeply rooted in our commonly shared nonacademic assumptions that it will inevitably remain relevant?

Among those working in RHM, there are various viewpoints on how tightly the field can be defined, or whether it can be restricted to certain methodologies. The view here is that there a need for ecological fluidity. If health and medicine resist fixed categories for examination, interpretation, and intervention, the same can be said of rhetoric, which has meant different things for different purposes across the centuries and within interdisciplinary spaces—and this suggests that the unfolding of time should not be counted on to eliminate the ambiguities. Medicine and health are partly about science, partly about practices, and partly about culture. *Humanities* may not have the same meaning it once did, but it comes to the fore when we need to signal that science does not have all the answers.

As these conversations suggest, C. P. Snow's famous "two cultures" narrative needs to be rethought in our own era. Even if it still seems apt in highlighting differences in the respective cultures of the sciences and the humanities (e.g., STEM vs. liberal arts) the "two cultures" trope has become just that—a rhetorical turn. We will also do well to deploy tropes that may give traction to *another kind* of "two cultures" perspective—the one in which academics and the general public coexist and in various ways interact. As we think about who might be our audiences, a healthy ecology for RHM might be conceived as one that generates productive conversation not only between research fields but also between academic and nonacademic audiences. Some version of a "third culture" model that emphasizes a cross-referencing of scientific, technological, and humanities-based research programs *as well as* professional and nonprofessional voices might be a part of the healthy ecology to which RHM should aspire (Lyne, 2005, 2010). In a dynamically evolving culture, the resources of rhetoric and the innovations of RHM may be especially helpful in making sense of fluid discursive patterns, and in moving from what *is* toward what might be *otherwise*.

REFERENCES

Elliott, C. (2003). *Better than well: American medicine meets the American dream.* New York, NY: Norton.

Erdbauer, J. (2005). Unframing models of public distribution: From rhetorical situation to rhetorical ecologies. *Rhetoric Society Quarterly, 35*(4), 5–24.

Lyne, J. (2005). Science, common sense, and the third culture. *Argumentation & Advocacy, 42*(1), 38–42.

Lyne, J. (2010). Rhetoric and the third culture: Scientists and arguers and critics. In M. Porrovecchio (Ed.), *Reengaging the prospect of rhetoric* (pp. 132–152). New York, NY: Routledge.

Melonçon, L., & Scott, J. B. (Eds.). (2018). *Methodologies for the rhetoric of health and medicine.* New York, NY: Routledge.

Wittgenstein, L. (1973). *Philosophical investigations* (3rd ed.). Pearson.

SECTION 2

REPRESENTATIONS AND ONLINE HEALTH

CHAPTER 4

Enactments of Self

Studying Binaries and Boundaries in Autoimmunity

MOLLY MARGARET KESSLER

> Long story short: Our bodies are fighting a Civil War with themselves.
> —Sheridan Watson, contributor, *Buzzfeed Health*

> My identity is very much so tied to my ostomy and
> how it gave me my life back.
> —Jessica Grossman, contributor, *Uncover Ostomy*

DISEASE IS commonly represented as an infiltrating invader, an enemy within the body that does not belong and therefore should be attacked and removed, as the opening epigraph so cogently uses the concept of civil war to describe a disease as it moves into a body. We fight diseases, win wars against illnesses, blame our bodies for having minds of their own, and sometimes have to deal with others placing conditions all in our heads. Present in all of these common framings are none other than binaries—that is, Cartesian dualities between mind and body, self and nonself, human and nonhuman. Rhetorical scholars have noted the persuasive power of such divisions in enabling patients to draw productive lines between notions of the self and nonself (disease), as well as between the mind and the body (see, for example, Segal, 1997; Sontag, 2001). Such separations empower patients to fight these invading entities and to compartmentalize the involuntary conditions of the body and/or mind as something beyond patients' control.

Autoimmune conditions, however, complicate these divides, challenging rhetorical and theoretical notions of bodies and boundaries. For instance, experiences like the one described in the opening epigraphs are no doubt familiar to many patients with autoimmune disease. Bodies attacking themselves, struggles with identity, and the necessity of medical technologies characterize life with an autoimmune disease. Typically, the immune system works as an internal defense mechanism to identify and destroy cells that do not belong in the body (e.g., a virus or bacteria). However, as the prefix *auto* indicates, autoimmune diseases occur when *oneself* is under attack by *oneself*. In other words, autoimmune diseases behave such that a person's immune system attacks the body's own cells and tissues. When this happens, a chain of physiological reactions transpires, and depending on the type of cells targeted, a range of destructive and even life-threatening symptoms manifest. In the words of Sheridan Watson (2016), the bodies of autoimmune patients are "fighting civil wars with themselves."

Additionally, the opening epigraphs demonstrate that boundaries regarding bodies and identities can differ across patients. Watson (2016) experiences divisions *within* her self and body (as would need to be the case for a civil war to commence). In contrast, Jessica Grossman's (2013) bodily and identity boundaries encompass her ostomy—a surgically created opening in her abdomen that is covered by a technology to collect digestive waste. Examining lived, embodied experiences with autoimmune disease in this chapter, I aim to address the following questions: How do patients experience and represent autoimmune diseases when they are unlike most conditions that are actually invaders in the body? Where and how are boundaries surrounding bodies and identities determined and represented when the body is both self and nonself? When technologies and/or prosthetics are introduced to help treat or cope with autoimmune conditions, where do borders between self, technology, body, and mind lie?

These question challenge the rhetoric of health and medicine (RHM) to find approaches that can adequately attend to messy, chaotic patient experiences in which various boundaries and divisions come into being and are represented. Through an analysis of lived experiences with autoimmune disease as represented in online spaces, I argue that boundaries such as those between mind and body or self and nonself are not inherent but certainly are possible. In other words, my goal in this chapter is to show how boundaries are *enacted* within rhetorical contexts for patients, specifically those with autoimmune diseases. Specifically, I advocate for inquiry into diverse patient practices to fully understand how embodied activity of autoimmunity influences the ways in which boundaries and binaries are experienced in patients' lives. This chapter queries *The Mighty* and *Uncover Ostomy*—two online blogs and support forums for people with a range of conditions including autoimmune diseases—and draws on Karen Barad's notion of intra-activity (2007) to argue that boundaries (and sometimes binaries) are embodied and enacted through lived practices.

This focus on "enactments" serves *as* a theoretical underpinning with which RHM can examine a range of entities that participate in people's lived experiences. Such an approach, I argue, enables rhetoricians of health and medicine to account for the diversity of boundaries, binaries, and entanglements of bodies, matter, disease, discourse, sites of practice, and culture that are at work in rhetorical situations. Importantly too, this approach shifts the work of rhetoricians of health and medicine away from examining how language *represents* patients' bodily and identity boundaries toward how *representational practices* participate along with other practices (physiological, symptomatic, technological, etc.) and influence wide-ranging patient lived experiences. The advantage of this shift, as I will argue, is that it enables RHM research to more fully explore meaning-making within patients' lived experiences. Accordingly, I build on Barad (2007) to theorize how RHM can attend to diverse entities and practices that participate in meaning-making, specifically in the boundaries that are enacted regarding bodies, diseases, minds, selves, technology, and more.

In what follows, then, I situate my study of autoimmunity within ongoing debates, particularly between postmodernism and new materialisms, regarding how we should approach various binaries and boundaries. In outlining the scholarly conversation between those bodies of work, I hope to illustrate how theory that builds on the strengths of both areas is necessary to best address the problems of binaries. I then detail two cases of autoimmune patients in which boundaries are enacted in unexpected or atypical ways.

DEBATES OVER BINARIES

Concerns over the pervasiveness of modernist binaries have been at the forefront of humanistic inquiry for decades. As Haraway (1991) noted, "Certain dualisms have been persistent in Western traditions . . . Chief among these troubling dualisms are self/other, mind/body, culture/nature, male/female" (p. 177). While a variety of theoretical solutions to these divisions have been proposed, scholarship categorized under postmodernism presumptively settled these debates by dismantling binaries into matters of the social, cultural, and discursive (see, for example, Butler, 1999; Haraway, 1991; Jordan, 2004; Selzer & Crowley, 1999; Wells, 2010). Postmodernist attention to binaries was a reaction to the modernist privileging of objects over subjects, nature over culture, bodies over minds. In response, postmodernism challenged these epistemologies and argued that objects and materiality are culturally meditated and socially constructed. This postmodern effort aimed to shift power and give due to the entities that had been ignored through modernism.

Much of this work, particularly in rhetorical studies, grew from an increasing recognition of the tension between materiality and discourse as "one of the most familiar and powerful" binaries (Wilson & Lewiecki-Wilson, 2001, p. 2). For instance, the scholarship featured in Selzer and Crowley's *Rhetorical Bodies* (1999) presents a variety of approaches for balancing or deconstructing dualisms, particularly those between language and matter, including Celeste Condit's (1999) "proto-theory of linguistic materialism" that "seeks to bridge the gap between the 'idea' and the 'material' realm—between the mind and the body" (p. 351) and Dickson's (1999) "material rhetoric" that offers a "mode of interpretation that takes as its object of study the signification of material things and corporal entities" (p. 297). According to this work, binaries are artifacts of a flawed epistemology, and divisions between mind and body, male and female, subject and object, self and other are constructions designed to subjugate entities within these binaries (e.g., female, mind, subject, other). As such, postmodern approaches, with their focus on social construction and cultural mediation, set out to "expos[e] the human motives and discursive forces operating behind the illusion of nature" and, I would add, the objects and bodies (Pender, 2018, p. 44). In so doing, many theories and approaches with postmodernism claimed to overcome or side-step the issues of Cartesian binaries.

Recently, however, a growing body of scholarship has reopened the Pandora's box of dualisms, calling for a reconsideration of postmodernist constructionism (see, for example, Barad, 2007; Graham, 2015; Mol, 2002; Pender, 2018). Much of this scholarship, often operating under the broad umbrella of "new materialisms," claims that the postmodern project actually reinscribes dualisms by privileging subjects over objects, selves over others, culture over nature, and so on (Barad, 2007; Graham, 2015; Gronnvoll, 2013). Essentially, new materialisms argue that postmodernist theories have inverted modernism. As Graham (2015) argued, "The postmodernists have been claiming to [overcome binaries] for years without actually accomplishing that aim" (p. 217). Despite postmodernist alternatives and solutions to binaries, these critiques argue, binaries have simply become a "habit of mind" (Barad, 2007, p. 4).

Furthermore, noting concerns with the postmodern project and emphasis on discourse, Gronnvoll (2013) wrote, "The linguistic turn launched a tsunami of scholarship, of many disciplinary flavors, leading inevitably to a tipping point where discourse began to be privileged over reality. The latter was sometimes dismissed as entirely constructed by language" (p. 98). Similarly, Graham (2015) contended that "where modernism privileges the real object over the perceiving subject, postmodernism recasts the object as an extension of the subject's perception, and the object becomes an epiphenomenon of the subject" (p. 19). According to this wave of critiques, overcoming binaries by reversing which entity in these binaries takes precedence (language over matter, for example) does little to resolve the modernist legacy and can be unproductive and damaging in real-world contexts.[1] For instance, scholars including Jay Dolmage (2014), Tobin Siebers (2001), and Marita Gronnvoll (2013) contend that when we privilege illness, language, and narrative, the physical, material experiences of bodies are elided. Dolmage (2014) explained:

> The postmodern model remains influential, often to the chagrin of disabled people who feel their experiences of disability are undermined. There certainly are dangerous implications for the issues of agency when a focus on individual empowerment and bodily reclamation cedes to discussions of social construction—particularly when a common assumption among "abled-bodied" bigots is that people with disabilities are faking it anyhow, or that they should just try harder to overcome their impairment and cure themselves. (p. 96)

Similarly, Gronnvoll (2013) contended that when the body becomes matter upon which discourse gives meaning, bodily experiences are lost, she said, "erasing the body, or rewriting it as a passive substance upon which discourses are sketched, also [brings] harm. To ignore the body is to ignore the fact that *bodies* experience violence, injustice, and pain" (p. 103).

For rhetoricians, this is especially complicated considering that our focus on language is often positioned as a defining feature of our field. However, one potential solution among the new materialist critiques of postmodernism is to shift from treating language as representational to positioning representational practices among many practices (including but not limited to discursive practices). In particular, Graham (2015) suggested that rhetorical studies would benefit from inquiry that "focuses not on what texts mean but rather on how representational activity articulates within and contributes to a deeper ecology of practices" (p. 69). This might at first seem a matter of semantics, but this shift from representations to representational practice is critical to avoiding a slide back to Cartesian binaries and the privileging of particular entities. When we focus on representations, we tend to also subscribe to the following premises: (1) linguistic artifacts are intrinsically separate from these deeper ecologies, and (2) particular binaries and boundaries are assumed at the outset of inquiry. That is, we perpetuate ontological categories in which subjects represent objects, language represents matter, minds represent bodies, and we concentrate on the accuracy, ethics, and constructions of those representations. To avoid reifying modernist dualisms, I argue in alignment

---

1. See for example, Graham's (2015) work on the two-world problem; Mol's (2002) discussion of the disease/illness dichotomy; or Siebers's (2001), Gibson's (2006), or Wilson and Lewiecki-Wilson's (2001) critique of postmodernism in relation to disability and embodiment.

with others, including Graham (2015), Mol (2002), and Pender (2018), that we attune our analyses to practices in order to avoid further calcifying assumed divisions and to better attend to boundaries and divisions as they emerge in specific rhetorical situations.

BINARIES WITHIN HEALTH AND MEDICINE

Moreover, many scholars have highlighted the specific problems that arise with our current approaches to binaries for health and medicine contexts. For example, in her research examining the stakeholders and practices associated with atherosclerosis, Annemarie Mol (2002) argued that as postmodern theorists have worked to make a way for themselves in the study of medicine, they have sequestered patient perspective/voice (illness) as their domain, leaving physicalities and bodily practices (disease) to biomedical experts. Ironically, this dichotomy at least partially emerged in an effort to give attention and authority to patient narrative, which is often subordinated to physical markers of disease (e.g., signs or symptoms made visible through examinations, MRI scans, blood tests). Yet, despite the effort to use a disease/illness dichotomy to encourage biomedical experts to attune themselves to patient experience, the dichotomy disempowers patient narratives by granting biomedical experts special access or even a justification to focus on the physical, materiality of the body (Mol, 2002, p. 9). Mol further argued, "In a world of meaning, nobody is in touch with the reality of diseases, everyone 'merely' interprets them" (p. 11).

Similar arguments have been made by rhetoricians of health and medicine as well, pointing both to the relevance of and concern over distinctions between disease and illness. Segal (2005) explained, "The physician is expert in disease, and the patient in illness; the physician in nosology, the patient in experience" (p. 147). Echoing these sentiments, Graham (2015) contended:

> The disease/illness dichotomy so popular in critical/cultural studies of medicine, it turns out, reinforces the line of demarcation between patient and physician, further enfranchising the singular "reality" of the disease over the manifold "perceptions" of the illness. (p. 217)

In other words, in splitting illness from disease, disease comes to align with an objective, verifiable reality, whereas illness (patient narrative) is deemed subjective and therefore less reliable or valuable within the domain of biomedicine. This disease/illness dichotomy, furthermore, indicates larger issues that arise out of postmodernist solutions to binaries (Graham, 2015; Mol, 2002; Pender, 2018).

Thus, the disease/illness dichotomy (and the subsequent divisions that follow) is of particular relevance for rhetoricians of health and medicine whose commitment to and focus on patient narrative or illness actually reinforces the very issues that RHM's goals (attending to and intervening in lived experiences) often work to overcome. If by focusing only on patient narrative, we excise patients' physical, bodily experiences from the linguistic representations of those experiences, it seems that rhetoricians of health and medicine ought to find new approaches by which we can work toward dismantling assumed binaries, particularly between disease and illness. Put simply, if, as a field, we focus exclusively on language, we actively uphold a binary that disempowers patients by positioning "what patients say" against "what bodies do."

Notably, though, some scholars have compellingly argued that binaries, although not pre-existing, can be quite productive for patients or certain bodies and identities (Krummel, 2001; Manderson, 2005). While examining how patients negotiate themselves after having life-altering surgery, Manderson (2005) identified the "need" for patients to separate themselves from their bodies, highlighting the "important and ongoing tension" that exists for "people who, on an everyday basis, have to deal with their bodies as objects" (p. 406). Additionally, in an autoethnographic piece regarding her own experiences with multiple sclerosis, Krummel (2001) explained that dealing with her condition has led to an "inevitable distrust of her own body, requiring her to rely more and more on her mind" (p. 68). In such examples, a tension exists between the theoretical or philosophical desires to overcome binaries and the lived divisions that scholars experience or observe. In a similar way, my analysis showcases the productive value in maintaining space for all boundaries that might be present in the lived experiences of people, especially those with autoimmune diseases.

To be sure, the opening epigraphs highlight that while binaries are not predetermined or inherent, divisions that we have come to recognize as Cartesian splits can actually have productive and persuasive power in certain contexts. This is to say that I agree with previous critiques of pre-existing binaries, but I resist the temptation to hybridize or subsume all entities into matters of social/discursive or materiality/nature. Instead, as the next section demonstrates, my goal is to build on theories that enable me to account for any entity and boundary that might emerge as meaningful.

Indeed, the work cut out for RHM, among all these debates and proposed solutions to binaries, is to find frameworks with which we can simultaneously engage the diverse boundaries, as well as the mix of discursive, material, cultural, and embodied entities at work within health and medical contexts. This is important to avoiding the many issues identified in both postmodernist and new materialist arguments regarding binaries. Equally, if not more, importantly, this is key for work in RHM that attempts to understand and empower patients who have lived experience that, to them, does not fit neatly into the binaries and boundaries of language/matter, mind/body, self/nonself, and so forth.

Intra-Active Enactments and Embodied Practices

Because autoimmunity complicates boundaries regarding self, nonself, mind, body, human, and nonhuman, a nuanced approach to examining how divisions and boundaries are established, dissolved, and maintained is necessary. Karen Barad's (2007) notion of intra-activity offers a way to capture and examine patient practices, boundaries, and identities without privileging any particular entity. Specifically, Barad asked many of the same questions I am posing throughout this chapter:

> What is entailed in the investigation of entanglements? How can one study them? Is there a way to study them without getting caught up in them? What can one say about them? Are there any limits to what can be said . . . how to responsibly explore entanglements and the differences they make? (p. 74)

Aiming to answer such questions, Barad (2007) theorized intra-action and intra-activity, which "enables us theorize the social and natural together, to read our best understandings of social and natural phenomena through one another in a way that clarifies the relationship between them" (p. 25). In other words, Barad suggested that the focus of inquiry should be on what phenomena or entities "become determinate" and "become meaningful" as they emerge in space and time (p. 139). Instead of studying how entities *interact*, which requires pre-existing, stable entities, Barad's intra-action enables a move away from pre-existing entities altogether.

Moreover, intra-activity provides an antidote to Cartesian dualisms. Within the framework of intra-activity, no entities are naturally separate in the world, but their separability is staged within intra-actions through what through specific "cuts." Drawing contrast with inherent, stable "Cartesian cuts," Barad (2007) offered *agential cuts*—distinctions that emerge through practices (p. 49). Critical to the idea of agential cuts is that what we reconsider the role of nonhuman entities without taking the distinctions between human and nonhuman as "foundational" or given (p. 32). Through intra-actions, specific agential cuts are enacted; in one intra-action a cut between (so-called) subject and object might be enacted, while in another a different cut that unifies subject and object might be enacted. Consequently, intra-activity requires demands that we focus on what becomes determinate "in the enactment of an agential cut" (p. 337). As Barad reminded, "boundaries and properties are *only* determinate within a given phenomenon through the *enactment* of an agential cut" (p. 345; emphasis added).

The significance of this attunement to intra-activity is that the world is no longer made up of pre-existing objects, subjects, cyborgs, minds, or bodies, and that the need to overcome or uphold binaries is no longer necessary. Under Barad's (2007) rubric, the entities previously understood as binaries or hybrids only emerge through their activities *within* enactments. As such, different practices stage different agential cuts, and we can begin to see enactments of mind/body divisions and mindbody unification as agential cuts that are rhetorically enacted in time and space. Instead of assuming or reinscribing "hardwired" divisions in the world, intra-activity provides a way for scholars to make sense of how phenomena come into being through practices. Accordingly, I attune the lively, agentic processes and practices that stage different enactments of boundaries surrounding patients' lived experiences, bodies, and identities.

Importantly too, the site or space of lived experiences has been demonstrated to be influential in the types of entities and boundaries represented through practices (Graham, 2015; Graham & Herndl, 2013; Mol, 2002). Put another way, sites of practice play a role in how entities we might call body, mind, self, nonself, human, technology, and so forth are articulated and represented. For instance, Barad (2007) reviewed an example of a textile shop floor to explore the role of spatiality and temporality within intra-actions. She argued that "the entangled, contingent, material conditions of the shop floor" intra-act with the "workers, machines, managers" to "constitute one another" (p. 239). Similarly, space plays an important intra-active role within enactments in health and medical contexts. In the doctor's office, boundaries between mind and body might emerge as a patient tells the doctor "my body has a mind of its own!" in an effort to distribute agency and control away from the patient. In contrast, when the famous track star Oscar Pistorius testified in the Court of Arbitration for Sport, his prosthetic legs were enacted and represented as part of his self, rather than as distinct entities enhancing his body, in an effort to qualify for the 2008 Olympic Games (Booher, 2010). These examples highlight that the site in which boundary-making practices occur—in a doctor's office, a court of law, a shop floor, or elsewhere—shapes where bodily and identity boundaries fall. In addition to a variety of discursive-material entities that might rhetorically engage in the meaning-making of patients (and their associated bodily and identity boundaries), the site in which meaning-making occurs powerfully participates.

Indeed, sites of practices have important implications for my examination of autoimmunity and enactments of boundaries. Over the last decade, a wealth of scholarship has shown the increasingly significant role of online spaces within patient experience. As this scholarship has noted, online spaces, especially support forums (Ginossar, 2008; Johnston, Worrell, Di Gangi, & Wasko, 2013; Oh & Lee, 2012; Wentzer & Bygholm, 2013) and social media (Househ, Borycki, & Kushniruk, 2014; Korda & Itani, 2013) have become incredibly popular and helpful spaces for patients to seek information and support regarding their conditions as well as to publicly represent various experiences and boundaries regarding their bodies and diseases. Accordingly, online spaces are especially rich sites for examining patient experiences and practices in which entities and boundaries are enacted and made meaningful. As my subsequent analysis argues, online spaces actively shape how various boundaries are enacted within lived experiences of autoimmune conditions.

Together, intra-activity, agential cuts, and enactments resonate productively with rhetorical work aiming to avert presumed binaries. That is, we can build on intra-activity within RHM to study what entities become both determinate and meaningful for patients and other stakeholders within health and medicine. In the following section, I illustrate how focusing on entities enacted through practices enables me to investigate how some within the autoimmune disease community experience civil wars within themselves while others live meaningfully with technologies as part of their identities.

Intra-Activity and Autoimmunity

An intra-active approach has profound ramifications for understanding the entities and boundaries enacted within the domain of autoimmune disease. Under an intra-active framework, different patients are engaged in different practices in which different agential cuts are enacted. Even more, online spaces enable particular agential cuts to be staged and represented. In particular, online spaces provide patients a site to represent and make public agential cuts that often contradict commonplace agential cuts regarding self, nonself, disease, immune system, and other entities. To explore this further, I offer two cases in which intra-activity allows me to account for the shifting entanglements that might emerge in autoimmune disease. As these cases will show, diverse boundaries are intra-actively enacted through representational practices in online spaces.

CASE 1: WHEN SELF BECOMES NONSELF

Sharilynn Battaglia is one of many contributors to *The Mighty*—a website that publishes "real stories by real people facing real challenges" in order to "face disability, disease, and mental illness together" ("Who We Are," 2016). Using one of Battaglia's articles as an exemplar case, I analyze her online representational practice regarding life with an autoimmune condition to demonstrate the common autoimmune patient's experience of living with self as nonself.

To begin, Battaglia (2016), who has been living with an autoimmune disease for over twenty years, describes having an autoimmune disease as "a lot like playing Jenga. Only we [autoimmune patients] are the tower." To help illustrate this comparison, Battaglia writes:

> When you first start playing, does the tower look like it's under attack? Does it look like it's in imminent danger of collapse? Of course not. But it is. It's exactly the same with us [people with autoimmune disease]. Why do you think they are called invisible illnesses? The attack is all happening on the inside, through the blood to whatever the target of the day is. But just because our diseases work quietly on the inside, and just because the effects of our diseases aren't as noticeable, that doesn't mean we aren't sick.

Even though autoimmune diseases do not necessary manifest visibly, Battaglia uses her online platform to share how these diseases "work quietly on the inside." Despite this containment within the confines of self, these diseases, at least according to Battaglia, are not self. It is perhaps a little odd to think about the internal activity of our body as nonself; after all, the external boundary of the body is commonly considered to be the skin. However, for Battaglia, what is happening inside of her—her autoimmune disease—is not self. Her immune system and its autoimmune "attacks" are separate entities that operate within her in ways that she does not control.

To explain further, she says that autoimmune patients' immune systems are "always on attack." Even more, she writes:

> [Autoimmune patients' immune systems] go after blocks of muscles or joints and push them out of balance, or they pull at blocks of nerves, creating rag-

gedy areas that send tremors through our whole structure . . . You see, a
healthy immune system knows what is foreign and what is not. You catch a
cold, it sees a virus, it attacks. End of story. With [us], it's not so easy. Our
immune systems are confused about what to attack.

Here, the practices enacted intra-actively shift Battaglia's immune system from
self to nonself, or, at the very least, her experiences with her autoimmunity are
enacted such that those specific "confused" responses within her body are not
her. Instead, she argues, such immune systems do not just "attack body parts";
instead they attack "*our* bodies. The bodies of people you know and love." A
division between "our" bodies, "our" selves, and the autoimmunity is enacted.
Importantly too, it's not just that immune systems are constantly confused;
instead, "just like in any war, troops take rest periods. So do our diseases. They
hide on us" (Battaglia, 2016). And, when autoimmune diseases decide to come
out of hiding, "they may pick and choose what to attack first in each person,
just like you choose which block to pull out when it's your turn in Jenga. But
eventually, the attack spreads and the tower falls . . . And it will happen over
and over." This sort of agentic, intentional behavior attributed to the autoimmune disease deepens the divide between conscious, controlled self, and non-
controllable, invading nonself.

Battaglia's emphasis on the nonself-ness of her immune system not only
demarcates the boundary between self and nonself but also relies on particular practices. That is, as Barad (2007) reminded us, "particular material
articulations of the world become meaningful" through intra-active entanglements emergent *in practices* (p. 139; emphasis mine). Accordingly, when
Battaglia's immune system "attacks," "hides," "picks and chooses," even as it
gets "confused," and when these practices are represented online, agential cuts
between Battaglia's self and nonself are enacted. In her embodied experiences
of autoimmunity, Battaglia's notion of self is under attack by what is enacted
as nonself.

Technically, autoimmunity is simply the immune system behaving in
such a way that is atypical, but this atypical behavior does not convert the
immune system to physiological nonself. The misbehaving immune cells are
still cells native to the body; however, when those misbehaving immune cells
lead to painful or unwanted experiences (e.g., symptoms), new agential cuts
may be enacted. In other words, it's not just that Battaglia represents the confused activity of her autoimmune disease as nonself, it's that she *experiences*
that confusion in ways that enable her autoimmune system to be agentially
cut from her self, and she consequently represents those cuts in her online

blogging practices. Ultimately, Battaglia's case highlights the fluidity of the boundaries surrounding self, nonself, body, and mind: specifically, when the intra-activity of autoimmune disease transforms self to become nonself.

CASE 2: WHEN NONSELF BECOMES SELF

For some patients with autoimmune disease, the use or integration of technologies as treatments becomes necessary. In particular, for patients with inflammatory bowel disease (IBD)—a category of autoimmune diseases in which the digestive tract is attacked by the immune system—a medical technology called the ostomy pouch is often required. Ostomy pouches are affixed to a person's abdomen and collect digestive waste that leaves the body through an end of intestine pulled to the surface of the skin called a stoma. Ostomy pouches and stomas are implemented when all or some of a patient's lower digestive tract must be removed due to inflammation, scarring, and/or progressive disease. For many people with ostomies, notions of self become increasingly complex. Is the ostomy pouch self? Is the self a cyborg? Can nonhuman become human? To examine these questions, I turn to Jessica Grossman, a contributor to *Uncover Ostomy,* an "online awareness campaign working to break the stigma surrounding ostomy surgery" ("About Us," n.d.).

Grossman blogs regularly on the Uncover Ostomy website, representing her personal experiences with IBD and ostomies and offering advice and support for others on topics ranging from clothing and exercising to dating and wedding planning via this online platform. For this analysis, I examine one of Grossman's posts, entitled "13 Years of Different: Bag-Mitzvah Edition," in which Grossman (2013) celebrates her thirteen-year ostomy anniversary. Reflecting on these thirteen years, she writes, "On January 30th, 2003, I was told that I needed to choose between life with an ostomy or death. 13 years later, I am here. Alive. Healthy. And celebrating . . . my 'Bag-Mitzvah.'" In addition to celebrating the life she was able to continue due to her ostomy, Grossman uses this post to offer thirteen bits of "wisdom" with readers.

Over the course of the thirteen points, Grossman specifically highlights the importance of acceptance, openness, and empowerment for people with ostomies. As I will show, through Grossman's points of advice, she not only highlights the importance of acceptance but describes her experiences in which the technology is enacted as self. Specifically, Grossman begins her list with the following sentiment: "There is no better choice that you can make in your life than to accept yourself for who you are." On this point, Grossman elaborates:

Having accepted my ostomy as part of who I am has given me the confidence to not only live my life, but to live it the way I want to live it. If there's one thing you take away from this whole post—do whatever it takes to get yourself to accept who you are.

Here, Grossman advocates for the acceptance of the previously non-self, nonhuman ostomy into her notion of self. Accepting the ostomy means accepting herself for who she is, the person/body that is enacted through her lived experiences, and she recommends that others with ostomy pouches do the same.

Building on this acceptance of self, Grossman then recommends that people with ostomies must educate others about their "difference" because people "won't understand what your difference really is." To support this point, she offers her own experience:

I was able to explain that the ostomy is a lifesaving surgery and that, without it, I would be dead. I can explain that it's *not* gross, it *is* weird, but *it's me* and I damn proud to be alive. (author's emphasis)

Grossman explicitly identifies the ostomy as self in this passage, which suggests that her intra-action with the ostomy is such that the boundary between self and technology dissolves. For Grossman her ostomy is part of her self. Note, Grossman explains that the ostomy "is me," not "I decided the ostomy is part of me" or "I talk about my ostomy as if it's part of me." The declarative sense that the ostomy becomes self through practices that involved Grossman, but were not controlled by her, aligns with the idea that these entanglements become determinate and meaningful through embodied intra-actions and practices (Barad, 2007, p. 333).

In addition to reminding readers to "not let [your] difference stop you from doing what you want to do," Grossman specifically tells readers that being different, having an ostomy, makes them "special" and that specialness is not only valuable but tied to identity and self. Reflecting on her personal experience, Grossman offers, "My fiancé treats me like gold because he loves everything about me—including my stubbornness *and* my ostomy. It makes me who I am and that's all he cares about" (author's emphasis). It is *because* her self includes an ostomy that she is special, unique, and loved. Because such "boundaries do not sit still" and materialize in practice, Grossman's boundary of self can be expanded to include her ostomy. The borders of her body and self are not limited to the boundaries of her physical body (e.g., skin); instead, the intra-activity emergent in Grossman's case enables what we might presumptively categorize as nonself (the ostomy) to actually become self. Too, Grossman's intra-actions are made publicly represented and shared through her online site; such a space not only enables Grossman's representational practices but allows her to reach a much wider and more public audience than would otherwise be possible. Grossman's case, like Battaglia's, supports intra-activity as a productive approach to binaries, even though the boundary for each of these women emerges differently.

CONCLUSION: LIVED EXPERIENCE AND PRODUCTIVE BINARIES

I include Grossman's case in juxtaposition to Battaglia's because these two offer what I would consider limit cases of embodied intra-activity. On one hand, in Battaglia's case an agential cut is enacted within what we might typically characterize as self—her self (immune system) becomes nonself. For Grossman, on the other hand, the agential cut enacted extends the notion of self as her ostomy pouch (nonself) becomes self. Together, these cases demonstrate that entities like self, nonself, human, nonhuman, mind, and body are not inherent entities in the world; much less are they inherently divided into binaries. Instead, in accordance with Barad's (2007) theory of intra-activity, these entities and the boundaries that create them are enacted in specific practices, whether those practices represent acceptance, symptomatic embodied experience, or otherwise.

These cases, too, offer critical insight regarding how we might overcome the problems of inherent binaries but maintain space for divisions to be enacted productively along binary lines. My analysis of Battaglia and Grossman highlights that we don't necessarily need a better theory to do away with binaries. Instead, we need a robust framework in which we can more adequately understand how boundaries and binaries are intra-actively enacted in diverse ways through diverse practices. Importantly, I'd like to emphasize that the focus on enactment I advocate for throughout this chapter does not do away with binaries altogether. Under Barad's (2007) rubric of intra-activity, any enactment can emerge and become meaningful. Key here is that preexisting binaries do not exist but that a division between what a patient might articulate as mind and body is indeed possible. In turning to Barad and an enactment approach, I'm working to account for the possibility of enactments of ostomy as self and enactments of immune system as nonself.

In either of these cases, boundaries and entities are enacted through the intra-action of disease, self, nonself, bodies, technology, and perhaps more, and *in* specific practices. Approaching boundaries in this way situates rhetoricians of health and medicine to better understand patients' practices and in turn better help patients navigate the complexities of their embodiment and patienthood. What's more, analyzing the cases in this chapter as representational practices further allowed me to avoid "reduc[ing]" Battaglia and Grossman's experiences to discourse (Graham, 2015, p. 8). Reducing their bodily practices and embodied experiences to discourse risks not only reifying the disease/illness dichotomy but also positioning those practices and experiences as somehow less real or valid. Additionally, the boundaries enacted regarding entities like self and nonself risk becoming artifacts of language and symbols, rather than embodied experiences and realities. When reduced to discourse, entities remain stable, the way we talk about them changes. However, as Battaglia and Grossman illustrate, entities themselves transform with intra-actions and lived experiences, and representational practices are an important element of these entanglements.

Additionally, by examining online representational practices in health and medicine like Battaglia and Grossman, it becomes clear that boundaries are enacted in diverse ways to make meaning of bodily experience and patienthood. The online space enables these patients, and others like them, to represent the diverse bodily and identity boundaries experienced in their everyday lives. As Battaglia mentions, autoimmune conditions are often characterized as "invisible" because they do not manifest in easily visible ways (e.g., like the way that crutches visually represent an injury). These patients capitalize on online space to enable enactments that would otherwise be difficult to represent in the public sphere. Blogs, social media sites, pictures, forums, and other online mediums provide these patients a way to represent their diverse boundaries and experiences and challenge assumed boundaries regarding self, nonself, technology, human, and more.

Examining autoimmunity and its associated experiences as enacted through intra-actions toward various rhetorical ends provides a way in which we can more adequately account for and balance the roles of these agents (e.g., discourse, matter) as they come into being and play a part in rhetorical practices. I hope the insights of this chapter demonstrate the ever-pressing need for rhetoricians of health and medicine to examine patient narrative as a resource for investigating patients' lived experiences and as part of larger systems of meaning-making in which a range of practices shape the enactments that become meaningful for patients. Focusing on enactments, ultimately, *is* a way for rhetoricians of health and medicine to broaden the types of practices we consider rhetorically powerful in patients' lived experiences. In this way, enactments can orient our research toward meaning-making practices within peoples' lives and help us find ways to intervene in those meaningful experiences.

REFERENCES

About Us. (n.d.). Retrieved from http://uncoverostomy.org/about-us/

Barad, K. (2007). *Meeting the universe halfway: Quantum physics and the entanglement of matter and meaning.* Durham, NC: Duke University Press.

Battaglia, S. (2016). Why having an autoimmune disease is like playing Jenga. Retrieved from https://themighty.com/2016/01/why-having-an-autoimmune-disease-is-like-playing-jenga/

Booher, A. K. (2010). Docile bodies, supercrips, and the plays of prosthetics. *IJFAB: International Journal of Feminist Approaches to Bioethics, 3*(2), 63–89.

Butler, J. (1999). Bodily inscriptions, performative subversions. In J. Pirce & M. Shildrick (Eds.), *Feminist theory and the body: A reader* (pp. 416–422). New York, NY: Routledge.

Coole, D., & Frost, S. (2010). Introducing the new materialisms. In D. Coole & S. Frost (Eds.), *New materialisms: Ontology, agency, and politics* (pp. 1–43). Durham, NC: Duke University Press.

Condit, C. (1999). The materiality of coding: Rhetoric, genetics, and the matter of life. In J. Selzer & S. Crowely (Eds.), *Rhetorical bodies* (pp. 326–356). Madison, WI: University of Wisconsin Press.

Derkatch, C., & Segal, J. Z. (2005). Realms of rhetoric in health and medicine. *University of Toronto Medical Journal, 82*(2), 138–142.

Dickson, B. (1999). Reading materiality materially: The case of Demi Moore. In J. Selzer & S. Crowely (Eds.), *Rhetorical bodies* (pp. 297–313). Madison, WI: University of Wisconsin Press.

Dolmage, J. (2014). *Disability rhetoric.* Syracuse, NY: Syracuse University Press.

Gibson, B. E. (2006). Disability, connectivity and transgressing the autonomous body. *Journal of Medical Humanities, 27*(3), 187–196.

Ginossar, T. (2008). Online participation: A content analysis of differences in utilization of two online cancer communities by men and women, patients and family members. *Health Communication, 23*(1), 1–12.

Graham, S. S. (2015). *The politics of pain medicine: A rhetorical-ontological inquiry.* Chicago, IL: University of Chicago Press.

Graham, S. S., & Herndl, C. (2013). Multiple ontologies in pain management: Toward a postplural rhetoric of science. *Technical Communication Quarterly, 22*(2), 103–125.

Gronnvoll, M. (2013). Review essay: Material rhetorics meet material feminisms. *Quarterly Journal of Speech, 99*(1), 98–113.

Grossman, J. (2013, January 30). *13 years of being different: Bag-Mitzvah edition.* Retrieved from http://uncoverostomy.org/2016/01/30/13-years-of-different-bag-mitzvah-edition/

Haraway, D. (1991). *Simians, cyborgs, and women: The reinvention of nature.* New York, NY: Routledge.

Househ, M., Borycki, E., & Kushniruk, A. (2014). Empowering patients through social media: The benefits and challenges. *Health Informatics Journal, 20*(1), 50–58.

Johnston, A. C., Worrell, J. L., Di Gangi, P. M., & Wasko, M. (2013). Online health communities: An assessment of the influence of participation on patient empowerment outcomes. *Information Technology & People, 26*(2), 213–235.

Jordan, J. W. (2004). The rhetorical limits of the "plastic body." *Quarterly Journal of Speech, 90*(3), 327–358.

Korda, H., & Itani, Z. (2013). Harnessing social media for health promotion and behavior change. *Health Promotion Practice, 14*(1), 15–23.

Krummel, M. A. (2001). Am I MS? In J. C. Wilson & C. Lewiecki-Wilson (Eds.), *Embodied rhetorics: Disability in language and culture* (pp. 61–78). Carbondale, IL: Southern Illinois University Press.

Kuehl, R., & Anderson, J. (2015). Designing public communication about doulas: Analyzing presence and absence in promoting a volunteer doula program. *Communication Design Quarterly, 3*(4), 75–84.

Manderson, L. (2005). Boundary breaches: The body, sex and sexuality after stoma surgery. *Social Science & Medicine, 61*(2), 405–415.

Melançon, L., & Frost, E. A. (2015). Special issue introduction: Charting an emerging field: The rhetorics of health and medicine and its importance in communication design. *Communication Design Quarterly Review, 3*(4), 7–14.

Mol, A. (2002). *The body multiple: Ontology in medical practice.* Durham, NC: Duke University Press.

Oh, H. J., & Lee, B. (2012). The effect of computer-mediated social support in online communities on patient empowerment and doctor–patient communication. *Health Communication, 27*(1), 30–41.

Pender, K. (2018). *Being at genetic risk: Toward a rhetoric of care.* University Park, PA: Pennsylvania State University Press.

Segal, J. Z. (1997). Public discourse and public policy: Some ways that metaphor constrains health (care). *Journal of Medical Humanities, 18*(4), 217–231.

Segal, J. Z. (2005). *Health and the rhetoric of medicine.* Carbondale, IL: Southern Illinois University Press.

Selzer, J., & Crowley, S. (1999). *Rhetorical bodies.* Madison, WI: University of Wisconsin Press.

Siebers, T. (2001). Disability in theory: From social constructionism to the new realism of the body. *American Literary History, 13*(4), 737–754.

Sontag, S. (2001). *Illness as metaphor and AIDS and its metaphors.* New York, NY: Macmillan.

Watson, S. (2016). 18 things you should know about people with autoimmune disease. Retrieved from https://www.buzzfeed.com/sheridanwatson/people-with-autoimmune-diseases

Wells, S. (2010). *Our Bodies, Ourselves and the work of writing.* Palo Alto, CA: Stanford University Press.

Wentzer, H., & Bygholm, A. (2013). Narratives of empowerment and compliance: Studies of communication in online patient support groups. *International Journal of Medical Informatics, 82*(12), 386–394.

Who We Are. (2016). Retrieved from https://themighty.com/who-we-are/

Wilson, J. C., & Lewiecki-Wilson, C. (Eds.). (2001). *Embodied rhetorics: Disability in language and culture.* Carbondale, IL: Southern Illinois University Press.

CHAPTER 5

"Did you have sex today?"

Discourses of Pregnancy and Big Data
in Fertility-Tracking Apps

AMANDA FRIZ AND STACEY OVERHOLT

IN THEN President Barack Obama's 2015 State of the Union address, a "new era of medicine" was declared, one that ostensibly will "give all of us access to the personalized information we need to keep ourselves and our families healthier," a sentiment that seems to endorse a proliferation of bodily data in order to maintain and monitor health. Transforming the human body and its health and wellness into discrete, measurable information first requires processes of quantification, a task accomplished passively (through wearing wireless sensors like the Fitbit, for example) or actively (by entering data into an app like a calorie counter, for example). Embracing and bolstering this logic of health attained via bodily quantification, measurement, and monitoring is the so-called quantified-self movement, a collection of enthusiastic technophiles who employ all manner of health-tracking devices (from Fitbits to Apple watches) to discipline their bodily movements and functions into conforming to and achieving a higher ideal of the self (Ajana, 2018; Johnson, 2014; Lupton, 2015; Schüll, 2016; Swan, 2012, 2013). These technologies, be they apps, websites, social media platforms, or other wireless sensors, lie at the center of a Gordian knot that combines the interests of private industry, health care, and government to produce a moral imperative that directs citizen-consumers to buy and use these self-surveilling technologies in order to expeditiously and efficiently quantify, measure, and share health practices and statuses.

Medical data and statistics are not new to the practice of medicine in the US. Starting in roughly the early 1800s, "the collection, study, and application of numerical data became one of the central characteristics of American medicine" (Cassedy, 1984, p. vii) and remain prominent in medical practice today via pushes for "evidence-based medicine" (see Weisz, 2005, for a tracing of this connection). Rather, we see the proliferation of sensors, apps, algorithms, and aggregators as an intensification of this centuries-old logic of quantifying health, developments that merit attention from a rhetorical perspective. As rhetorician Jeanne Fahnestock (2009) argued, "The role of mathematics as a persuasive language in itself and a source of perhaps unique topoi deserves more rhetorical attention" (p. 189). Mathematics can persuade through their presentation as self-evident, objective facts (Porter, 1996). And yet, to count something is also to make a rhetorical determination that the observed phenomenon "counts as" or belongs to a particular category. Quantification and counting have rhetorical effects in that they enable judgments of having too much or not enough of something, determinations that easily map onto conceptions of illness or health.

Therefore, we propose thinking about the rhetoric of health and medicine (RHM) through a lens of "quantification-as-representation." What distinguishes RHM as a field is that rhetorical scholarship reveals not just how humans talk about or perceive health but how we practice it. Whether one is "healthy" is, in today's world of wireless sensors, biostatistics, and big data analytics, in part determined by how and what health data are generated and measured, which in turn depends on how the body is converted into measurable quantities. Blood pressure, cholesterol levels, fasting glucose—one's health or illness is in part defined by how these data points "measure up" against statistical norms. Health in the rhetoric of quantification is neither absence of disease nor a state of being one achieves; it is never a noun one possesses ("to have health") but a verb one performs ("to do health") via generating and tracking data.

In this chapter, we trace the discourses advanced by creators and users of health-tracking apps that constellate a particular conception of "health" as synonymous with surveillance, discipline, and quantification to encourage the adoption of particular behaviors and attitudes that optimize the gathering of health data for the ultimate benefit of for-profit companies. We see this push toward bodily quantification as a key strategy for enacting "health" as the performance of a digitized, disciplined, and docile body in order to aid the collection and analysis of bodily quantities. Health-tracking apps are a prime case study for unpacking the rhetoric of health as the quantification of the body. These apps represent the body by figuring quantification as the prime means of knowing not just the body (through its data) but also oneself (via comparisons with other users' data). Quantification thus (re)presents the body as numerical measurements and simultaneously (re)defines "health" in terms of gathering and analyzing data. It is "healthy" to cultivate behaviors that make one's body easier to monitor and thus quantify so that algorithmic analysis might yield somatic insights, no matter how minute. Further, such data profiles come to (re)present our "selves" as well; we are our data (see, for example, Ajana, 2018; Lupton, 2015; Schüll, 2016).

Because smartphone apps are increasingly being developed for such data gathering and tracking (Johnson, 2014; Lupton, 2013; Swan, 2012, 2013), in this chapter we examine one such app as a rhetorical artifact whose very existence relies upon and reifies extant health citizenship discourses that encourage self-surveillance via quantifying and measuring minute bodily changes. Prominent among these health-monitoring apps are period-tracking apps, which assist (female) users in avoiding pregnancy, becoming pregnant, or dealing with fertility issues by gathering myriad data points from users' input. Much like with the familiar Fitbit, the data produced by users are rendered intelligible only by algorithms and other practices of big data analytics, and information produced by these devices is bought and sold in the burgeoning data economy (Federal Trade Commission, 2014).

With this in mind, this project examines a particular period-tracking app, Eve, part of a suite of ovulation, pregnancy, and birthing apps created by Glow, Inc. As a health surveillance technology, Eve is situated at the intersection of online surveillance and the quantified-self movement. Using Foucauldian articulations of biopolitics as a theoretical frame, this project explores the broader discourses that enable and mobilize notions of authenticity, expertise, and moral duty in order to encourage a particular kind of performative consumerism that aligns with neoliberal mandates to know and care for oneself through surveillance and discipline.

Specifically, we argue that Eve constructs an identity of an empowered, knowledgeable, and knowable self for consumers through three key moves: shifting the medical gaze from the purview of health-care professionals to individual consumers, advocating the use of big data, and resituating pregnancy as not just a woman's responsibility but as something women can and must have control over. Furthermore, we argue that in its usage, Eve asserts that you can best know yourself—perhaps even only know yourself—through your data, thus encouraging female users to discipline their bodies into potentially maternal bodies. This injunction to discipline, surveil, and "know" oneself is refracted through a neoliberal lens of autonomy, self-responsibility, and moral consumerism, creating a framework of discipline and conformity.

This chapter proceeds in four parts. We begin with a description of Eve and justify the focus on this app over other fertility or pregnancy apps. Next, we lay out our theoretical framework, which draws on Foucauldian articulations of biopolitics and critical approaches to big data, and our methodological framework, which is grounded in rhetorical criticism. This is followed by a close analysis of Eve and its extant discourses. Finally, we conclude with a discussion of future directions and implications for RHM as a field, specifically how thinking about quantification and potentially maternal bodies as health guides rhetoricians' scholarship, as well as how the rhetoric of health is in practice an examination of the ways (re)definitions of health do work in the world.

"FROM PERIOD TO PARENTING!": THE GLOW ENTERPRISE AS AN OBJECT OF STUDY

Started in 2012 by PayPal co-founder Max Levchin, Glow, Inc., is the result of Levchin's aspiration to apply "Silicon Valley innovation" to improving health-care delivery and lowering health-care-related costs (Manjoo, 2013). In promoting Glow's big data analytics as an advantage over other apps on the market at the time, Levchin said, "We see so many opportunities to improve the state of health and wellness through data science. Deeper insights will result in more informed diagnostics and decisions, earlier treatments and ultimately cheaper, more informed healthcare" (as quoted in Adams, 2013, n.p.). Beginning with its flagship app, Glow (an ovulation tracking app, website, and attendant social media platform), Glow, Inc., has been recognized as one of the best health and fitness apps available, and is a free download on both Apple and Android operating systems ("Glow," 2015). Reflecting its popularity with users, Glow, Inc., has expanded into a suite of apps that take users "from period to parenting" through "an ambitious enterprise that uniquely applies the power of data science to health" ("About Glow," 2016). All Glow, Inc., apps—including Glow, Glow Nurture, Glow Baby, and Eve by Glow—are connected and funneled together such that a user's data and profile carry over from one app to the next, taking a user from avoiding pregnancy through conception to the ultimate goal of having a baby. A key part of this enterprise is Eve by Glow (hereafter referred to as Eve), an app designed to track users' menstrual cycles, sexual activity, and birth control use in the service of avoiding pregnancy and empowering users to know their own bodies. Featuring a period-tracking calendar, a sex and health log—in which users input their moods, PMS symptoms, sexual activity and experiences, exercise activities, and the like—contraceptive information, and sexual activity quizzes, the app encourages women to provide a comprehensive profile of their physical and emotional lives. Unlike the other apps in the Glow, Inc., suite, Eve is marketed to women who do not want to become pregnant; it therefore poses a rich opportunity to study how fertility apps might pivot to enroll users who are monitoring their bodies not for better conception rates and reproductive outcomes but for the very opposite reason. We argue that Eve's users are nevertheless positioned as having "potentially maternal bodies," that is, bodies that could become pregnant (if not imminently, then at least eventually) and whose docile submission to biomedical surveillance must be trained early in service to that inevitable pregnancy.

In using the phrase *potentially maternal body* we echo and build from feminist scholarship that explores the *maternal body* as a concept (see Ettorre, 2002; Lupton, 2011, 2012, 2013, 2015). The maternal body as a concept addresses maternity as an embodied subjectivity in which pregnant women and mothers are encouraged to place the health and well-being of their children, including (and especially) children still in utero, above their own desires and even well-being (Lupton, 2011, 2012, 2013). The maternal body is often constructed in contrast with the in-utero fetal body, as Lupton (2012) described: "The maternal body is represented as dangerously permeable, open to medical view and intervention. In contrast, the foetal body is represented as more bounded and contained within the maternal body" (p. 332). Furthermore, the concept of maternal bodies in feminist scholarship also encompasses those bodies which *are not yet* pregnant but are *trying to become* pregnant. For example, Ettorre (2002) argued that technological and medical advances over the past twenty years have created "a feminized regime of reproductive asceticism and involvement in a discourse on shame" (p. 246) for women who are trying to conceive.

Building on this literature, we see similar logics applied to women who are not currently pregnant and who are not trying to conceive, but who hypothetically *could* become pregnant. The discourses and cultural logics of reproductive asceticism, shame, personal responsibility, and self-sacrifice that infuse maternal subjectivity have been extended and applied, via apps like Eve, to all bodies that could potentially bear children and therefore have *the potential to become pregnant.* Just as reproductive asceticism has been extended from gestational practices to practices during attempts at conception (such as taking prenatal vitamins while trying to conceive), so has this asceticism extended even further via Eve by requiring similar vigilance and practices even of women who *are not yet* trying to conceive. We explore and support this argument throughout this chapter; in the next section we explain the biopolitical imperatives that undergird this extension of surveillance and vigilance beyond maternal bodies to potentially maternal bodies.

THE BASIS OF BIG DATA DISCOURSE:
BIOPOLITICS AND BIOMEDICALIZATION

We see apps such as Eve as technological manifestations of big data discourses that valorize self-surveillance and bodily quantification. Such discourses are grounded in shifts toward biomedicalization logics and biopolitical imperatives. In this section, we outline how the interrelationships between these three discourses function to constellate a (re)definition of "health" and ensuing enactments thereof, starting with biopolitics as the guiding schema undergirding the turn to big data analytics.

Inherent in our focus—and Foucault's theorizing—is an understanding of knowledge as produced via particular discursive and power relations among subject-positions. From this perspective, power is not necessarily always already oppressive but rather is "a total structure of actions brought to bear upon possible actions" (Foucault, 1983, p. 220). Thus, power should be considered for its productivity as well as its oppression. This power often manifests through particular disciplining, which can be achieved through quantification and measurement. "Quantitative measures are a key mechanism for the simplifying, classifying, comparing, and evaluating that is at the heart of [Foucauldian] disciplinary power" (Espeland & Stevens, 2008, p. 414).

Nowhere is this productivity of power more evident than in biopolitical discourses that serve to "make live and let die." For our discussion of Eve we read Foucault's concept of *biopolitics* through the notion of biomedicalization (both elaborated below) because, as Rose (2006) argued, contemporary enactments of biopolitics are often wrapped up in biomedicalization discourses that privilege a keen focus on and examination of the body via attendant developments in medical technology (in our case, health-tracking apps).

Biopolitics hinges on norming populations and disciplining individual bodies to adhere to those population norms. This "norming" process is usually achieved through the vast resources at the disposal of the state to advance the state's long-existing interest in the health of its citizenry. Central to this biopolitical regime is an articulation of the purpose of sex as solely for reproduction in order to contribute to the capitalist economy by increasing the population of workers and consumers (Foucault, 1976/1980). Concern over birth rates compared with death rates, who is or is not "fit" to reproduce, incentives to encourage reproduction (e.g., the tax deductions that US parents receive for dependent children comes to mind)—these have traditionally been the purview of the state's biopolitical apparatus.

In turning to health-monitoring apps like Eve, we note a shift in the locus of biopolitical power, not only wielded by the state to control its citizens but harnessed as a cultural logic by private corporations for the control of their customers. Foucault (1975/1995) argued that the state has always had an interest in creating docile, conformist, and (re)productive bodies, an interest that only applied to capitalism as far as an ethics which "accords a particular moral virtue to the search for profit through the management of life" (Rose, 2006, p. 8). Because the state's interest in the regulation of populations is so tied to the needs of the market, capitalism is always already implicated in biopolitics, but apps like Eve even further entangle the state and the market by situating the responsibility for generating, monitoring, and adhering to population norms squarely on the shoulders of individuals.

Whereas Foucault's theorizing flows from spatially limited surveillance (i.e., the panopticon), we argue alongside scholars like Espeland and Stevens (2008), who see such surveillance and requisite bodily docility being extended across space and time today via new digital technologies. In particular, big data analytics permit a refinement in this translation between population norms and individual compliance with such norms by enrolling masses of users in the collecting of data points via promises of personally tailored "health insights" that simultaneously contribute to the healthy population through aggregated data. Indeed, part of biopower's productivity lies in its ability to "define what is appropriate, normal, and to what we should aspire, [. . . and] which kinds of persons should be subjected to which forms of knowledge, applied by which groups of experts" (Espeland & Stevens, 2008, p. 414). Everyone has their part to play in making the body healthy—a part nonetheless limited to submitting oneself to constant biomedicalized surveillance and analysis.

Biomedicalization can be understood as an intensification of the insertion of medical expertise into everyday aspects of life as well as a refocus on the interior of the body. Per Clarke, Shim, Mamo, Fosket, and Fishman (2003), biomedicalization is marked by widely available and normalized self-surveillance health technologies that shift the duty of medicalized surveillance from the purview of the medical professional to the self-surveillance of the neoliberal patient. Foucault (1963/2003) pointed out that such intense visual focus on the body is not new but rather is the foundation of modern medicine. This "medical gaze," or the trained ability to see the body as always already transitioning from healthy to ill, and to read such illness as a text in itself, has far-reaching implications for knowledge-power regimes such that available health discourses become circumscribed by what is viewable on or in the body.

In our biomedicalized age, the impetus to gaze upon the body is operationalized via neoliberal imperatives that urge self-knowledge via self-surveillance. Lupton (2012) noted an intense attention to "self-regulation in the context of a neoliberal political environment in which individuals are required to take personal responsibility for their actions, and in the case of pregnant women or mothers, for the health and wellbeing of their children" (p. 336). Discourses that urge women to have "healthy pregnancies" and "healthy babies" by performing specific behaviors (doctor's visits, prenatal vitamins, abstention from alcohol and certain foods, etc.) presume the pregnant body to be in a state of risk and in need of discipline (Lupton, 2011, 2012; Salmon, 2011). Within this neoliberal environment, however, the common pressures to become pregnant remain invisible, and thus any woman of childbearing age must bear the personal responsibility for potential fetuses. In this way, Eve and similar apps draw from and reinscribe a cultural logic that places responsibilities for the reproduction of the citizenry primarily on women.

As an apparatus of biopolitics, biomedicalization is implemented through the application of big data analysis techniques to the daily monitoring and profiling of health and wellness. Reformulations of biomedicalization have brought various aspects of life—for example, pregnancy and the avoidance thereof—under the jurisdiction of medicine, and thus position reproductive health as a commodity to be managed, produced, and earned (often through self-surveillance; Clarke et al., 2003). A primary avenue through which consumers partake in self-surveillance of the body is through health-focused apps (e.g., Glow) or wearable technologies (e.g., Fitbit; Lupton, 2012). Examining apps like Glow and Eve necessitates sensitivity to their material and technological elements (Latour, 1992) and how they function to assign and circumscribe power under the auspices of contributing to optimal health, especially as the data produced contribute to the product and practice of the proliferating data market (Puschmann & Burgess, 2014).

As boyd and Crawford (2012) explain, the significance of big data centers on the ability "to search, aggregate, and cross-reference large data sets" rather than merely the presence or absence of data (p. 663), thus demonstrating the significance of Glow's and Eve's decision to wield control of the data generated by the apps to produce generalizing research about the reproductive and menstruation habits of users (Chenette & Martinez, 2014). By doing so, these apps produce generalized representations of their users, a daunting practice that (falsely) assumes that all consumers are genuine in their social media self-disclosure (Manovich, 2011). The profiles created by consumers of apps and other technologies (e.g., grocery store club cards) allow for and prompt an extensive process of surveilling that users are socialized into, thus normalizing the process and practice of inputting extensive data into these technologies (Elmer, 2003).

If biomedicalization discourses supply the impetus to surveil oneself, big data analytics and monitoring technologies supply the means. Continuous tracking and data input are most easily enabled by wearable devices such as the Fitbit. Such devices sit at the nexus of the logics of big data analytics and biomedicalization, wherein "health" is attainable only through constant surveillance and the execution of complicated algorithms (Schüll, 2016). This "data for life" (Schüll, 2016) is a digital addendum to Foucault's (1963/2003) concept of the medical gaze, in which clinicians' senses are trained to detect disease. In this intersection of big data analytics, sensor technology, and biomedical surveillance, the locus of the gaze is not illness but "health" as "quantitative variations, greater or lesser according to corresponding physiological phenomena" (Canguilhem, 1989, p. 42). "Health" is not a matter of the absence of disease but of the deviation in measurable quantities from biopolitically motivated population norms.

In this way, big data discourses are predicated upon and feed back into biopolitical imperatives. Big data analytics and the algorithms used to observe and categorize users based on their data input constitutes what John Cheney-Lippold (2011) termed a "soft biopolitics" that utilizes "algorithmic inference as a mode of control" (p. 166) by demanding constant input from users. Whether that input comes from passive sensor technology (like the Fitbit) or active user entry (like with Eve), the need to gather and analyze this data is the unquestioned premise, reinforced by the logics of biomedicalization and biopolitics.

ADAM ANALYSIS AND EVE: KNOWING AND QUANTIFYING THE SELF

The following analysis speaks to the cultural discourses and logics surrounding the power of data collection and amalgamation that are prevalent in our society. By examining how Eve shifts the medical gaze onto consumers, advocates the use of big data, and perpetuates the notion of controlling the (potentially pregnant) body, we argue that this app masks invasive profiling as empowering monitoring, which is emblematic of a cultural trend toward quantifying the self in order to better know the self, thus encouraging female users to consider their bodies as always already potentially maternal bodies. Through neoliberal imperatives of self-responsibility and moral consumerism, this injunction to discipline, surveil, and "know" oneself quantitatively creates an urgent pressure to shape one's body and behavior to conform to biomedicalized and biopolitical directives.

Shifting the Biomedicalized Gaze from Doctors to Consumers

Previously the domain of medical experts and empirical evidence, the medicalized gaze has been resituated as a biomedical imperative that citizens must manage and maintain in order to align with the institutional level of goals of healthism and personal responsibility. Enabled and expanded by the advances in big data collection and mining, this gaze now operates at the level of the individual while operating at the behest of those in power. Eve, as part of the larger Glow enterprise, reconfigures relationships between fertility doctors and patients by decentering the authority of the doctor's knowledge by applying algorithms to a woman's sexual life. A doctor might know about female bodies generally, but Eve knows about your body specifically, even if those data are extraneous or ultimately unimportant. When the app is first downloaded and opened, a home screen appears, announcing Eve by Glow as "your period positive squad," "your body positive squad," and "your sex positive squad," all references that underscore Eve's focus on the physical and emotional spheres of a woman's existence (as well as scoring pop culture cache in utilizing the currently fashionable term *squad* to refer to the capabilities of the app). This screen interpellates users as proactive experts on their own bodies, able to monitor and track themselves in ways that doctors track patients (e.g., maintaining records of menstrual cycles and diet and exercise patterns). The login screen for Eve underscores the app's attention to the physical and emotional spheres of a woman's life by interpellating users as not only body-positive but as members of a similarly minded community (see https://apps.apple.com/us/app/period-tracker-eve/id1002275138).

Thus, users are encouraged to act in ways that remove the immediate necessity for a doctor by participating in their own self-monitoring and relying on Eve as both a diagnostic tool and a corrective for noncompliant behavior (e.g., reminders about the start of one's fertility window). This trend of silencing the medical doctor is inherent in the transition to biomedicalization such that "'medicine' itself has also been transformed. It has become technomedicine, highly dependent on sophisticated diagnostic and therapeutic equipment. [. . .] Doctors have lost the monopoly of the diagnostic gaze and of the therapeutic calculation" (Rose, 2006, p. 11). When one's bodily knowledge consists solely of data entered into and displayed on a smartphone, the role of doctors is minimized and obfuscated insofar as they are only called upon when the app fails the consumer (e.g., a user gets pregnant).

Users of Eve are navigated through a series of screens in which they create a basic profile for themselves, starting with basic information (name, email address, password, and full date of birth). Next are a calendar widget with which the user indicates the start and duration of her last period, and a health profile that details her birth control usage, relationship status, and health statistics (e.g., height and weight). As the introduction to Eve, this sign-up interface is important in socializing new users into the norms and practices of the app, as well as "a moment in which the site engineers inscribe their imagination of who the user is through [. . .] design conventions and structures" (Friz & Gehl, 2016, p. 690). Eve's first screens orient and train the new user in the app's conventions, values, and uses through its structure of menus, input fields, buttons, and rules. So what conventions, values, and uses are inscribed in Eve's sign-up interface? A valorization of monitoring one's body in accordance with a specific subject-position.

That subject-position is a disciplined, self-surveilled one, in which "the voluntary turn of the gaze upon oneself for one's own purposes" (Lupton, 2015, p. 446) is key. Indeed, in line with Foucault's (1983) concept of the technology of the self, Eve's injunction to discipline, surveil, and manage one's body becomes an internalized ambition. Rather than erasing the necessity for the medical gaze, Eve reifies the need for it by shifting its locus from a small coterie of medical professionals to the hands of its entire user base. In ostensibly replacing physicians' expertise with its own quantified knowledge about individual users, Eve does not abolish or even reduce the purview of the medical gaze but expands it. Thus, at the level of the individual, Eve promises scientific ways of knowing oneself. The app essentially functions like a full-body, full-life scan every day, requiring users to chart the slightest change in their weight, mood, exercise habits, sexual activity, and so on. Users can feel justified in claiming to be the best source of information on themselves not because they live in their bodies but because they have turned the medical gaze upon themselves, gathered the requested data, and permitted the app to run statistical analyses on it. Indeed, the linchpin of this valorized, intensified medical gaze is the data it yields and the prospect of "big data analytics" as a utopian tool in which problems of the body can be identified and potentially even solved through the mere application of math. By vaunting big data analytics as a means of answering scientific questions about reproduction at the level of the individual, Levchin and the Glow enterprise advance the idea that for-profit companies can research fertility science better than practicing physicians (hence his aforementioned assertion that thousands of data points will allow us to finally understand infertility). It is this necessary role of big data in producing knowledge about reproduction at the level of the population that fosters the biomedical gaze and serves to perpetuate and reinforce the need for self-surveillance. As such, we now turn to this promotion of big data.

ADVOCATING THE USE OF BIG DATA

The emergence and subsequent refinement of big data analytics has ushered in new schematic approaches for understanding health writ large. Effectively fulfilling the biopolitical imperatives to oversee and manage the well-being of the population, data collection and mining visualize the public generally—and the individual specifically—in ways that extend and align with the perceived expertise of the patient fostered by biomedicalization. Health technologies— smartphone applications serving as an exemplar—adhere to and fulfill these interrelated interests by assuming that personal-level data exists in service to population-level needs. In advertising the Glow enterprise as a cutting-edge means to answering questions that institutional reproductive science is unable to address (Manjoo, 2013), creator Levchin is targeting not just individual data sets but broader, population-level trends. "Health is a big information problem waiting for data analytics and wearable sensors [. . .] Once we have a few hundred thousand data points, we'll know a lot more about infertility" (Levchin, as quoted in Williams, 2013, n.p.). Indeed, Glow purports to have access to a "critical mass" of data whose sheer quantity can control for "noise" and triangulate truth. A very large user base is necessary for Glow's predictions to work and to advance knowledge about reproduction and fertility. Thus Eve is necessary for expanding the app's user base by recruiting a group of women who might not otherwise use the other apps in the Glow enterprise. Women who ostensibly might not be interested in obsessively tracking minute bodily changes,[1] perhaps because they are already using a form of birth control whose effectiveness does not rely on such monitoring, are nevertheless interpellated as owners of "potentially maternal bodies." Users might be trying to avoid pregnancy for now, but because they are physically *able to get pregnant* they must remain ever-vigilant: either in preventing pregnancy or in caring for their bodies *just in case they do become pregnant*. In this either-or trap, users need to remain "healthy," a state achieved via tracking all manner of data.

---

1. Basal body temperature, for example, is measured to the one-hundredth-degree Fahrenheit because changes of just a few degrees might indicate ovulation.

These discourses draw from and reinscribe centuries-old logics that presumes pregnancy and motherhood as default desires for all women and the "natural" course for a woman's life (for a detailed tracing of the pervasiveness of these discourses from the thirteenth century onward in Western thought, see Federici, 2014). Even though all women are implicated in Eve's injunctions to prepare for motherhood, not all women want or are able to conceive children. Instead, they are absorbed into a biomedicalized, neoliberal system wherein performing "healthy woman" means attaining a greater degree of discipline over one's body and conformity with other bodies—as measured by their frequency of using Eve and the number of data points they store in the app.

Several features of the app function to reinforce the creation and disciplining of this potentially maternal body. Throughout the tutorial, users are given words of encouragement for every datum they enter: "Well done!" and "Nice!" the app proclaims to the user. Depending on how many of the daily log input fields the user fills in, an icon of a heart with a percentage (corresponding to the number of questions answered) is displayed on the user's home screen. This icon is labeled "Today's health awareness." "Awareness" is thus positioned not as a qualitative value one can experience but as a quantitative measure directly connected to the completeness of a form. This "awareness" is communicated to the user via alerts, which have their own default screen that proclaims "We are so excited you have chosen to use Eve to track your cycles and take control of your reproductive health! Please remember the more you log, the more accurate Eve becomes." If users have internalized self-surveillance as an important moral injunction, they will be likely to continue compliantly inputting data daily into the app in order to obtain ever more accurate information and thus self-knowledge. This central focus on obtaining self-knowledge is highlighted when the app is first opened: a rotating banner describes the benefits Eve can offer users: "Eve gives you highly accurate cycle predictions every day" and "The more you log, the more you learn about yourself." From these screens and continuous stream of data entry, then, Eve's value is framed as offering users unprecedented access to knowing their true selves through the interface of the app.

These discourses and promises of increased self-knowledge in exchange for users' voluntary self-profiling are not new; countless online companies and services prompt consumers to rate commodities in exchange for better predictions and targeted advertisements (e.g., Amazon and Netflix ask users to rate products and movies / television shows in order to align suggested products with consumer interests and tastes). In the case of Eve, the app taps into the fact that its users have likely already been socialized into the cultural logic that normalizes the production and sharing of such preferences and personal information with essentially unknown entities in order to receive "improved" services and products. However, what sets Glow apart from other big data and social media endeavors are the stakes involved. Whereas a poor Netflix recommendation could simply result in an unpleasant viewing experience, a poor Eve experience could result in an unwanted pregnancy or failure to conceive. As such, women who use Eve and need its produced information to achieve their reproductive goals must partake in the logic of big data analytics and (inadvertently or not) advance the idea that profiling and disciplining yourself into a daily data-gathering routine is the way to know yourself. This utopian discourse is how an acceptance and internalization of the medical gaze is enacted.

As boyd and Crawford (2012) point out, it is not necessarily the gathering of such data that is inherently problematic but rather how it is being used. In the case of Eve, the data not only are used for more accurate predictions for the entire user base but also are distributed to both private clinics and advertisers for running statistical analyses on everything from matters of reproductive science to potential purchasing trends. In partnership with some private clinics, Eve has even begun publishing papers based on correlations made with its users' data. The first such paper, "Synchronization of Women's Cycles: A Big Data and Crowdsourcing Approach to Menstrual Cycle Analysis," found a correlation between the start of menses and the cycles of the moon, arguing that a significant proportion of users across the Glow apps generally have their period around the full moon.[2] The authors conclude by vaunting the quantity of data to which the Glow enterprise granted them access: "A big data approach to menstrual cycle analysis provides unique and powerful insights into population fertility, and potent opportunities for future study of menstrual cycle dynamics, and patient counseling on fertility, and fertility avoidance" (Chenette & Martinez, 2014, p. e250). The authors are industry scientists, working for a private fertility clinic in San Francisco and granted access to Glow's data through a special arrangement with the company. (Glow's data are otherwise not publicly available.) The broader use of these data, then, encourages users to accept a discourse that treats all female bodies as potentially maternal and in need of not just supervision but control. Thus, the need for this control—paradoxically facilitated by the emphasis on user-generated data and the attendant alienation of users from this form of labor—is normalized by the biopolitical imperatives that undergird the need to maintain health at the societal level.

---

2. The connection between cycles of the moon and cycles of menstruation has long been part of folk wisdom, but the authors of the paper claim that this knowledge was previously insignificant until Glow's large data set "proved" a correlation.

Biopolitical Imperatives to Control Pregnancy

Considering the rise of the biomedicalized gaze and the concomitant proliferation of big data analytics wielded for health-related reasons, the mechanism of policing the female body under the guise of maintaining the population's health is, perhaps, not entirely surprising. As the progenitors of the population, women's bodies are consistently situated under medical jurisdiction—only now the internalized need for self-surveillance relies on women acting on the imperative to self-monitor rather than in compliance with doctor's orders. As such, Eve deploys a discourse that valorizes self-knowledge in the form of quantified data, a valorization with a moral valence that not only urges users to produce volumes of data but that also positions them to be ideal maternal bodies, which themselves are little more than ideal fetal environments (Lupton, 2011). Some users might select the "avoiding pregnancy" mode, but they are not, in fact, given a choice to extricate themselves from an overall maternal track that is nonetheless preparing the body for potential pregnancies. Instead, the users can only ward off pregnancy until they change their minds or experience menopause. Eve users are always at risk of becoming pregnant in spite of concerted efforts to the contrary. The Glow enterprise is a perfect illustration of this, since users are seamlessly carried from tracking their periods via Eve to tracking their ovulation cycles to tracking fetal development during pregnancy, each with a different, yet interconnected, app. Of course, there are many more kinds of experiences of reproduction and fertility than even just the categories created by Glow, Inc.'s, different apps (none of the apps, for example, address miscarriage or stillbirth). By claiming to bring all aspects of pregnancy into one enterprise, users who are trying to avoid pregnancy are unavoidably interpellated into the "maternal track." Because the potentially maternal body is always looming in the background, ready to become actualized, the app necessitates the kinds of constant monitoring that pregnant bodies already receive.

In these ways, Glow, Inc., generally and Eve specifically draw from and reinforce a moral imperative to reproduce. Fertile bodies are portrayed as desiring reproduction, and it is only through daily supervision, the expertise of cutting-edge scientific techniques, and the innovation of Silicon Valley that such imperatives might be temporarily abated. These discourses emphasize reproduction as solely a women's issue, which Glow, Inc., reinforces and normalizes. Throughout the sign-up process, it is implied that a disciplined, medically surveilled body can and should be controlled, and that "new" statistical tools on "unprecedented" scales are the means of achieving such control. By disciplining their daily bodily movements so as to gather and enter large quantities of data about themselves, users might control their hysterical and potentially maternal bodies while simultaneously fulfilling their obligation to conform to societal standards of data production and sharing. And as Espeland and Stevens (2008) demonstrated, quantification disciplines human behavior: people react differently in response to measurement. Therefore, to measure is not neutral or passive but requires submitting to Foucauldian disciplinary power.

Of course, the means of this control are dubious at best. Body mass index (BMI), for example, is a highly contested (Nuttall, 2015) means of tracking and optimizing health, yet it is a common consideration in determining "healthy" pre-pregnancy and pregnancy weights, and it is a required data point that Eve users must input. The daily logs are likewise questionable as far as the actual information they yield. These fields are used to generate "health insights" available under the app's menu item "Genius." If a user enters that she feels stressed, for example, a corresponding "insight" is generated for her: "You are just as stressed as 28.4% of Eve users who logged stress today. Studies suggest the act of chewing gum can reduce cortisol levels, helping to alleviate stress." Of course, this "insight" does not tell the user much about her own stress: where it is coming from, whether it is at an unhealthy level, what physiological effects it might be having. It merely indicates that other users have also input similar data. This aggregation of data trends does not provide actual personal information, merely the illusion of insight and the promise of corporeal control. As such, we read Eve as symptomatic of a larger trend in which the biomedicalization of pregnancy gives way to a pathologization of the potentially maternal body as needing to be monitored and controlled at all times in all ways.

Further complicating Eve's claims to be providing users with self-knowledge and the tools to control their bodies is the fact that important fertility factors are obfuscated or outright omitted from the questionnaire. For example, it asks for the type of insurance plan that a user has but not whether it covers pregnancy or even whether the user has a regular doctor. The app prompts users to create daily logs of their emotional and physical states; "today's weight"; an accounting of their exercise, sleep, smoking, and drinking habits; and whether they have had sex that day. The daily logs and sign-up profile do not, however, ask for an accounting of geographic location or environmental pollution therein, socioeconomic status, or the kinds of access to health care available to them (someone who has physical access to and can afford a top hospital in their city will have a very different pregnancy experience from someone who only has access to a drugstore walk-in clinic). We read these larger external factors as having a much greater impact on reproductive health than internal factors such as mercurial moods and diet. Ultimately, however, the app functions to perpetuate healthism in order to deflect attention from political, social, environmental, and economic risk factors.

This exclusive focus on internal factors also perpetuates a notion that these factors are capable of being controlled. Users are "nudged" (Thaler & Sunstein, 2009) to adjust their mood and stress levels in much the same way that patients might be encouraged to adjust their diet, exercise, and sexual routines by doctors. But few, if any, of those internal factors can be changed. Can the 28.4 percent of users who were stressed lower their stress simply from having logged in? Should users who are trying to avoid pregnancy strive to raise their stress levels? The non sequitur nature of nudging users for the sake of (positive) change is ultimately overshadowed, however, by the app's overreliance on extensive data to protect the body and promote optimal (reproductive) health. This interrelationship of biomedicalization, big data, and biopolitics, then, positions users in a zero-sum game of technologized health: either users create, log, and monitor their data for the sake of maintaining optimal health, or they are bereft of health (and related knowledge) altogether, resulting in a complex of imperatives that render one phenomena indistinguishable from the next.

Untangling the Gordian Knot of Biopolitics, Biomedicalization, and Big Data

The mobilization of big data, biopolitics, and biomedicalization to interrogate Eve—as representative of Glow's larger tracking trajectory—suggests that the intersections between them hinge on the historical grounding of biopolitical approaches to managing populations and the collective health of the citizenry. This app implicitly relies on eighteenth-century sensibilities of normalized surveillance of the female (read: maternal) body that are central to modern understandings of health generally and to reproductive health specifically (Foucault, 1976/1980). The adherence to biopolitical imperatives—monitoring and making the body visible and malleable—that is prompted by Eve is rendered desirable through biomedicalization and enabled through big data aggregation, and thus this Gordian knot makes one apparatus nearly indistinguishable from the next. This knot further shifts the medical gaze from medical practitioners to medical consumers (a move heralded by Lupton and further articulated here) and ultimately positions consumers as necessarily in need of self-surveillance to learn about, understand, and shape their bodies. Thus, the idea that pregnancy can and should be controlled is generated from the two prongs of biopolitical imperatives and biomedicalization discourses: the former assumes not only the need but the right to monitor the reproductive health of the citizenry, while the latter asserts that any part of the body can be monitored once it is brought under the purview of medical supervision. As such, Eve serves as a way to both aggregate and monitor the health of all users in the process of situating the minutiae of (avoiding) pregnancy under the rubric of technologized medical jurisdiction.

Eve and those similar technologies that valorize the acquisition of self-knowledge through data collection and quantification exist within a cultural/social tension about representation such that users are prompted, molded, and reflected back in ways that promise and purport authenticity. Specifically, the body, the self, and states of health are reconfigured as best represented via quantifiable measurements of mucus, mood, menstruation. We, as rhetoricians and critical consumers of health technologies, need to think through how this now-perfunctory quantification is a new avenue for representation and how the aggregation of data creates new ways for users to be articulated in and by these technologies. Since Eve tells us that the only way to know oneself is to be quantified, repackaged, and legitimized as technological output, how might this alter our conceptualizations of what it means to be represented in technological and social spheres? This emphasis on legitimation via health data has implications for our understandings of corporeality and agency, particularly in light of these apps that blur the lines of distinction between object and subject, app and user. As technology continues to become more specialized and unique bodies become more generic and technologized, research on quantification-as-representation requires that we consider how ways of knowing and seeing the body have the potential to be fundamentally changed by the privileging of ones and zeros over feelings and experiences.

DISCUSSION AND IMPLICATIONS

Eve's appeal to—and use of—big data taps into larger cultural assumptions about the authority of numbers in and of themselves (Porter, 1996). The tracking of contraceptive use and sexual position is not a new technique, but Max Levchin is able to sell the idea of Eve—via the Glow enterprise—as representing "Silicon Valley innovation" because of the trust and power ascribed to numbers. The quantified female body (and possible subsequent pregnancy) is alluring precisely because it can make claims to objectivity and authority that qualitative experiences of pregnancy cannot. Indeed, Eve is part of a larger biomedicalization trend that demands the use of ever newer and more sensitive technologies to illuminate the interior of the body in order to control it. This connection between the quantified self and the authority of numbers will most likely become more prominent and thus worthy of greater attention from scholars, medical professionals, and patients in the years to come.

Given our preceding analysis, one implication for rhetorical scholarship is a reconfiguration of representation as something achieved via quantifying one's body and identity. Apps like Eve (re)present the body through analyzing data about it and the careful logging of that data, purporting to render the body (finally) transparent. These apps produce an imperative not only to monitor oneself but also to create impressive and extensive profiles that ultimately feed back into the personal information and neoliberal capitalist economy (Elmer, 2003). Through the production of such profiles, health-monitoring apps purport to (re)present their users more perfectly than human perception alone can achieve, even as users' bodies are reduced to only those physiological phenomena that can be quantified.

Following scholars such as Cheney-Lippold (2011) and Ajana (2018), we argue that health-monitoring apps advance the argument that "you are your data profile." If Ajana (2018, p. 3) is correct that we live in a "metric culture" that encourages individuals "to voluntarily quantify themselves and their lives more than ever before, happily sharing the resulting data with others and actively turning themselves into projects of (self-) governance and surveillance," then we see health-tracking apps, especially period-tracking apps like Eve, as important tools that afford such self-surveillance projects. The days that you menstruate, ovulate, feel certain emotions, exercise, orgasm—these data are sought out for the way they tell you something about yourself that you might not know without quantification, monitoring, and tracking. These apps heighten this quantification-as-representation through redefining "health" as not something one has but as something one does. The frequency and accuracy with which one surveils oneself is both how one practices health and how health knowledge is obtained. Apps like Eve and the Glow suite posit that we cannot obtain this health knowledge without first quantifying ourselves.

Quantification-as-representation is thus a key strategy for (re)defining "health," with clear ramifications for the field of RHM. Different modes of bodily representation enable different definitions of "health," shaping not only perceptions of our very bodies but also subsequent behaviors and ways of inhabiting our bodies. Our analysis of Eve reveals how the (re)definition of "health" as the ready submission to biomedicalized surveillance and the voluntary conformity to biopolitical imperatives in the name of reaping the "insights" of big data analytics channels users' perceptions and actions toward particular performances of health, such as daily bodily monitoring and data entry. According to apps like Eve, "health" is not a default state (i.e., the absence of illness) but a state of knowledge; it is an active goal that one achieves through disciplined behaviors and constant bodily monitoring. Ultimately, such apps position users as always already consumers of technology in lieu of attending to one's holistic health and well-being.

Our case study illustrates how quantification-as-representation articulates a (re)definition of health—how theories of what health means (e.g., the quantification of health) become enacted in how health is practiced (e.g., the disciplined entering of data into apps). At the level of rhetorical practice, RHM enacts a definition of "health" as adherence to statistical norms and compliance with constant data generation and monitoring. Connecting practice to theory, we can think of the rhetoric of health via rhetorics of quantification, which would guide our field to focus on the tracing of discourses that constellate the measuring and statistical norming of "health." We believe RHM thus is uniquely positioned to unpack the inherent rhetoricity of quantification.

REFERENCES

About Glow. (2016). Retrieved from https://www.glowing.com/about

Adams, J. (2013). PayPal co-founder Levchin's fertility crowdfunding app is born. *Payments Source,* August 9. Retrieved May 5, 2015, from https://www.paymentssource.com/news/paypal-co-founder-levchins-fertility-crowdfunding-app-is-born

Ajana, B. (Ed.). (2018). *Metric culture: Ontologies of self-tracking practices.* Bingley, UK: Emerald.

boyd, d., & Crawford, K. (2012). Critical questions for big data. *Information, Communication & Society, 15*(5), 662–679.

Canguilhem, G. (1989). *The normal and the pathological.* New York, NY: Zone Books.

Cassedy, J. H. (1984). *American medicine and statistical thinking, 1800–1860.* Cambridge, MA: Harvard University Press.

Chenette, P., & Martinez, C. (2014). Synchronization of women's cycles: A big data and crowdsourcing approach to menstrual cycle analysis. *Fertility and Sterility, 102*(3), e250.

Cheney-Lippold, J. (2011). A new algorithmic identity: Soft biopolitics and the modulation of control. *Theory, Culture & Society, 28*(6), 164–181.

Clarke, A. E., Shim, J. K., Mamo, L., Fosket, J. R., & Fishman, J. R. (2003). Biomedicalization: Technoscientific transformations of health, illness, and U.S. biomedicine. *American Sociological Review, 68*(2), 161–194.

Elmer, G. (2003). *Profiling machines: Mapping the personal information economy.* Cambridge, MA: MIT Press.

Espeland, W. N., & Stevens, M. L. (2008). A sociology of quantification. *European Journal of Sociology, 49*(3), 401–436.

Ettorre, E. (2002). A critical look at the new genetics: Conceptualizing the links between reproduction, gender and bodies. *Critical Public Health, 12*(3), 237–250.

Fahnestock, J. (2009). The rhetoric of the natural sciences. In A. A. Lunsford, K. H. Wilson, & R. A. Eberly (Eds.), *The SAGE handbook of rhetorical studies* (pp. 175–195). Thousand Oaks, CA: SAGE.

Federal Trade Commission. (2014). *Data brokers: A call for transparency and accountability.* Washington, DC: Author.

Federici, S. B. (2014). *Caliban and the witch.* New York, NY: Autonomedia.

Foucault, M. (1976/1980). *The history of sexuality, volume I: An introduction.* (R. Hurley, Trans.). New York, NY: Vintage Books.

Foucault, M. (1983). Afterword: The subject and power. In H. L. Drefus & P. Rabinow (Eds.), *Michel Foucault: Beyond structuralism and hermeneutics* (2nd ed., pp. 208–226). Chicago, IL: University of Chicago Press.

Foucault, M. (1975/1995). *Discipline and punish: The birth of the prison* (2nd ed.). (A. Sheridan, Trans.). New York, NY: Vintage Books.

Foucault, M. (1963/2003). *The birth of the clinic: An archelogy of medical perception.* (A. Sheridan, Trans.). Abingdon, England: Psychology Press.

Friz, A., & Gehl, R. W. (2016). Pinning the feminine user: Gender scripts in Pinterest's sign-up interface. *Media, Culture & Society, 38*(5) 687–703.

Glow—Leading women's health platform from sexual wellness to period & ovulation tracker and pregnancy app. (2015). Retrieved August 12, 2015, from https://glowing.com/

Johnson, S. (2014). "Maternal devices," social media and the self-management of pregnancy, mothering and child health. *Societies, 4*(2), 330–350.

Latour, B. (1992). Where are the missing masses? The sociology of a few mundane artifacts. In W. E. Bijker & J. Law (Eds.), *Shaping technology/building society: Studies in sociotechnical change* (pp. 225–258). Cambridge, MA: MIT Press.

Lupton, D. (2011). "The best thing for the baby": Mothers' concepts and experiences related to promoting their infants' health and development. *Health, Risk & Society, 13*(7–8), 637–651.

Lupton, D. (2012). "Precious cargo": Foetal subjects, risk and reproductive citizenship. *Critical Public Health, 22*(3), 329–340.

Lupton, D. (2013). Infant embodiment and interembodiment: A review of sociocultural perspectives. *Childhood, 20*(1), 37–50.

Lupton, D. (2015). Quantified sex: A critical analysis of sexual and reproductive self-tracking using apps. *Culture, Health & Sexuality, 17*(4), 440–453.

Manjoo, F. (2013). Glow vs. stick: A much-hyped new fertility aid reveals the limitations of data-tracking apps. *Slate,* August 8. Retrieved from http://www.slate.com/articles/technology/technology/2013/08/new_fertility_app_glow_it_wants_to_know_absolutely_everything_about_you.single.html#return1

Manovich, L. (2011). Trending: The promises and the challenges of big social data. In M. K. Gold (Ed.), *Debates in the digital humanities* (pp. 460–475). Minneapolis, MN: University of Minnesota Press.

Nuttall, F. Q. (2015). Body mass index: Obesity, BMI, and health: A critical review. *Nutrition Today, 50*(3), 117–128.

Obama, B. (2015, January). Remarks by the President in State of the Union Address. Washington, DC. Retrieved from http://www.whitehouse.gov/the-press-office/2015/01/20/remarks-president-state-union-address-january-20-2015

Porter, T. M. (1996). *Trust in numbers: The pursuit of objectivity in science and public life.* Princeton, NJ: Princeton University Press.

Puschmann, C., & Burgess, J. (2014). The politics of Twitter data. In K. Weller, A. Bruns, J. Burgess, M. Mahrt, & C. Puschmann (Eds.), *Twitter and society* (pp. 43–54). New York, NY: Peter Lang.

Rose, N. (2006). *The politics of life itself: Biomedicine, power, and subjectivity in the twenty-first century.* Princeton, NJ: Princeton University Press.

Salmon, A. (2011). Aboriginal mothering, FASD prevention and the contestations of neoliberal citizenship. *Critical Public Health, 21*(2), 165–178.

Schüll, N. D. (2016). Data for life: Wearable technology and the design of self-care. *BioSocieties, 11*(3), 317–333.

Swan, M. (2012). Sensor mania! The internet of things, wearable computing, objective metrics, and the quantified self 2.0. *Journal of Sensor and Actuator Networks, 1*(3), 217–253.

Swan, M. (2013). The quantified self: Fundamental disruption in big data science and biological discovery. *Big Data, 1*(2), 85–99.

Thaler, R. H., & Sunstein, C. R. (2009). *Nudge: Improving decisions about health, wealth, and happiness.* New York, NY: Penguin.

Weisz, G. (2005). From clinical counting to evidence-based medicine. In G. Jorland, G. Weisz, & A. Opinel (Eds.), *Body counts: Medical quantification in historical and sociological perspective* (pp. 377–393). Montreal, Canada: McGill-Queen's University Press.

Williams, F. (2013). Max Levchin wants to get you pregnant. *Slate,* June 20. Retrieved from https://slate.com/human-interest/2013/06/glow-fertility-app-max-levchin-will-pay-if-you-dont-get-pregnant.html

CHAPTER 6

Theorizing Chronicity

Rhetoric, Representation, and Identification, on Pinterest

SARAH ANN SINGER AND JORDYNN JACK

IMAGINE A YOUNG WOMAN, newly diagnosed with fibromyalgia. Let's call her Cathy. For years, Cathy has experienced debilitating symptoms that her doctors have dismissed, including physical symptoms, such as swollen, stiff joints; persistent fatigue and insomnia; and psychosocial symptoms, such as anxiety and depression, that stem from missing deadlines at school and social engagements with friends. Cathy hopes that a diagnosis will finally help her to at least cope with her condition. Imagine how she feels, now that she finally has a diagnosis, when she logs on to her computer, types "living with chronic illness" in her search engine, and comes across advice from official sources that tell her she simply needs to adjust to a "new normal"—the same thing her doctor told her earlier that day. The "Living with Chronic Illness—Dealing with Feelings" page on MedlinePlus, for instance, attempts to sound understanding:

> You may feel like you are not a whole person anymore. You might be embarrassed or ashamed that you have an illness. Know that, with time, your illness will become part of you and you will have a new normal. (Vorvick, Zieve, & Ogilvie, 2016, para. 3)

Reading on, however, our newly diagnosed patient reads advice that seems simplistic. To deal with stress, the website suggests that Cathy should, "go for a walk," "try yoga, tai chi, or meditation," or "spend time with a friend" (Vorvick et al., 2016, para. 11). Eventually, the website continues, you will "learn how to live with your chronic illness" by learning more about it, and although "at first it might seem like it is controlling you, but the more you learn and can do for yourself, the more normal and in control you will feel" (Vorvick et al., 2016, para. 13).

At first glance, this advice seems sound and even empowering, but to Cathy it is not helpful. She already tried a yoga class but found that the challenging poses exacerbated the pain in her joints. She barely has enough energy at the end of the day to make dinner, let alone take a bus to an art class halfway across town. She doesn't want this to be her "new normal." She doesn't want to accept that, at twenty-four, she is resigned to a life of explaining to her friends why she is too tired to go out or to her doctor that yoga is not going to solve all her problems.

Distraught, Cathy wanders over to Pinterest, one of her favorite social media platforms, and types in "chronic illness." There, she sees hundreds of posts, or "pins." Some of them are humorous—ironic images of 1950s housewives that call attention to the challenges of living with a chronic illness while presenting, publicly, the face of a polished, put-together woman. Others are more emotional—visual metaphors, such as digitally modified photographs of a woman's naked back, covered in purple and blue bruises to signify the physical pain that is normally invisible for people with chronic illnesses. There are silly memes, how-to tips written by patients, life hacks, and lots of images of spoons (for reasons we explain later).

Cathy starts pinning some images to her own Pinterest board. They represent aspects of her experience with illness and diagnosis with chronic illness in a way that other sources, such as pamphlets about fibromyalgia or the MedlinePlus website, have not. The images illustrate everyday challenges that Cathy and other people with chronic illness face that are invisible to others. Even though Cathy has fibromyalgia, she notices that some of her favorite pins have been added to boards for specific conditions like multiple sclerosis, Lyme disease, and endometriosis, as well as generic boards called "Chronic Pain" or "The Struggle is Real." For the first time since becoming ill, she feels less alone. It is comforting to know that she has people with whom she can identify, even if they have different diagnoses, especially since her friends and family don't understand her diagnosis anyway. She shares some pins with close friends on Facebook. At least, she thinks, maybe these will help people understand what I'm going through.

In this chapter, we argue that Cathy's experience can be better understood as a problem of representation that is addressed by chronicity, which we define as a process of rhetorical identification. We define chronicity *as* a rhetorical, multilayered process of identification that depends on available representations of chronic illness and how individuals engage with them. When people find dominant representations of their experiences lacking, they may turn to alternative representations as they seek to understand themselves and their experiences. While medical understandings of chronicity view it as a primarily biological process, and psychological understandings view it as a detrimental process of overidentification, a rhetorical view suggests that chronicity (and identification in general) is not necessarily a problem but is a necessary part of dealing with a chronic condition. Our analysis of Pinterest boards and pins related to chronic illness demonstrates that chronicity can be enacted through an ongoing process of selecting, sharing, and collecting that is rendered visible on social media.

In turn, individuals like Cathy are left to negotiate these limited and limiting rhetorics of chronic illness on their own. During this process, questions about identity arise: Do I see myself as a chronically ill person? Does my diagnosis (or lack thereof) define me? Does my chronic illness help me relate to certain groups of people more than to others? To answer these questions, Cathy and others must draw on available representations, ranging from the MedlinePlus website to Pinterest. We describe this rhetorical process of identification (with self and others), which we call chronicity, in the next section.

CHRONICITY *AS* IDENTIFICATION

Scholars of the rhetoric of health and medicine (RHM) can use the term *chronicity* to better understand the rhetorical process of identifying with chronic illness. We borrow this term from researchers in medical anthropology, who understand chronicity as a process of identification, but we would like to extend their definitions to emphasize the rhetoricity of that process and its productive dimensions.

Medical anthropologists equate chronicity with shifts in identity that can be problematic for patients, especially when that identification becomes totalizing. Estroff (1989) suggested that chronicity "consists of *a fusion of identity with a diagnosis,* a transformation of self to self and with others" that engenders an "unauthorized but nonetheless *demoralizing* change of self from a person who has an illness to someone who is an illness or diagnosis" (p. 251; emphasis added). Similarly, Manderson and Smith-Morris (2010) argued that chronicity is "the process of identification with one's disease—the movement from having a disease to *being a person inhabited by that disease*" (p. 25;

emphasis added). And moreover, Honkasalo (2001) noted, "Chronicity may result in patients *fusing their identities with their diagnoses*" (p. 321; emphasis added). In these definitions, we see a concern that an individual may be overcome by a total identification with illness, especially if they remain ill for a long time. Implicitly, then, these medical anthropologists suggest that resisting identification is important for people with chronic conditions.

As rhetoricians, we believe that we can more comprehensively understand chronicity through Kenneth Burke's (1969) concept of identification, which he defined as "the ways in which members of a group promote social cohesion by acting rhetorically upon themselves and one another" (p. xiv). Burke (1969) recognized that this process of identification helps explain individual identity as well: "The individual person, striving to form himself in accordance with the communicative norms that match the cooperative ways of society, is by the same token concerned with the rhetoric of identification. To act upon himself persuasively, he must variously resort to images and ideas that are formative" (p. 39). Burke (1969) suggested, then, that everyone forms identifications based on "formative" images and ideas—the representations available to them.

From Burke's (1969) perspective, though, this process is not necessarily a totalizing one. Identification is unavoidable, but so is division (p. 22). Due to what Burke (1969) called "the paradox of substance," though, one can never fully identify with someone or something else: one is both "consubstantial" with the other and yet separate (p. 21). From Burke's understanding, then, we need not fear total identification, as division always remains. While he recognized the perils of identification,[1] Burke also recognized that that same overidentification would be viewed as positive in another context (such as a compliant patient in a hospital). Thus, Burke's emphasis on identification as a necessary condition for human identity and human relations makes it a suitable term with which to understand chronicity.

We argue that chronicity is a rhetorical *process of identification* that depends on available representations and that often takes the form of "not wholly deliberate, yet not wholly unconscious" (Burke, 1969, p. xiii) affinities between an individual, images, and ideas, that allow them to round out an identity and form identifications with others. Existing understandings of chronicity seem to assume that a diagnosis is singular and stable and that illnesses unfold in a linear fashion. Instead of "being inhabited by" a health condition, as Manderson and Smith-Morris (2010) suggested, or engaged in the act of "fusi[ng] of identity with a diagnosis," in Estroff's (1989) terms, we

---

1. See Jack (2004) for additional insight into the "piety of degradation" as exemplified in the scrupulous identifications of the drug fiend.

understand identity to be constituted through an ongoing, always incomplete, yet potentially productive rhetorical process of identification.

Identification can help us understand why and how individuals meld their existing identities with new identifications and do so repeatedly over time. In the case of chronic illness, which is so often invisible and indescribable, chronically ill people are not only choosing to identify with a particular diagnosis. As we show, chronicity is a rhetorical *process* of identification, so that individuals who post on Pinterest may do so either because it reflects how they already understand illness or because it offers new, useful ways of understanding a chronic condition. Theorizing chronicity accounts for the presence of multiple chronic conditions, the lack of clear diagnosis, and other identities that overlap with chronic illness. Theorizing chronicity in this way positions users as active, empowered agents instead of compliant or "adherent" patients.[2]

REPRESENTATIONS OF CHRONICITY

As a theory, chronicity could offer many directions for RHM scholars, including interview- or survey-based studies of how individuals come to identify with chronic illness. Here, we focus on one approach to the study of chronicity by examining how people represent chronicity in digital contexts and how those representations offer rhetorical resources for identification.

Scholars such as Kim Hensley Owens (2015) have called upon researchers in RHM to shift their studies to "examine a wider, messier circle of both influence on and output by individuals across technologies" (p. 137). Such work often includes studies of representation—how health, illness, and disability are depicted in popular and scientific texts (Dubriwny, 2012; Graham, 2015; Johnson, 2014) as well as how different actors characterize themselves and are characterized by others (Jack, 2014; Keränen, 2010; Koerber, 2013; Stormer, 2002). Extending this research, Mara Mills (2015) argued that representations "do not simply reflect broader patterns of discourse"—they do not simply depict health issues. Mills claimed that representations are rhetorical in that they "create new symbolic associations, disseminate terminology, translate affect, and discipline practices of looking" (p. 176). It is this capacious view of representation that we take up here in relation to chronicity. That is, as a theory, chronicity highlights the rhetorical process of identification with or against a chronic condition. In practice, chronicity helps us illuminate how representa-

---

2. See, for example, Arduser (2017) for critique of compliance.

tions of chronic illness allow individuals to share these symbolic associations and create relationships with others. This practical view of chronicity is necessary because dominant representations of chronic illness can form rhetorical barriers for the individuals who experience them. In particular, chronically ill people face three specific rhetorical problems. First, individuals must confront the negative and/or stereotyped rhetorics of chronic illness. Individuals with chronic illness frequently encounter misperceptions, which persist and have become complex cultural rhetorics, such as the argument that people with type 2 diabetes have brought their illness upon themselves through poor lifestyle choices. For individuals with lesser-known or mysterious conditions such as myalgic encephalomyelitis / chronic fatigue syndrome (ME/CFS), the lack of understanding is even more intense. The representations that do exist draw on long-held stereotypes or idealistic narratives that narrow what constitutes a chronic condition and how it can be treated. Indeed, representations may function as "caricatures and stereotypical portrayals that depend more on gesture than complexity" (Thomson, 1997, p. 11). For instance, individuals with ME/CFS may be depicted as lazy housewives. Such representations persuade people to adopt limited or even problematic views of chronic illness, which means that individuals with chronic illness must work against those representations to form positive, alternative representations.

Second, representations of chronic illness are limited because symptoms are often invisible and variable over time, so that people who have those conditions must therefore describe their symptoms persuasively in order to be believed. Many chronic illnesses can be considered "rhetorical disorder[s]" (Segal, 2005, p. 74), which means that sufferers must rely on rhetorical acts to convince health-care providers (and others) that their suffering is real. Individuals who have a chronic illness are often met with the assumption that, because they appear normal, they must not be in pain, that they are lazy, or that they are exaggerating or even making up their condition. Chronic illness symptoms, such as fatigue and pain, may wax and wane based on the weather, daily activities, amount of rest, diet, treatment, and stress level, and thus they may be more visible at certain times and nearly invisible at others. As Georgia Kleege (2015) noted, chronically ill people may be "doubly stigmatized" since they must "disclose impairments that are not visually apparent and therefore rouse suspicions about the authenticity of the claim" (p. 184). This is especially a problem for individuals experiencing the ambiguous symptoms of many chronic conditions, such as fatigue, brain fog, and pain, which, as Elaine Scarry (1985) argued, "destroy language" and therefore "resist expression" (p. 54). For this reason, such individuals are placed in the rhetorical situation of having to convince others that "they really are disabled, not seeking some special—unfair—advantage," in N. Ann Davis's (2005) terms (p. 154). Additionally, so-called symptoms of treatment from chronic illness—negative side effects caused by medications used to treat illness—may also wax and wane, and acute problems may require faster or more intense attention than the underlying chronic condition, which is thus re-rendered.

Third, individuals with chronic illness must confront continuously changing medical rhetorics of chronic illness that may actually exacerbate these problems because of the shifting nature of medical knowledge and practices. Conditions that count as chronic have shifted over time. Emerging medical advancements overturn stable diagnoses, complicate established treatment plans, and, in turn, shift rhetorical identifications. For instance, ME/CFS was at one time considered psychiatric, but emerging evidence suggests that it may be related to gut bacteria or to autoimmune conditions. Such diagnostic changes can also shift rhetorical identifications. It is a very different thing to consider oneself as having an autoimmune condition than to be perceived as a crazy woman who is making it all up. Individuals with one chronic condition are statistically more likely to acquire other chronic conditions because of advancing age, genetics, or so-called symptoms of treatment that themselves become chronic. Moreover, many people are chronically ill yet live without a clear or stable diagnosis, and thus choose to identify (or not) with multiple communities. As Wall (2005), a writer, noted in her memoir about living with ME/CFS, these individuals become part of an "invisible community" and lack the "benefit of diagnosis, validation, medical support, or treatment" (p. 11).

CHRONICITY *IS* IDENTIFICATION: CURATING THE SELF ON PINTEREST

Recent research by Elena Gonzalez-Polledo (2016), an anthropologist, suggests that social media sites are being used as "health devices" that enable people to share their experiences with living with chronic illness in a way that is "normalized and made newly visible" (p. 2). She argued, "Social media invite us to think about pain not as a one-off, catastrophic lifechanging event, but as a way of being in the world with a difference" (p. 2). In other words, social media can showcase how chronicity is an ongoing process of identification. As individuals post, share, tag, and comment on social media, they engage in this process; in essence, they curate a self by drawing on available representations and sometimes creating their own.

For this study, we chose to focus specifically on one social media site, Pinterest, that we find especially compelling because it largely depends on individuals collecting and sharing "pins" (typically, images with short captions that may or may not link to an external website) to "boards." While it draws on the metaphor of the bulletin board, Pinterest might more closely resemble a virtual scrapbook or commonplace book in which individuals collect images and then share them with others. Users pin everything from recipes to outfit ideas to workout tips. Most users have multiple boards, which reflect multiple aspects of their identities, including chronic illness.

Pinterest is an interesting site of rhetorical action for a variety of reasons. First, its interface and modes of content generation may offer "alternative ways of producing knowledge" (Lui, 2015, p. 129) and features "fragmented identity stories" that may not be told otherwise. On Pinterest one can browse images and re-pin them to one's own boards with the click of a mouse. It does not require sustained effort or activity and, in turn, captures the experiences of chronically ill people who may not have the ability to share their stories in narrative form. Unlike textual forms such as illness narratives, which draw on the resources of language to vividly convey experience, often through realism, the visual images we find on Pinterest function more obliquely, through repeated rhetorical figures such as irony, metaphor, and simile.

Pinterest is not as exclusive as other social media sites dedicated to a single chronic condition (such as MyFibroTeam, a social media platform for people with fibromyalgia, or a dedicated Facebook group such as Diabetes Support or Diabetes Daily). Participants can pin the same pins to multiple boards (i.e., a "spoonie" image might appear on a multiple sclerosis board, a chronic illness board, and an endometriosis board), thus identifying and disidentifying with chronic illness on their own terms. And since boards are personal, other participants do not question the legitimacy of users' experiences. Other illness communities on social media sites such as Facebook function as "safe" spaces for sharing private medical information and resisting biomedical authorities. In turn, participants who wish to join are often tested to ensure that they are legitimately ill with that particular condition. Moreover, these groups are often private, and therefore rendered unsearchable; new users must be invited to join by current participants. On Pinterest, participants can re-pin any pins located on public boards, and the curation framework invites invention instead of criticism. A simple search for "chronic pain" or "fibromyalgia" turns up thousands of pins with new content added continually. Although there are chat features available, users are primarily expected to share and re-pin pins as they please without regard for other users. All of this might help explain why chronically ill individuals turn to Pinterest as a means of identification and representation.

Between August and December 2016, we collected 587 pins about chronic illness on a public Pinterest board, "Chronicity," available at http://pin.it/ TKiGT3j. We used search terms such as *chronic illness, spoonie, fibromyalgia, chronic fatigue syndrome,* and *Lyme disease* to gather our first set of pins; then, the Pinterest algorithm suggested similar pins for us that we added to our board. We focus on Pinterest as a place where people primarily engage in visual or visual/verbal representations of chronic conditions that forge identifications with the self and others. Pinning and sharing images constitutes part of a process of identification with a particular chronic illness or as part of a larger group of people with chronic illness writ large. The representations we examine here work primarily against the divisions created by the stigmatizing and silencing representations of chronic illness that individuals encounter elsewhere in their lives. While the range of pins related to chronic illness number in the thousands, our analysis identified four repeating types of images that we focus on here: 1950s housewives, spoons, cats, and bodies that make invisible ailments visible. There is no necessary correlation between the various items featured in the images; they cohere because they owe their persuasiveness to their repetition over time and across genres. Each pin contains a number of identifications, in Burke's (1969, p. 55) terms, and we offer several possible, overlapping interpretations of what they might mean for the process of chronicity. Together, these pins critique the societal expectations that help construct chronic illness, particularly for women: in a society where women are still expected to manage all domestic duties, even while working a full-time job, chronically ill people face multiple disadvantages.

In what follows, we examine how representations of chronic illness shared on Pinterest, to borrow Mills's (2015) words again, "create new symbolic associations, disseminate terminology, translate affect, and discipline practices of looking" (p. 176). Here, we focus on kinds of pins shared frequently to boards related to chronic illness that perform these four functions. Each of these types of pins helps us demonstrate how chronicity is a rhetorical process of identification in which individuals curate an identity based on these available representations.

Creating New Symbolic Associations: 1950s Desperate Housewives

One type of pin that we found frequently features images of 1950s housewives with witty or ironic statements superimposed on them. These images, we think, help create new symbolic associations for people who have chronic illnesses. Mainstream advice for people with chronic illness tends to use a bootstraps approach, like the MedlinePlus website we opened with, encouraging people to take control, become empowered, and soldier on. Pins featuring the 1950s housewife point out that beneath the facade of someone who is keeping it together, who appears to be in control, lies someone who is struggling with mental and physical pain. The 1950s housewife can be understood as an avatar, a character that individuals use to represent themselves and their experiences. Identifying (ironically) with the 1950s housewife, as one commonly available avatar, then, constitutes part of the process of chronicity-as-identification.

The housewife pins seem to capture this attempt at passing and to poke humor at it while revealing its impossibility. The housewife images on Pinterest typically feature perfectly coiffed, neatly dressed women with text superimposed on them that features an ironic comment. The images appear to be repurposed either from vintage advertisements or from newer images evoking that style. These pins are recognizable as 1950s housewives because of culturally constructed ways of viewing them, or what Burke (1984b) referred to as a sense of piety, or "what properly goes with what" (p. 74). The 1950s housewife is represented in these images, first and foremost, by the shirtwaist dress, the iconic style that came to represent domesticity and femininity in that period and that continues to be used to index "1950s housewife" in period films and television shows today. As Vaughan (2009) explained it, the shirtwaist dress emerged after World War II and is typically credited to Christian Dior's "New Look." The look also demanded high heels and pearls to be complete. In magazines and television shows, this outfit was worn for doing housework—vacuuming and washing dishes—and not just for outings. The shirtwaist dress, with its nipped-in waist, full skirt, and fitted bodice, emphasized a feminine shape. Notably, as Vaughan showed, that shape was only achieved through uncomfortable foundational garments, including longline bras, girdles, petticoats, and shoulder pads. In contrast to utilitarian styles popular during World War II, the "New Look" signaled a return to traditional values. As Cowan (1983) argued, these expectations persisted long past the 1950s era, even as more women joined the workforce and were no longer responsible only for domestic duties.

Of course, in practice few women in the 1950s lived up to the ideal represented by the image of the woman in the shirtwaist dress. Thus, nor do the users pinning those images on Pinterest today mean to literally represent themselves as disillusioned housewives. Instead, they are forming "symbolic associations" (Mills, 2015) between those elements that symbolize the 1950s housewives and the experience of chronic illness. One possible interpretation of that association is that images of 1950s housewives seek to call viewers' attention to the difficulty of maintaining a facade while managing a chronic illness. Pinterest users may be saying that they struggle with the expectations that women, in particular, should always look good, maintain a neat and tidy home, and put a hot meal on the table for dinner, all with a cheerful smile. One pin makes this connection rather directly; in it, a 1950s-era woman wearing a full face of makeup, complete with red lipstick and matching manicured nails, applies mascara as she smiles at the viewer. The text reads: "I don't look like I'm in pain? Thank you!! It only took 5 layers of makeup and really strong painkillers." Thus, the 1950s housewife may represent, to these users, the masterful ability to conceal pain beneath a smile and polished appearance—even if it takes powerful drugs to do so. In other words, the stereotype of the 1950s housewife arises due to the unrepresentability of chronic illness itself; the discomfort that the 1950s housewife faced while doing housework in a dress and heels stands in metaphorically for the discomfort that women face today while managing the competing demands of femininity and chronic illness. Another pin featuring a similar image of an aproned housewife reads: "Another day of outward smiles and inward screams." The discomfort referenced in housewife images is emotional as well as physical. Betty Friedan (2010) famously captured the disillusionment many housewives faced in *The Feminine Mystique*, where she describes the unfulfilled desires of many women to do something beyond managing a household and children. This dissatisfaction ran so deep among women in the 1950s and 1960s that, according to Friedan, many resorted to tranquilizers just to get through the day (p. 31). The 1950s housewife may have become an emblem of chronic illness, then, because she encapsulates that disconnect and allows for multiple users to identify with it. The 1950s housewife thus constitutes a new symbolic association that allows pinners to speak back to dominant representations of chronic illness and gender that limit their ability to share their experiences.

Disseminating Terminology: Spoons

Images of spoons appear on Pinterest in photographs, infographics, graphs, and illustrations. These spoons function as visual representations of a new term used to forge identifications among individuals who identify with chronicity: *spoonie.* By pinning and sharing these images, individuals help disseminate that terminology. For pinners, the term *spoonie* indexes a now-famous essay written by Christine Miserandino (2003) while she was a student at Hofstra University seeking to explain her experience with an autoimmune disorder to a friend. The essay relates how Miserandino was out one evening at a diner with her friend, who asked what it was like to live with a chronic illness.

To illustrate, Miserandino grabbed a bunch of spoons and handed them to her friend. Then, Miserandino explained how each activity of the days—starting with waking up—took one "spoon"—a unit of time and energy. Miserandino described the work that goes into something as simple as getting dressed; for a person with an autoimmune disorder, getting dressed might involve choosing clothing that does not require buttons if her hands are sore, finding a long-sleeved shirt to cover bruises, or putting on a sweater if she has a fever that day. Each activity uses up another spoon. Whereas healthy people seem to have an unlimited quantity of spoons at their disposal, for people with a chronic illness the number may be limited. Thus, one must carefully plan their daily activities knowing that there are never enough spoons to cover everything. Accordingly, impossible choices emerge—between eating dinner, say, and being able to clean up afterward. Since Miserandino's original post, the idea of *spoon theory* has been taken up by others who have chronic conditions. The many images of spoons on Pinterest speak to the spread of this idea.

The spoon exemplifies how chronicity functions as a process of identification because those who share these images often describe themselves as spoonies, a term suggesting that the idea has gone beyond a metaphor to become an identity. One reason for the popularity of this identity may be that it transcends any particular illness and can be adopted by anyone who relates to the phenomenon of chronicity that it represents. *Spoonie,* in other words, helps constitute a new type of identification by disseminating a new term.

To take just a few examples, one pin features an image of three green plastic spoons with this text superimposed on top: "If you understand this post I am very sorry." This pin assumes that spoons offer a code for others who have a chronic illness, and that healthy individuals will not understand the reference. Other pins feature infographics that chart how each daily task requires a certain number of spoons. In one chart, for instance, "going out for coffee" is illustrated with four spoons, while taking a shower requires two spoons and getting out of bed requires one spoon. These images visualize the mental calculus involved in planning one's day with a limited stock of energy. The spoon metaphor is literalized in jewelry, often linked to on Pinterest but sold on Etsy. These include bracelets made out of spoons and engraved with sayings such as "live one spoon at a time," or a necklace with a tiny spoon encased in a glass vial with a tag that reads "in case of emergency break glass." The spoons reflect a culture in which people with illnesses are expected to try to maintain a daily schedule that includes school or work, household tasks, and personal care without much assistance from others.

Translating Affect: Chronic Illness Cat

Mills (2015) suggested that representations work not only to transmit meaning but also to "translate affect." Frequently, pinners share images that do precisely that; most often, they seek to evoke humor, poking fun at the experience of living with a chronic condition. One particularly common denizen of Pinterest, in this regard, is Chronic Illness Cat, a meme that features the stoic face of a Siamese cat with light blue eyes against a geometric blue background. Chronic Illness Cat personifies, or speaks for, a person with a chronic condition. By pinning and sharing these images, people are of course not literally identifying as a cat but are identifying with the sayings juxtaposed onto the picture of that cat.

Of the hundreds that have been pinned, here are a few that epitomize the nature of the meme:

- "PAIN LEVEL: Bargaining with God"
- "I got 99 Problems and a decent painkiller would solve 17 of them";[3]
- "That stupid moment when you have your pill bottle in front of you but you can't remember if you already took it or not";
- "Did you hear that? That's the sound of your chronic illness laughing when you make plans";
- "Looks up side effects of meds / OH GOD."

These memes speak to serious problems that accompany chronic illness—managing seemingly unmanageable pain, memory loss, side effects, and making decisions about the future despite illness—but they do so using humor.

Using cats, of course, is a common trope in internet memes in general, as exemplified by the "I Can Haz Cheezburger" cat meme or the broader phenomenon of LOLcats that began in the mid-2000s. Cats function to translate humor about chronic illness because they have already been established in internet communities as being humorous. When we see an image of a cat online, we can bet that humor is the emotion being evoked: the cat itself evokes an expectation among viewers.

Notably, Pinterest users may not only pin and re-pin available memes but can also generate their own by using meme generators such as Imgur.com or MemeGenerator.net, digital tools that offer readymade templates for Chronic Illness Cat and other popular memes. Meme generators provide the

---

3. This meme references Jay-Z's 2003 chart-topping rap song, "99 Problems."

standard backdrop of Chronic Illness Cat against the blue background. In fact, users can go to https://imgflip.com/memegenerator/25162854/Chronic-illness-cat to create a Chronic Illness Cat meme without additional search-ing. To create a meme, users simply type their desired text into the generator and it appears on the image in the standard font, Impact, which is commonly used for memes. In this way, meme generators offer a degree of rhetorical freedom for users, who can work within those constraints to craft a message. In a similar way, we might consider how the available images on Pinterest offer a diverse, but bounded, set of representations, mostly re-pinned and repurposed from various online sources, to users seeking to curate their own online identity.

On the one hand, it may be easy to dismiss these humorous cat memes as frivolous but otherwise insignificant for an understanding of chronicity-as-identification. On the other hand, we can interpret these pins as performing valuable rhetorical work for participants. Through humor, pinners enact what Burke (1984a) referred to as the "comic frame," or the ability to "be observers of themselves, while acting" and to "'transcend' himself by noting his own foibles" (p. 171). Indeed, the tagline on the Facebook page associated with Chronic Illness Cat reads:

A note to members before commenting: A lot of our Chronic Illness Cat members have life altering genetic diseases to which there are NO supple-ments, no research, no drugs, and often they feel there is no hope. There IS NO Recovery when your body alters from the normal 46 perfect chromo-somes. . . . A lot of our members face shortened life spans due to the impact of their drugs, or choosing not to use drugs prescribed for them. A lot of them face genetic diseases that are slowly killing them or forever altering their ability to walk, drive, write or live independently. Some face life long mental illness to which they feel there is no Hope. So arguing for a positive mental attitude is useless when they feel so utterly hopeless. So please, watch what you say in this community. If you read the memes you would under-stand WHY allowing people to accept their own reality is so, so important. If you've found healing, that's great, but this is not an outlet for telling others how to heal. (Chronic Illness Cats)

By employing a comic frame, this post suggests, those who share Chronic Illness Cat memes are doing very real and important work in their lives, iden-tifying themselves with images and sayings that employ humor to come to terms with chronic illness. Humor does serious work. Humor can also ease identification between those who have a chronic condition and those who do not; by sharing an affect with others, pinners may hope to convey a difficult message in a way that is less threatening to others.

Disciplining Practices of Looking

As we described above, representing chronic illness can be challenging because symptoms are often invisible. For one, people may dismiss those symptoms through false equivalency. As Wall (2005) put it, "If I tell someone I have chronic fatigue syndrome, they're likely to say, 'Yeah, I'm tired all the time, too,' or 'Yeah, my friend had that, but I think she was depressed'" (p. 12). For Wall, this is a false form of identification that fails to really address what the suffering person experiences. Alternatively, people may dismiss symptoms outright—"But you don't look sick!" For these reasons, Wall, a memoirist, writes that she often finds herself trying to illustrate her experience through comparisons with physical objects such as a car with one piston and a brain filled with sand (p. 12). On Pinterest, we frequently found posts that try to do the same work through visual metaphors. These images seek to "discipline practices of looking" (Mills, 2015) by suggesting to viewers that they need to look deeper, past a normal-looking surface to "see" (or at least try to understand) the pain and suffering that may lie underneath. To do so, pinners attempt to create identifications between the kind of pain that is readier at hand, easier to grasp, and the kind of pain that is less apparent to others.

Frequently, these images use a woman's back as a canvas on which to represent invisible pain. One such image features a photograph of a person's back with purple and blue bruises painted on it and the caption, "If you could see my invisible illness, would you finally believe I'm in pain?" A similar pin shows a woman sitting on a bed with a gaping wound on her back, spine exposed, with red and purple bruising radiating outward; this one is captioned, "If you could see how it feels, would you judge me so quickly?" A third image of this type features a grayscale image of a woman's bare back. The woman is embracing herself, and we see her hands gripping her shoulder and upper back, but we also see a second set of hands pressing outward against the flesh of her back and the outline of another, smaller woman trapped inside, pushing outward.

These images function on a much different affective level from the humorous cat or housewife pins, and they seem to do so by challenging viewers' assumptions about what they see (and what they don't see) when they look at someone who has a chronic condition. They seem to operate on a visceral level, evoking shock on the part of the viewer. Here, pinners seem to be communicating the frustration they feel when faced with others who either do not believe they are ill or seek to minimize their feelings, as well as the nature of that pain itself. By relating that pain to a shocking but recognizable image (bruises, bleeding, etc.), pinners hope to forge identifications with those who might otherwise not see the kind of pain they experience.

Unlike other types of pins on Pinterest (such as pins for recipes, child-rearing tips, home decor ideas, or fashion inspiration), these pins frequently do not lead to an article or website (or they lead to dead links). This suggests that the pins are being shared not because they lead to useful content but because the pins themselves are the message. If the experience of chronic illness, and of pain specifically, challenges representation, then these images can be understood as an attempt to capture visually what cannot be easily expressed linguistically, to discipline viewers into looking more deeply at the experience of pain.

CONCLUSION

Overall, the types of pins we identified in our analysis represent four ways that identification can occur through representation: as a way of creating new symbolic associations (as in the 1950s housewife pins); as a way of disseminating terminology (as in the spoonie pins); as a way of translating affect (as in humorous cat pins); and as a way of disciplining ways of looking (as in visual metaphors that depict pain). These forms of identification can be understood as a non-exhaustive list of the ways that chronicity functions in digital contexts through acts of curating from available representations. When we consider rhetorics of health and medicine as chronicity, we focus attention on how the multiple rhetorics surrounding chronic illness enable identification through available representations of illness. We see at least three paths forward for scholars seeking to engage chronicity from an RHM perspective.

1. As researchers, we should continue to focus on how individuals with illnesses and disabilities represent themselves, an approach exemplified in work by Arduser (2017), De Hertogh (2015), and Owens (2015).

We contend that RHM scholars must legitimize chronically ill and disabled individuals as rhetors and not merely examine their rhetoric to complement or refine studies of professional rhetorics. By paying attention to representations generated by patients (including narrative writing, blog posts, forums, and social media sites), RHM scholars can develop a better understanding of how those individuals generate counterrepresentations—thereby theorizing chronicity—in ways that trouble dominant depictions of chronic conditions in biomedicine. Such an approach follows Michael Bérubé's (2015) advocacy for self-representation in disability studies, which limits the circulation of "severe misunderstandings of disability" and "literally and allegorically demeaning depictions of people with disabilities" (p. 153). In this way, chronicity serves in the "as" framework to extend scholarly research in RHM to engage with chronic conditions as a place from which to theorize identifications and representation.

2. As educators, we should ask our students to compose and analyze vernacular representations alongside professional scientific and medical texts.

While many teachers incorporate illness narratives into health communication and health humanities courses, the images posted on Pinterest allow students to see how patients respond to medical advice by incorporating it into an identification with (or sometimes against) a diagnosis. Students might analyze social media posts (such as Pinterest boards) to better understand the readers for a document they are composing—how they interpret and understand their condition, whether and how they identify with that condition. Through this practice, we can highlight issues of gender, disability, power, and production: Who produces certain representations and why? How do these representations shape chronicity—and, in turn, identification? Alternatively, students might compose material to be pinned and shared on social media sites, an exercise that would lead them to consider rhetorical forms of identification and not just concerns about finding the right information or adapting technical information for nonspecialist readers. Here, chronicity functions in the "is" perspective as a tool for pedagogical application.

3. As cross-institutional collaborators, we might ask whether producing and sharing rhetorical products—from Pinterest pins to blog posts to essays— might benefit individuals with chronic illnesses by encouraging a positive process of identification with illness.

In other work (Edwell, Singer, & Jack, 2018), we partnered with an endocrinologist, anthropologist, and occupational therapist to conduct workshops for people with diabetes that focused primarily on written compositions (letters, case reports, and more). This study prompts us to think about whether future interventions might also incorporate a wider range of traditional and nontraditional composing activities and how those activities might encourage participants to reflect on their own processes of identification with diabetes. Extending this approach, we and other RHM scholars might inquire into the effectiveness of social media compositions in interventions related to patient education, health literacy, or shared decision-making, all spaces in which patients with chronic conditions are encouraged to take an active role in their own course of treatment. Far from functioning only in a negative way, we see identification as a key element in those sorts of interventions but one that is seldom considered from a medical standpoint. In this manner, chronicity can serve in the "is" perspective as a practical means of engagement with patient communities.

Ultimately, we hope that our chapter serves as an example for how rhetoricians might articulate how rhetorical tools can help chronically ill people and other stakeholders communicate about their experiences of illness. As a theoretical framework, chronicity calls attention to the rhetorical processes of identification that enable (or constrain) identity-formation for individuals with chronic illnesses. As a practical method, chronicity focuses attention on representations of chronic illness as one site for analysis or, possibly, productive interventions in which RHM scholars can engage.

REFERENCES

Almjeld, J. (2015). Collecting girlhood: Pinterest cyber collections archive available female identities. *Girlhood Studies, 8*(3), 6–22.

Arduser, L. (2017). *Living chronic: Agency and expertise in the rhetoric of diabetes.* Columbus, OH: The Ohio State University Press.

Bérubé, M. (2015). Representation. In R. Adams, B. Reiss, & D. Serlin (Eds.), *Keywords in disability studies* (pp. 151–154). New York, NY; London, UK: New York University Press.

Burke, K. (1969). *A rhetoric of motives.* Berkeley, CA: University of California Press.

Burke, K. (1984a). *Attitudes toward history.* Berkeley, CA: University of California Press.

Burke, K. (1984b). *Permanence and change.* Berkeley, CA: University of California Press.

Chronic Illness Cats. [2011, September 1]. In *Facebook* [Community page]. Retrieved September 16, 2016, from https://www.facebook.com/ChronicIllnessCat/about/?entry_point=page_nav_about_item

Cowan, R. S. (1983). *More work for mother: The ironies of household technology from the open hearth to the microwave.* New York, NY: Basic Books.

Davis, A. N. (2005). Invisible disability. *Ethics, 116*(1), 153–213.

De Hertogh, L. B. (2015). Reinscribing a new normal: Pregnancy, disability, and health 2.0 in the online natural birthing community, Birth Without Fear. *Ada: A Journal of Gender, New Media, and Technology, 7,* https://doi.org/10.7264/N3Z899PH

Dubriwny, T. N. (2012). *The vulnerable empowered woman: Feminism, postfeminism, and women's health.* New Brunswick, NJ: Rutgers University Press.

Edwell, J., Singer, S. A., & Jack, J. (2018). Healing arts: Rhetorical techne as medical (humanities) intervention. *Technical Communication Quarterly, 27*(1), 50–63.

Ehrenreich, B., & English, D. (1978). *For her own good.* Garden City, NY: Anchor.

Estroff, S. E. (1989). Self, identity, and subjective experiences of schizophrenia: In search of the subject. *Schizophrenia Bulletin, 15*(2), 189–196.

Friedan, B. (2010). *The feminine mystique.* New York, NY: Norton.

Friz, A., & Gehl, R. W. (2016). Pinning the feminine user: Gender scripts in Pinterest's sign-up interface. *Media, Culture & Society, 38*(5), 686–703.

Gonzalez-Polledo, E. (2016). Chronic media worlds: Social media and the problem of pain communication on Tumblr. *Social Media + Society, 2*(1), 1–11.

Goodman, R. A., Goodman, R. A., Posner, S. F., Huang, E. S., Parekh, A. K., & Koh, H. K. (2013). Defining and measuring chronic conditions: Imperatives for research, policy, program, and practice. *Preventing Chronic Disease, 10,* 1–16.

Graham, S. S. (2015). *The politics of pain medicine: A rhetorical-ontological inquiry.* Chicago, IL: University of Chicago Press.

Hand, M. (2017). Visuality in social media: Researching images, circulations and practices. In L. Sloan & A. Quan-Haase (Eds.), *The SAGE handbook of social media research methods* (chap. 14). Los Angeles, CA; London, UK: SAGE.

Honkasalo, M. L. (2001). Vicissitudes of pain and suffering: Chronic pain and liminality. *Medical Anthropology, 19*(4), 319–353.

Jack, J. (2004). "The piety of degradation": Kenneth Burke, the Bureau of Social Hygiene, and permanence and change. *Quarterly Journal of Speech, 90*(4), 446–468.

Jack, J. (2012). Gender copia: Feminist rhetorical perspectives on an autistic concept of sex/gender. *Women's Studies in Communication, 35*(1), 1–17.

Jack, J. (2014). *Autism and gender: From refrigerator mothers to computer geeks.* Urbana, Chicago, and Springfield, IL: University of Illinois Press.

Johnson, J. (2014). *American lobotomy: A rhetorical history.* Ann Arbor, MI: University of Michigan Press.

Keränen, L. (2010). *Scientific characters: Rhetoric, politics, and trust in breast cancer research.* Tuscaloosa, AL: University of Alabama Press.

Kleege, G. (2015). Visuality. In R. Adams, B. Reiss, & D. Serlin (Eds.), *Keywords in disability studies* (pp. 182–184). New York, NY; London, UK: New York University Press.

Koerber, A. (2013). *Breast or bottle? Contemporary controversies in infant-feeding policy and practice.* Columbia, SC: University of South Carolina Press.

Lui, D. (2015). Public curation and private collection: The production of knowledge on Pinterest. com. *Critical Studies in Media Communication, 32*(2), 128–142.

Manderson, L., & Smith-Morris, C. (2010). *Chronic conditions, fluid states: Chronicity and the anthropology of illness.* New Brunswick, NJ: Rutgers University Press.

Mills, M. (2015). Technology. In R. Adams, B. Reiss, & D. Serlin (Eds.), *Keywords for disability studies* (pp. 176–179). New York, NY; London, UK: New York University Press.

Miserandino, C. (2003). The Spoon Theory. Retrieved from http://www.butyoudontlooksick. com/articles/writtenby-christine/the-spoon-theory/

Owens, K. H. (2015). *Writing childbirth: Women's rhetorical agency in labor and online.* Carbondale, IL: Southern Illinois University Press.

Scarry, E. (1985). *The body in pain: The making and unmaking of the world.* New York, NY: Oxford University Press.

Scott, B., Segal, J. Z., & Keränen, L. (2013). The rhetorics of health and medicine: Inventional possibilities for scholarship and engaged practice. *Poroi, 9*(1), Article 17.

Segal, J. (2005). *Health and the rhetoric of medicine.* Carbondale, IL: Southern Illinois University Press.

Stormer, N. (2002). *Articulating life's memory: US medical rhetoric about abortion in the nineteenth century.* Lanham, MD: Lexington Books.

Stuckey, Z. (2014). *A rhetoric of remnants: Idiots, half-wits, and other state-sponsored inventions.* Albany, NY: SUNY Press.

Thomson, R. G. (1997). *Extraordinary bodies: Figuring physical disability in American culture and literature.* New York, NY: Columbia University Press.

Vaughan, H. A. (2009). Icon: Tracing the path of the 1950s shirtwaist dress. *The Journal of American Culture, 32*(1), 29–37.

Vorvick, L. J., Zieve, D., & Ogilvie, I. (2016, 3 September). *Living with a chronic illness: Dealing with feelings.* Retrieved from https://medlineplus.gov/ency/patientinstructions/000601.htm

Wall, D. (2005). *Encounters with the Invisible: Unseen Illness, Controversy, and Chronic Fatigue Syndrome.* University Park, TX: Southern Methodist University Press.

An Analytic of and Beyond Representation for the Rhetoric of Health and Medicine

J. BLAKE SCOTT

THE RHETORICAL STUDY of representations in health and medical practices has been a generative topos or topology for our field, directing multiple lines of inquiry.[1] In conversation with other scholars of health and medicine, rhetoricians have directed our attention to the specific relationships, conditions of emergence, functions, and effects of representations, especially representations of patients and health publics. Among other dynamics of persuasion, rhetoricians have explored the following: how inaccurate representations (e.g., about lobotomy) historically shape meanings and stories that travel across cultural arenas (Johnson, 2014); how clinical constructions of patients (e.g., migraineurs) shift over time with medical treatments to shape physician–patient interactions (Segal, 2005); how health-care providers record "external representations" of their individual and collective memories of critical patient information (Angeli, 2015); how cultural representations of illness shape acts of self-doctoring (Emmons, 2010); how identity-based notions of risk stigmatize some groups and limit others' identification with risk (Scott, 2003); how patients attempt to use self-presentations of expertise (e.g., in birth plans) to shape their future clinical experiences in moments of "rhetorical disability" (Owens, 2015); how self-representations of (women's) bodies foster counter-

---

1. As Walsh and Boyle (2017) explained, a topology "traces the contours [including "unarticulated gaps and margins"; p. 10] of a discourse and may [opportunistically] fold it into a new configuration" (p. 4).

publics and shape embodied self-exploration and experiences with caregivers (Wells, 2010); and how public health representations of counterpublics (e.g., "vaccine refusers," "bug chasers") make generalizing and unproductive assumptions about people's values and motives (Lawrence, Hausman, & Dannenberg, 2014; Malkowski, 2014). This body of scholarship has generated new and more nuanced understandings of how representations can work as parts of entangled practices to unevenly constrain or facilitate health care, distort or affirm embodied experiences and perspectives, disable or enable identifications, and limit or empower forms of resistance and advocacy. Representations do not just signify or mean; they also make, configure, and instantiate. This matters as a starting premise for the rhetoric of health and medicine (RHM) because of the way our scholarship attends to high-stakes *inter-articulations of materiality and language*, from patient–provider encounters to biomedical research to personal health-care management practices. Further, as Lynch (2009), drawing on Stormer (2004), explained, attending to such inter-articulations can not only help account for the "flows of matter and energy" across "objects, bodies, and discourses" (p. 438); it can also *help determine how the process of inter-articulation can "foreground either material or symbolic being in order to enable certain types of activities" and impacts* (p. 437; emphasis added).

Rhetoricians of health and medicine have increasingly turned to examine representations in online spaces (e.g., Arduser, 2011; De Hertogh, 2015; Keränen, 2012; Moeller, 2014; Mogull & Balzhiser, 2015). Such studies have contributed to our understanding of the unique dynamics, affordances, and constraints of online health and medical practices. Like the larger body of scholarship referenced above, these studies also highlight how representations of bodies and embodied practices are key sites of rhetorical contestation, often involving alternative self-representations by marginalized people and counterpublics. These past conversations are extended and illustrated through the three chapters in this section.

In our introductory chapter to *Methodologies for the Rhetoric of Health and Medicine*, Melonçon and I (2018) claim that one of the defining (though not unique)[2] characteristics of our field is its careful attention to the "interanimation of the discursive and material . . . dimensions of health and medical practices, including what Hayles (1999) describes as a feedback loop between inscription and incorporation practices" (p. 6). The analytic focus we point to here—and that we hope continues to characterize our field—is not about making loose connections or broad claims about distinctions and relationships

---

2. Lynch (2009) made a similar claim about the direction of rhetorical criticism of science.

between representations and what they represent, bodies and embodiment, inscription and incorporation practices, discourse and materiality—but about careful, precise, and embedded attention to emergent, mutual conditioning and co-configuring processes.

One focal or rather nodal point in processes that co-configure representations and materiality, and one perhaps especially prominent in online representations, is technology or technological systems and environments. In "The Materiality of Informatics," Hayles (1993) argued that "one of the urgent needs in a field [e.g., rhetoric of health of medicine] that wants to understand how technology, discourse, and materiality work together is a theoretical framework that will not only give all these elements appropriate weight but will also indicate how they are interconnected through complex feedforward and feedback loops" (p. 170). Instead of informational loops in closed systems or environments, *these are loops in which embodied experiences, discursive constructions, and technology mutually condition and co-determine interfaces with one another in contingent, emergent, and open processes.* As Hayles (1999) explained, "changes in experience of embodiment," which she described as enmeshed in contexts (which include technological spaces, actants, and constraints), "bubble up in language," including bodies as cultural constructs, and, at the same time, "discursive constructions [including those in online and other technology-conditioned environments] affect how bodies move through space and time" (pp. 206–207). Relatedly, the processes of inscription and incorporation are in interplay, though both bodies and forms of embodiment shape incorporating practices. Hayles (1999) also pointed to the roles of technology in co-configuring incorporation, arguing that "when changes in incorporating practices take place, they are often linked with new technologies that affect how people use their bodies and experience space and time" and adding that "embodiment mediates between technology and discourse by creating new experiential frameworks that serve as boundary markers for the creation of corresponding discursive systems" (p. 205). So, *technologies do not just mediate the relationships in feedback loops; they interact with discourse and experiential frameworks to co-figure the interfaces, boundaries, and instantiations of health and medicine's actants and phenomena.*

The three chapters in this section make compelling additions to and raise important questions about how to study rhetoric in terms of open feedback loops involving technologies, representations, and material experiences. In what follows I discuss the contributions of these chapters in extending and in some ways disrupting our field's readings of representations. I also position these chapters in a larger argument about the usefulness and limitations of an analytic of representation, drawing on Barad (2007) and others to discuss how an alternative analytic of performativity, which focuses on how rhetorical and other entities materialize rather than what they represent and mean, could offer new insights about the rhetorical phenomena we study. At the same time that the field has continued to examine the meaning-making functions and effects of rhetorical constructions or representations, including their roles in complex inscription–incorporation feedback loops, it has also begun to shift away from such a focus toward one on the "processes of materialization" (Coole & Frost, 2010, p. 2); this shift and new focus on materialization rejects distinctions between rhetorical constructions and any pre-existing entities they are assumed to represent, instead exploring how various material-discursive entities mutually emerge through their entangled intra-actions.

In discussing the implications of this shift for the field, I take the Sophistic stance that *both representational and performative analytics offer promising directions for the field*—including its study of online and digital health and medical practices—in part because, as Lynch (2009) explained, representations and their meanings often get foregrounded through articulation processes. Finally, I make the meta-argument that we also attune a performative attention to materialization to our own research and analysis practices, in order to more intimately account for these practices as embedded and emergent.

ACCOUNTING FOR THE INTER-ANIMATED WORK OF REPRESENTATIONS IN FEEDBACK LOOPS

One takeaway from these three chapters and the field's conversations they enter is that rhetorical studies of health and medicine can treat the mutually conditioning relationship between language and materiality as a premise or starting point rather than as a key finding or conclusion. This enables the chapters to pose and explore more specific questions about what this mutual conditioning looks like and what it configures; such questions get at more than configurations of meanings but also embodied experiences and material conditions, including those of online spaces. In her "epidemiology of signification" of AIDS discourses, Treichler (1999) similarly encouraged moving from the premise that representations shape meaning-making practices and embodied experiences to more precise and interesting questions about how representations "develop and flourish, taking hold in cultural discourse," how "discursive realities" are entangled with and enacted through "material practices and performances," and how "linguistic, social, and cultural constructions . . . interact with the phenomena that we call *data, facts,* and even *experience*" (p. 327).

In examining the inter-articulation and mutual conditioning of discursive representations and embodied experiences, all three chapters in this section ask more specific questions about how representations function to normalize and resist subject formation—through identification, self-perception, self–other boundaries, and (counter)public formation. In doing so, the chapters illustrate ways that rhetoricians of health and medicine can examine these roles as parts of complex feedback loops that shape embodied, contextualized, health-related practices.

In their study of Pinterest pins and shares by women with chronic illness (e.g., chronic fatigue syndrome, fibromyalgia), Sarah Singer and Jordynn Jack (this volume) offer the analytic framework of chronicity that "calls attention to the rhetorical processes of identification that enable (or constrain) identify-formation for individuals with chronic illnesses" through "social media compositions" (p. 140). While most of their analysis examines how the texts and images pinned by these women "index" their experiences in ways that counter stereotypical cultural depictions—itself a useful observation about the representation-embodiment inter-animation—Singer and Jack also explain how the social curation of such self-representations creates new opportunities for positive identification and, by extension, forms of social cohesion. Like Brouwer's (2006) analysis of the counterpublicity by activist HIV/AIDS zines, this analysis shows how self-representations, including ones that depict "modes of corporeality," can help constitute counterpublics "through explicit and implicit identifications and disidentifications" (p. 355). As Singer and Jack suggest, the pinned images can affect the social and individual experiences of women as self-advocates, which can, in turn, shape their and others' (including medical providers') expressed understandings and engagements of people with chronic illness, forming a version of the feedback loop between bodies (as normalized constructs) and forms of embodiment (as contextualized instances that resist normalization) that Hayles (1999) described and about which our field is making ever-interesting observations. We might relate the self-advocacy that Singer and Jack study to Emmons's (2010) "rhetorical care of the self," which involves questioning how the language of medicine interpellates us as particular types of gendered patients, and reconsidering our embodied, contextualized symptoms and other experiences (p. 17). In this case, the rhetorical care of the self would apply not only to individual patients but also to a *social collective* that emerges through networked Pinterest actions, which adds another layer of feedback between social and individual advocacy experiences.

In their chapter, Friz and Overholt (this volume) also focus on technology's role in a body–embodiment feedback loop, explaining how fertility tracking apps such as Eve enact new ways of "quantifying one's body and identity" and a new "definition of 'health' as adherence to statistical norms and compliance with constant data generation and monitoring" (p. 119; p. 120). "We, as rhetoricians and critical consumers of health technologies," they write, "need to think through how this now-perfunctory quantification is a new avenue for representation and how the aggregation of data creates new ways for users to be articulated in and by these technologies" (p. 118). In their case, these mutually conditioning functions are connected to quantification and biomedicalization, the latter "an intensification of the insertion of medical expertise into everyday aspects of life" (p. 107). This concept provides a framework for identifying new connections between data production and health maintenance, and for tracking some of the concrete ways users of these apps are implicated in and affected by a feedback loop between embodied data-based user profiles and self-surveillance practices (or, more generally, between body-focused representations and embodied experiences). Friz and Overholt connect this loop with a Foucauldian knowledge–power loop, noting that "if users have internalized self-surveillance as an important moral injunction, they will be likely to continue compliantly inputting data daily into the app in order to obtain ever more accurate information and thus self-knowledge" (p. 113). Ultimately, Friz and Overholt argue that this process is a concrete and internalized manifestation of a neoliberal imperative of health citizenship emphasizing "self-responsibility and moral consumerism" (p. 103), but that we need alternatives to this technology of the self. Again, we could look for how such alternatives might be informed by a rhetorical care of the self, or we might imagine more collective repurposings of embodied technologies, including wearables (see Boyle, 2016).

Beyond teasing out the relationships between representations and other actants, and between representations and embodied experiences, as the other chapter authors do, Molly Kessler (chapter 4, in this volume) more pointedly blurs distinctions between representations and other entities involved in *rhetorical enactments*. In examining how patients narrate and conceptualize in online spaces their experiences with autoimmune conditions, including the ways they call into question metaphorical and experiential boundaries of self and embodiment (p. 84), Kessler provides an example of how to navigate a rhetorical care of the self in the face of less empowering knowledge–power loops enacted through technology. In this way, Kessler's study employs more of the performative analytic advocated by Barad (2007), treating patient's self-representations as co-actants in and products of emergent boundary-shaping practices, showing how representational and performative analytics can be usefully combined in RHM research.

In contrast to the self-images of immune systems that Martin (1994) discussed in *Flexible Bodies*, the women studied by Kessler blur and reconfigure self–other boundaries, pointing to instances where self—their immune systems—becomes nonself and where nonself—embodied treatment technologies—become self. Kessler's analysis emphasizes how such boundaries are not predetermined or only discursive constructions but emerge through intra-active experiences involving a range of agents. Kessler draws on Barad's (2007) performative framework of agential realism to call on rhetoricians of health and medicine to shift from "examining how language *represents* patients' bodily and identity boundaries toward how *representational practices* participate along with other practices (physiological, symptomatic, technological, and so on) and influence wide-ranging patient lived experiences" (p. 84). Barad (2007) rejected the idea that phenomena are shaped by pre-existing entities and apparatuses (including patient narratives, self-constructions, form of embodiment) that interact, instead using the word *intra-action* to capture how such entities and their properties and relationships are enacted or materialized through boundary-making phenomena or "differential patterns of mattering" (pp. 139–140). For Kessler, rhetorical enactment, which we can read in terms of intra-action, is more than how representations shape meanings (including perceptions of our own identities and bodies) and even embodied experiences as a patient—instead, it captures how representations and their meanings co-emerge through their entanglements with other agents. We could say that this understanding collapses any feedback loop between bodies and embodiment.

Collectively, the three chapters in this section raise questions and invite further research about the roles of technology and online spaces in the rhetorical enactments they study, and about how rhetoricians can contribute to ameliorating marginalizing dynamics to which representations contribute. If rhetoricians of health and medicine want to identify not only what representations mean and constitute but also how they emerge and function in complex feedback loops involving embodiment and technology, then we need to ask more specific questions about how online spaces, medical devices, and other technologies intra-act in these loops. In her study of the Virtual Human Project, Waldby (2000) offered an example of such research, showing how biomedical images "are not simply re-presentations of pre-existing objects but rather . . . 'operative images,' images or trace systems which are in-themselves technologies, able to effect transformations in the bodily tissues" (p. 27). Instead of mediating entities, Waldby engaged images as operative ones that co-enact. Following this approach, we might replace the concept of mediation with that of interface,[3] which Drucker (2011) described in terms of "specific relations between properties and affordances" of technology "within a system of codependent relations of production" (p. 3). With such an understanding, rhetorical studies of online health and medical practices would treat the technologies and spaces involved not as contextual backdrops for or mediators of rhetorical enactments but as co-shapers, with discourse and other elements, of interfaces and their boundaries and cominglings.

The three chapters also usefully raise open questions about how our studies of feedback loops and/or intra-actions can contribute better understandings of health and medical practices, and how they can identify opportunities for more empowering forms of boundary-making. As I have advocated elsewhere, examining feedback loops of bodies and embodiment, inscription and incorporation, knowledge and power, can be crucial to pinpointing places to productively rupture or redirect such loops (Scott, 2014). Kessler's analysis demonstrates how patients' "boundaries and entities are enacted through the intra-action of disease, self, nonself, bodies, technology, and perhaps more"—including "representational practices"—a focus that can help us "better understand patients' practices and in turn better help patients navigate the complexities of their embodiment and patienthood" (p. 98).

SHIFTING TO PERFORMATIVITY

Kessler's chapter, in particular, begins to articulate an alternative to an analysis focused on representations that holds promise for rhetorical studies of health and medicine. Though they have taken various forms, calls by rhetoricians to move beyond representation are not new; for example, we can point to Greene's (1998) proposal nearly twenty years ago for a new materialist rhetoric that replaces a logic of representation with a logic of articulation "to better account for how rhetorical practices distribute different elements into a functioning network of power" (p. 21),[4] a shift that Stormer (2004) and Lynch (2009) extended, the latter for rhetorical studies of science.

---

3. Although Hayles (1999) used the term *mediate* to describe technology's roles, the approach I'm advocating avoids this metaphor, as the idea of mediation can reinforce and even add another layer to unproductive distinctions and pre-existing relationships among constructions and practices, information and materiality, nature and culture. Barad (2007) argues that "the notion of mediation has for too long stood in the way of a more thoroughgoing accounting of the empirical world" (p. 152).

4. I should note that Greene's (1998) proposal, unlike Barad's, maintained distinctions "between rhetoric and other material elements" (p. 39).

Like Kessler, I find Barad's theoretical framework of performativity (which draws from Haraway, Butler, and others) a promising resource for moving beyond a representational analytic. In her essay "Posthumanist Performativity," Barad (2003) defined representationalism as "the belief in the ontological distinction between representations and that which they purport to represent; in particular, that which is represented is held to be independent of all practices of representing" (p. 804). This belief contrasts with what Barad (2003) called a "performative understanding" of discourse and discursive-material enactments (p. 804).

Such an approach does not overlook discourse in the same way that a focus on representations can fade material conditions and practices into the background or consider them as secondary sources or effects. Instead, it shifts the understanding of discourse from "what is said" to "that which constrains and enables what can be said," and what otherwise comes into being (Barad, 2003, p. 819). That is, a performative analytic still pays attention to representations but focuses on different questions about them, moving beyond what they mean to the processes through which they are shaped. Treichler (1999) similarly encouraged cultural critics to "concentrate . . . on understanding the rules of discourse whereby truth in various universes is produced, sustained, deeply experienced, or contested" (p. 272).

Barad (2007) took this orientation further. Beyond being inter-animated by the material, she argued, discourse is always already part of material phenomena; discursive practices are "ongoing material (re)configurings of the world" (p. 152). In addition to understanding discursive practices as material, this framework understands materiality as discursive, as "matter [that] emerges out of and includes . . . the ongoing reconfiguring of boundaries" through "apparatuses of bodily [including rhetorical] production" (Barad, 2003, p. 822). Applying this bidirectional inter-animation of the material and discursive to Friz and Overholt's discussion of fertility apps, such apps might not, as they conclude, "render the body (finally) transparent" (p. 119) (a claim that accounts for only the discursive rendering of the material), but might instead function as co-agents that emerge from, and that help both bodies and material forms of embodiment emerge from, intra-actions in particular ways.

A performative reading of rhetorical enactments, Barad (2003) posited, "shifts the focus from questions of correspondence between descriptions and reality . . . to matters of practices/doings/actions" (p. 802). Further, this shift understands performativity as more than enacted through iterative chains of discursive citations, as Butler (2006) imagined, but more fundamentally as "*iterative intra-activity*" (p. 822). The "boundaries and properties of the 'components' of phenomena" emerge out of and "become determinate through" their intra-actions, which are both discursive and material in their effects. To illustrate, I (Scott, 2003) support an intra-active understanding of risk in my rhetorical-cultural analysis of risk-identified HIV testing practices, drawing on Patton's (1996) analogic model of queer cruising to redefine risk from a pre-existing quality tied to particular identities and managed through representations to a quality "emerging from situated action and movement" (p. 234). Because cruising is enacted through an intra-action involving timing, space, the *movement* of bodies, discursive and embodied codes, the risk that emerges from it is fluid and contingent (Scott, 2003, p. 234). Although, like Butler, Barad rejected the idea of pre-performative entities, she helped us shift from approaching performativity as discursive citationality to a performative process of co-figuration from which discursive and material entities co-emerge.

Like Kessler, Graham (2015), Teston (2016, 2017), and others have enlisted Barad's (2007) theory of agential realism as well as other new materialist frameworks, such as multiple ontologies theory, to study and foreground the ways that health and medical practices *matter*, in both senses of that word, through entangled intra-actions (p. 209). We could describe this shift as moving from representations to enactments and meanings to practices, but we could alternatively describe it as reversing the causal relationship of pre-existing agents shaping phenomena to intra-active phenomena shaping these entities. Such a shift requires rhetoricians to ask how rhetorical enactments emerge and what makes them possible. Consider, for example, Teston's (2016) study of what she called "evidentiary shadow work" in lab-based genetic testing: "When genetic scientists translate results from intra-acting phenomena into something that resembles actionable evidence," she explained, "they do so based on comparisons to reference material," adding that the "ontological intra-actional yield (of technologies, actants, actors, discourses, sites, activities, and so on) is compared with reference material (which is, as well, a result of ontological intra-actions, but from an earlier time), and from those comparisons evidential inferences are made" (p. 7). In this case genetic "results" and the reference material on which they are based are not representations but "intra-actional yields" that enact rhetorical and material force. They emerge from and become co-shapers of performative intra-action.

Although I see the value of turning from a representational to a performative analytic, I am not arguing that rhetorical studies of health and medicine should abandon the analytic notion of representation altogether. Instead, I prefer to take the Sophistic stance that both approaches can be useful at times, particularly because wicked problems in health and medicine (e.g., patient "noncompliance") resist easy or one-dimensional solutions. Many health and medical practices—such as public health campaigns, treatment protocols, clinical testing, patient advocacy—are largely staged by, understood as, and enacted through representations. In addition, as standpoint theory has taught us, it is sometimes politically necessary to argue for the primacy of some types of representations and forms of embodiment over others. Singer and Jack instructively point to rhetoricians' ethical obligation to help privilege self-presentations of patients, in their case people with disabling chronic illnesses, that can create more accurate understandings and empowering identifications. Even the pragmatic constraints of our research practices sometimes depend on assuming pre-existing subjectivities (e.g., in securing IRB approval for working with subjects at risk) and on distinctions between representations and embodied subjects (e.g., in the ethical principle to accurately represent participants' perspectives and voices in our write-ups). Working within a representational framework, we can still, as Hayles (1999) proposed, treat "the overlap between the enacted and the represented bodies" as a "contingent production" that can be shaped and studied with rhetoric (p. xiv).

ACCOUNTING FOR OUR RESEARCH PRACTICES AS PERFORMATIVE

In her chapter, Kessler calls for focusing on "enactments," informed by Barad's (2007) agential realism, "*as* a theoretical underpinning with which RHM can examine a range of entities that participate in people's lived experiences." Although I share her goal of better accounting "for the boundaries, binaries, and entanglements of bodies, matter, disease, discourse, sites of practice, and culture," (p. 84) I want to extend her call to argue for adding our own theory-building and other analytic practices to this accounting. If we are to account for performative intra-actions, we have to include our analytic and other research practices as also emerging from these intra-actions rather than underpinning and revealing them. In addition to the "as" of who we are as defined by our theoretical and methodological framework, we must also attend to the "is" of how we enact our field and its boundaries through implementing these frameworks in our research practices. Such practices (including theory-building) do not just reveal or explain or elucidate—they participate, emerging along with other discursive-material agents out of the phenomena in which we are enmeshed. Barad (2007) similarly proposed that we recognize "not merely that knowledge practices have material consequences but that practices of knowing are specific material engagements that participate in (re)configuring the world" (p. 91).

Another characteristic that Melonçon and I (Scott & Melonçon, 2018) attribute to research in the RHM is a "methodological mutability," or a "willingness and even obligation to pragmatically and ethically adjust aspects of methodology to changing exigencies, conditions, relationships" (p. 5). This mutability requires careful attunement and attentive responsiveness to the emerging contexts and dynamics of which we are part, and it entails our approaches to identifying, analyzing, and theorizing about the practices we study. In her field research of health communication involving new mothers in neonatal intensive care units, Bivens (2017) enacted such mutability through rhetorical listening that attuned her to participants' changing embodied responses to her presence as a researcher. This practice of attunement enabled Bivens to notice how contextual intra-actions were shaping relationships between observation and experience, researcher and participant. She noticed, for example, how new mothers signaled their emergent desire to stop participating through such embodied acts as closing a curtain or avoiding eye contact with her (see pp. 140–141, 149–150). Rhetorically listening *with* rather than *for* intent (Ratcliffe, 2005, p. 28) was not something Bivens applied from a critical distance but something that emerged, and that disrupted, the entangled, unfolding intra-actions at the research site. Although she had, of course, secured each mother's consent to participate in the study, the discomfort she felt by the emergent embodied stances of some participants toward her presence prompted her to change her in situ (and future) research practices. Specifically, she stopped observing women who nonverbally signaled their desire for privacy, and she adjusted her informed consent process to allow for a more continuous attunement to participants' wishes.

This methodological mutability applies to theory-building as part of or in addition to other types of research. Gouge and I (Scott & Gouge, 2019) advocate for approaching theory-building as a performative form of care for RHM. Also indebted to Barad's framework, such an approach treats theorizing, like experimentation, as a material practice (Barad, 2007, p. 5), and theories as "living, breathing reconfigurations of the world" (Barad, 2012, p. 207). More than a tool or lens to engage the world and its phenomena, theory emerges from and participates in intra-action that manifests symbolic constructions and forms of embodiment. Theories are responsive but also performative, transforming and being transformed by phenomena they feed back into and intra-act with. To return to Bivens (2017), she developed the concept of "microwithdrawals of consent" out of the material-symbolic enactments of her research, and she used this concept to argue for and enact an ethical process of attuning and responding to participants' changing needs and desires, sometimes subtly and nonverbally expressed (see pp. 152–155).

Accounting for ourselves and research methodologies in the intra-actions we study can be a useful corrective to studying online spaces as mediation or as spaces we can observe from a safe distance. For instance, a performative analysis of chronicity in online spaces might identify, as Singer and Jack do, how the rhetorical practices of participants in such spaces shape counteridentifications, but it might also account for the rhetoricians' own chronicity and concordant acts of identification, asking how these emerged from and shaped what they noticed about the Pinterest practices as resistant and affirming self-presentations, and how these might affect rhetoricians' support of participants' social media compositions in workshops or other contexts.

Studying Rhetorical Enactments in Online Environments—Emergent Possibilities

The chapters in this section and larger body of rhetorical work on health and medical representations raise and offer tentative answers to a number of questions about the processes and environments of rhetorical enactments in and beyond online spaces. These questions include the following: What are the more specific roles of online spaces and the technologies that structure them in complex feedback loops involving representations and embodied acts of incorporation? How do such functions and larger processes foreground particular co-agents, boundaries, and emerging effects—be they representations, embodied experiences, and/or something else—that are both productive and limiting for health practices? Singer and Jack point to how such enactments shape both individual and collective forms of identification, enabling a counterpublic to form. We might extend this argument to ask how such identifications can operate as part of what Rice (2008) called affective economies, and how technological and sociocultural infrastructures can work together to support particular types of identifications in online environments (Scott, 2014). Friz and Overholt examine the normalizing functions of technology-enabled biomedicalization, in their case through online apps. Their analysis raises questions about how such technologies help configure interfaces that simultaneously amalgamate and personalize data, enabling multiscalar modes of surveillance. Like the chapters in the collection's final section, this chapter also suggests directions for a rhetorical care of the self that rejects neoliberal interpellations of health citizenship, and perhaps for a collective version of this that takes a moral (and not just informational) approach to what Boyle (2016) called "pervasive citizenship." Kessler's chapter takes up important questions about the agency of patients to opportunistically enact or disrupt distinctions between and boundaries of self/nonself and body/embodiment in more empowering ways.

This collection's "As/Is" framework invites us to be more attentive to and reflexive about our emergent boundary-making practices around what we do and who we are, to ask *how* we are persuaded to recognize and value characteristics and boundaries that distinguish RHM. The performative analytic and examples of studies discussed here point to several possibilities for redirecting this attention vis-à-vis our analysis of representations:

1. view the co-emergence and mutual conditioning of bodies, embodied incorporating practices, frames of experience, technology, and other entities as a *starting and not an ending point* for our analysis so that we can get to more specific questions about the functions and effects of intra-actions;

2. more specifically, instead of approaching health and medical interfaces as discrete spaces, approach them as parts of intercontextual, interanimating processes through which health and illness are represented and instantiated;

3. similarly, treat technology and online spaces not as mediating forces or sites but instead as co-agents of intra-action so that we ask more concrete questions about how boundaries and properties of such entities are enacted and how we can pinpoint opportunities for rupture and redirection;

4. instead of assuming we can study online spaces and processes from a distance or through codified ethical standards, *embrace and ethically respond to "the entanglements materializations of which we are a part,* including new configurations, new subjectivities" (Barad, 2007, p. 384; emphasis added);[5]

5. extend a performative analytic to a *self-reflexive accounting of our methodologies, including theory-building, as also emergent* so that we can become better attuned to, more responsive to, and more reflexive about how our research intra-acts.

Regardless of the extended or new directions in which our analysis of rhetorical constructions and enactments take us, they will help us shape the contours of who we are by what we do. Just as acts of embodied incorporation resist the normalizing force of discursive constructs, I hope the "is" of what

---

5. On this point, Opel (2017) recommended that rhetoricians engaged in Health 2.0 research projects take a "process-based approach rather than a codified approach to research ethics" characterized by context-specific, "nuanced decisions about informed content, privacy and surveillance, and reporting" (p. 191).

we do enables our field to enact self-perceptions and boundaries that are useful but not stable.

REFERENCES

Angeli, E. L. (2015). Three types of memory in emergency medical services communication. *Written Communication, 32*(1), 3–38.

Arduser, L. (2011). Warp and weft: Weaving the discussion threads of an online community. *Journal of Technical Writing and Communication, 41* (1), 5–31.

Barad, K. (2003). Posthumanist performativity: Toward an understanding of how matter comes to matter. *Signs: Journal of Women in Culture and Society, 28*(3), 801–831.

Barad, K. (2007). *Meeting the universe halfway: Quantum physics and the entanglement of matter and meaning.* Durham, NC: Duke University Press.

Barad, K. (2012). "Matter feels, converses, suffers, desires, yearns, and remembers": Interview with Karen Barad. In R. Dolphijn & I. Van der Tuin (Eds.), *New materialism: Interviews & cartographies* (pp. 48–70). London, UK: Open Humanities.

Bivens, K. M. (2017). Rhetorically listening for microwithdrawals of consent in research practice. In L. Melconon & J. B. Scott (Eds.), *Methodologies for the rhetoric of health and medicine* (pp. 138–156). New York, NY: Routledge.

Boyle, C. (2016). Pervasive citizenship through #SenseCommons. *Rhetoric Society Quarterly, 46*(3), 269–283.

Brouwer, D. C. (2006). Counterpublicity and corporeality in HIV/AIDS zines. *Critical Studies in Media Communication, 22*(5), 351–371.

Butler, J. (2006). *Gender trouble: Feminism and the subversion of identity.* New York, NY: Routledge.

Coole, D., & Frost, S. (Eds.). (2010). *New materialisms: Ontology, agency, and politics.* Durham, NC: Duke University Press.

De Hertogh, L. B. (2015). Reinscribing a new normal: Pregnancy, disability, and Health 2.0 in the online natural birthing community, Birth Without Fear. *Ada: A Journal of Gender, New Media, and Technology, 7,* https://doi.org/10.7264/N3Z899PH

Drucker, J. (2011). Humanities approaches to interface theory. *Culture Machine, 12,* 1–20.

Emmons, K. (2010). *Black dogs and blue words: Depression and gender in the age of self-care.* New Brunswick, NJ: Rutgers University Press.

Graham, S. S. (2015). *The politics of pain medicine: A rhetorical-ontological inquiry.* Chicago, IL: University of Chicago Press.

Greene, R. W. (1998). Another materialist rhetoric. *Critical Studies in Mass Communication, 15*(1), 21–40.

Hayles, N. K. (1993). The materiality of informatics. *Configurations, 1*(1), 147–170.

Hayles, N. K. (1999). *How we became posthuman: Virtual bodies in cybernetics, literature, and informatics.* Chicago, IL: University of Chicago Press.

Johnson, J. (2014). *American lobotomy: A rhetorical history.* Ann Arbor, MI: University of Michigan Press.

Keränen, L. (2012). "This weird, incurable disease": Competing diagnoses in the rhetoric of Morgellons. In T. Jones, D. Wear, & L. D. Friedman (Eds.), *Health humanities reader* (pp. 36–49). New Brunswick, NJ: Rutgers University Press.

Lawrence, H. Y., Hausman, B. L. & Dannenberg, C. J. (2014). Reframing medicine's publics: The local as a public of vaccine refusal. *Journal of Medical Humanities, 35*(2), 111–129.

Lynch, J. A. (2009). Articulating scientific practice: Understanding Dean Hammer's "gay gene" study as overlapping material, social and rhetorical registers. *Quarterly Journal of Speech, 95*(4), 435–456.

Malkowski, J. (2014). Beyond prevention: Containment rhetoric in the case of bug chasing. *Journal of Medical Humanities, 35*(2), 211–228.

Martin, E. (1994). *Flexible bodies: Tracking immunity in American culture from the days of Polio to the age of AIDS.* Boston, MA: Beacon.

Moeller, M. (2014). Pushing boundaries of normalcy: Employing critical disability studies in analyzing medical advocacy websites. *Communication Design Quarterly, 2*(4), 52–80.

Mogull, S. A., & Balzhiser, D. (2015). Pharmaceutical companies are writing the script for health consumerism. *Communication Design Quarterly, 3*(4), 35–49.

Opel, D. S. (2017). Ethical research in "Health 2.0": Consideration for scholars of medical rhetoric. In L. Melonçon & J. B. Scott (Eds.), *Methodologies for the rhetoric of health and medicine* (pp. 176–194). New York, NY: Routledge.

Owens, K. H. (2015). *Writing childbirth: Women's rhetorical agency in labor and online.* Carbondale, IL: Southern Illinois University Press.

Patton, C. (1996). *Fatal advice: How safe-sex education went wrong.* Durham, NC: Duke University Press.

Ratcliffe, K. (2005). *Rhetorical listening: Identification, gender, whiteness.* Carbondale, IL: Southern Illinois University Press.

Rice, J. E. (2008). The new *new*: Making the case for critical affect studies. *Quarterly Journal of Speech, 94*(2), 200–212.

Scott, J. B. (2003). *Risky rhetoric: AIDS and the cultural practices of HIV testing.* Carbondale, IL: Southern Illinois University Press.

Scott, J. B. (2014). Afterword: Elaborating health and medicine's publics. *Journal of Medical Humanities, 35*(2), 229–235.

Scott, J. B., & Gouge, C. (2019). Theory building in the rhetoric of health and medicine. In A. Alden, K. Gerdes, J. Holiday, & R. Skinnell (Eds.), *Reinventing (with) theory in rhetoric and writing studies: Essays in honor of Sharon Crowley* (181–195). Logan, UT: Utah State University Press.

Scott, J. B., & Melonçon, L. (2018). Manifesting methodologies for the rhetoric of health and medicine. In L. Melonçon & J. B. Scott (Eds.), *Methodologies for the rhetoric of health and medicine* (pp. 1–23). New York, NY: Routledge.

Segal, J. Z. (2005). *Health and the rhetoric of medicine.* Carbondale, IL: Southern Illinois University Press.

Stormer, N. (2004). Articulation: A working paper on rhetoric and taxis. *Quarterly Journal of Speech, 90*(3), 257–284.

Teston, C. (2016). *Rhetorical ontographies of evidentiary shadow work.* Paper presented at the Conference on College Composition and Communication, Houston, TX, April.

Teston, C. (2017). *Bodies in flux: Scientific methods for negotiating medical uncertainty.* Chicago, IL: University of Chicago Press.

Treichler, P. A. (1999). *How to have theory in an epidemic: Cultural chronicles of AIDS.* Durham, NC: Duke University Press.

Waldby, C. (2000). *The Visible Human Project: Informatics bodies and posthuman medicine.* London, UK: Routledge.

Walsh, L., & Boyle, C. (Eds.). (2017). *Topographies as techniques for a post-critical rhetoric.* London, UK: Palgrave Macmillan.

Wells, S. (2010). *Our bodies, ourselves and the work of writing.* Palo Alto, CA: Stanford University Press.

SECTION 3

HEALTH CITIZENSHIP AND ADVOCACY

CHAPTER 7

Rhetoric *as* Rhetorical Health Citizenship

Rhetorical Agency, Public Deliberation, and
Health Citizenship as *Rhetorical Forms*

REBECCA A. KUEHL, SARA A. MEHLTRETTER DRURY,

AND JENN ANDERSON

THIS CHAPTER'S PURPOSE is to conceptualize rhetoric *as* rhetorical health citizenship. We do so through connecting concepts such as rhetorical agency, public deliberation, and health citizenship to explain how rhetoric *is* a praxis of deliberative decision-making processes. To support this claim, we analyze two deliberative case studies about health issues in two different midwestern communities.[1] We suggest that rhetorical health citizenship *is* a useful way to conceptualize the interactions of these concepts in praxis and suggest ways to apply this concept to other health issues and contexts.

In what follows, we examine literature about rhetorical agency, public deliberation, and health citizenship. We then describe the rhetorical methods and contexts of our deliberative case studies. We analyze how rhetorical agency, public deliberation, and health citizenship are present in discourse about two health issues of breastfeeding support and substance abuse. We suggest conceptualizing rhetoric *as* rhetorical health citizenship, which brings together these existing rhetorical forms to illustrate how rhetoric *is* operating

1. The Brookings Supports Breastfeeding project was funded by a Bush Foundation Community Innovation grant. The authors wish to acknowledge the Brookings Supports Breastfeeding team members Lois Tschetter, Mary Schwaegerl, Marilyn Hildreth, Charlotte Bachman, Heidi Gullickson, Julia Yoder, and Jamison Lamp. For the Montgomery County Community Conversation project, the authors wish to acknowledge collaborators Jennifer Abbott, Jeffrey P. Mehltretter Drury, and Todd McDorman for their contributions to the project.

in praxis through deliberation about health issues. Farrell (1993) wrote: "Rhetorical form is situated in an ongoing tension between the creative insights of self . . . and the generality of afflictions we share with our community of others" (p. 139). Although Farrell referred to classic rhetorical forms such as epideictic rhetoric, we suggest here that rhetorical agency, public deliberation, and health citizenship also function *as* rhetorical forms situated between self and community. We rely on rhetorical agency, public deliberation, and health citizenship as individual rhetorical resources for communication but also recognize their necessity and connections to a larger shared community, especially regarding health issues.

RHETORICAL AGENCY, PUBLIC DELIBERATION, AND HEALTH CITIZENSHIP *AS* RHETORICAL FORMS

Rhetorical agency refers to the capacity to exert influence or act on public issues (Campbell, 2005; Foss, 2006). Foss (2006) explained that agency "is the means through which rhetors use symbols to construct the world" (p. 378). Usually, speakers or rhetors are attempting to instill rhetorical agency within their audience in persuading them to take action, but agency is also a necessary condition for speakers or rhetors (Campbell, 2005; Foss, 2006; Geisler, 2004; Miller et al., 2016). Often, this capacity to act is connected to politics (Greene, 2004). This model of rhetorical agency has limitations; some rhetorical scholars have instead advocated for a materialist approach (Cooper, 2011; Ewalt, 2016; Greene, 2004) that reconceptualizes agency within people's lived experiences and material conditions. Agency is simultaneously located within individuals (Cooper, 2011) and in the interactions between individuals, in a collective or communal sense (Campbell, 2005; Hanchey, 2016), and through social networks (Campbell, 2005; Geisler, 2004; Greene, 2004).

In a postmodern turn, rhetorical scholars have promoted a view of agency that prioritizes its interactive characteristics that move beyond a static agent or subject (Geisler, 2005). Notably, in turns to subaltern agency (Hanchey, 2016), nonhuman agency (Jansen, 2016), and spatial agency (Ewalt, 2016), rhetorical scholars have developed a more nuanced approach to studying how and why social change develops within and across diverse contexts. Enactment and movement become important characteristics for explaining how agency occurs (Cooper, 2011; Ewalt, 2016; Jansen, 2016). Foss (2006) argued that agency is located in the interplay between an agent and a structure toward which that agent is directing an action. The tension between rhetorical agency as something to critique in public discourse versus rhetorical agency as something to create or produce in citizens (Geisler, 2004) is at the heart of many discussions about rhetorical agency in rhetorics of science (Miller et al., 2016), medicine, and health.

Public Deliberation

The praxis of public deliberation works to empower the rhetorical agency of members of a community. Deliberative rhetoric, as a genre of discourse and rhetorical form conceived by Aristotle (Farrell, 1993) and theorized by many rhetorical scholars since, represents discursive exchanges that engage questions of the future, resulting in judgment (Hauser & Benoit-Barne, 2002). As used here, the term *public deliberation* refers to a particular form of deliberative rhetoric whereby community members come together to discuss an issue of common concern in depth, focusing on understanding alternative pathways for action, weighing trade-offs and tensions of possible solutions, with the ultimate goal of coming to shared—though not necessarily consensus-based—judgment (Asen, 2015; Nabatchi, 2012). From a rhetorical perspective, this communal, embodied civic engagement is critical, as public deliberation's process of coming together encourages new understandings and innovative outcomes (Hauser & Benoit-Barne, 2002).

Numerous forms of deliberation have been used in health contexts, including brief citizen deliberations, community deliberations, citizens' panels, and online deliberative polling (Carman et al., 2018). Public deliberation on health topics increased participant knowledge of medical evidence and shifted their views on the value of knowing about medical evidence (Carman et al., 2018). Importantly, the deliberative process brings out vernacular discourses on health issues, using small group, public deliberation as an inclusive and productive way to address public values and concerns from people's lived experiences (Baum, Jacobson, & Goold, 2009; Hicks, 2002). The deliberative process enables citizens to discuss health citizenship and civic actions from a variety of stakeholders' perspectives.

Health Citizenship

Health citizenship, health activism, and *health advocacy* are related terms but have important distinctions. Health citizenship refers to understanding individuals as citizens who make health decisions rather than viewing them as patients or consumers (Rimal, Ratzan, Arntson, & Freimuth, 1997).

This approach also draws attention to the social and institutional contexts in which individual health decision-making occurs (Rimal et al., 1997). Individual action in public health can also be characterized as "health activism" (Zoller, 2005, p. 341). Whereas health citizenship is concerned with the rights and responsibilities of an individual with respect to their health (Rimal et al., 1997), health activism is concerned with issues of power and conflict in health contexts. Individuals and communities engaged in health activism develop what Zoller (2005) called an "oppositional consciousness," which challenges social structures that influence individual health experiences and outcomes (p. 352).

In contrast to health activism, which works *against* social structures and a biomedical model of health care, health advocacy works *within* existing structures (Brown et al., 2004). Zoller (2005) wrote that "advocates tend to rely on expert knowledge rather than insert lay knowledge into expert systems" (p. 344). Whereas health activists value lay knowledge and ground-up community organizing, health advocates value expert knowledge and work within biomedical models of care. As we conceptualize rhetoric *as* rhetorical health citizenship, we suggest that health citizens enacting rhetorical health citizenship make myriad rhetorical choices that may be classified as activism, advocacy, or both. This contribution of rhetorical health citizenship *as* a mode of engagement with health allows citizens and scholars to broaden their scope of understanding how individuals engage localized social structures to improve public health. With an understanding of how the literature has articulated these rhetorical forms, we next discuss the choice of rhetorical methods and contexts of our deliberative case studies.

RHETORICAL METHODS AND CONTEXTS FOR RHETORICAL HEALTH CITIZENSHIP

In developing rhetoric *as* rhetorical health citizenship, we drew upon two case studies of public deliberation events on health issues. The first event took place in Montgomery County, Indiana, and focused on addressing substance abuse; the second, in Brookings, South Dakota, focused on promoting breast-feeding support. We included the two case studies to offer an argument for the significance of these concepts of rhetorical agency, public deliberation, and health citizenship *across* diverse health issues, locations, and stakeholder populations. We also included the two case studies out of convenience, since we are located as researchers and citizens in these two communities; however, as we spoke about our experiences, we realized that the case studies had similarities in terms of what we saw of rhetoric in praxis when it comes to conceptualizing rhetoric *as* rhetorical health citizenship. As we note in the conclusion, we advocate for more research to see whether these trends are consistent across additional health issues and contexts.

Rhetorical Methods

The collection and analysis of texts for this chapter follow the model of rhetorical fieldwork (Endres, Hess, Senda-Cook, & Middleton, 2016; McKinnon, Asen, Chavez, & Howard, 2016; Middleton, Hess, Endres, & Senda-Cook, 2015), which blends qualitative modes of inquiry with rhetorical approaches to analysis (Endres et al., 2016; Middleton et al., 2015) and focuses on understanding rhetoric in situ, or through direct participation in and observation of rhetorical performances as they happen in communities (Endres et al., 2016). In the cases explored for this project, rhetorical performances occurred during local public deliberations. The record of these performances, that is, table notes or transcripts from the public deliberations, serve as the texts for analysis (Endres et al., 2016).

We chose to analyze the table notes, facilitator worksheets, and participant worksheets from the Montgomery County public deliberation since the event was not audio-recorded because of the sensitive nature of the topic of substance abuse. For the Brookings public deliberation, we chose to analyze the ten audio-recorded and transcribed table conversations, since these transcripts provide a record of people's discussions about breastfeeding support. To ensure consistency across case studies, Kuehl and Drury analyzed the texts and worked together in the process of rhetorical analysis to compare and justify the use of textual evidence from the case studies that supported claims related to the three concepts of rhetorical agency, public deliberation, and health citizenship. Additionally, Anderson completed a final review once the case studies were integrated in the analysis to ensure that the aforementioned concepts fit with the textual evidence from both case studies.

Rhetorical fieldwork draws upon qualitative modes of data collection, but in the analysis, it maintains a focus on the ways that symbolic interactions constitute and influence our world, particularly in situations where meaning is contested through "deliberation, advocacy, and strategic communication in everyday public life" (Endres et al., 2016, p. 512). In this chapter, we use applied rhetorical criticism (Condit & Bates, 2009). Our analysis focuses on how participants talked about public health issues, with particular attention to discussions of possible individual, collective, and community actions in the context of each local deliberative public. By comparing across the two specific case studies, we theorize the topoi of rhetoric *as* rhetorical health citizenship.

The purpose of our study was to explore deliberative talk about health issues through community-based partnerships and representations of diverse stakeholders. We used public deliberation across two different health issues to explore the commonalities in rhetorical agency of participants as expressed in their deliberative discussions, how participants described enacting their health citizenship, and the different means used through public deliberation to express their views on both community issues of substance abuse and breast-feeding support. By comparing the two case studies, we learned that across diverse community contexts and seemingly disparate health issues, conceptually, rhetoric in praxis has shared characteristics of how rhetorical agency, public deliberation, and health citizenship emerge in deliberative talk about health.

Context of the Case Studies

The case studies of the public deliberations in Indiana and South Dakota have some similarities. Both are small, rural communities in the midwest region of the US: Montgomery County in Indiana has around 38,000 residents; Brookings County in South Dakota has around 32,000. Both are relatively contained communities, meaning that most people who live in the community work in the community. Institutions of higher education figure prominently in both communities, and both institutions have a commitment to using the universities' resources in partnership with local communities to improve overall health and well-being. We describe the communities' differences below.

Montgomery County, Indiana. In 2013, after seeking input on issues in need of public discussion, Drury and Abbott (2013) held a two-hour public deliberation on substance abuse in Montgomery County, Indiana. The composition of the research team for the Montgomery County public deliberation included communication faculty researchers and trained student and faculty facilitators, and community convening partners. The research team developed an issue-framing guide and video that articulated the specific, local health problem and outlined three approaches to addressing it, with each approach containing a list of actions, benefits, and concerns (Drury, 2015). To give you a little overview of who we are, the WDPD is a group of trained facilitators who work with community partners around the state to lead community conversations. Using trained facilitators to aid the deliberation, over 100 community members attended the public deliberation on substance abuse, based on the attendance count from event organizers. While specific demographic data were not collected due to the sensitivity of the topic, anonymous surveys were used to collect participants' insights at the public deliberation. At the public deliberation event, community members were invited to sit at tables where they did not know people; many individuals split up from groups they arrived with so as to encourage discussion across the community. In the end, more than 100 community members participated across ten tables (labeled A–J in the analysis), and seventy-eight participants completed post-event surveys (Drury & Abbott, 2013).

Brookings, South Dakota. In 2014 Kuehl et al. held a public deliberation about breastfeeding support in Brookings, South Dakota. The research team, which included researchers, hospital representatives, lactation consultants, and the Chamber of Commerce, followed a public deliberation process (Anderson et al., 2017) similar to that outlined above for Indiana. Early community input was formalized via three focus groups with breastfeeding mothers ($n = 28$) and three focus groups with business representatives ($n = 28$), and then used to create a deliberation framing guide (Kuehl et al., 2014). Both research teams for Montgomery County and Brookings engaged in a similar process of analysis of formative focus group or interview transcripts, to develop the deliberation framing guides for each event, which guided discussions among participants. The three-hour public deliberation was attended by approximately seventy people, including the facilitators, and, as in Indiana, community members were invited to sit with people whom they *did not* know or arrive with. Trained facilitators, including students and community members, led discussions at ten tables (labeled 1–10 in the analysis) and completed brief table notes. All table conversations were audio-recorded and transcribed.

Pre- and post-event surveys were completed at the public deliberation by thirty-eight participants. The sample represented key stakeholder groups, with many participants belonging to more than one group. The sample included thirty-two parents, twenty-two currently breastfeeding mothers, twenty-nine employees, four employers, three employees able to *make* policy, and seven employees able to *enforce* policy. The sample was made up predominantly of women (84%, $n = 32$); all but one woman had breastfed ($n = 31$). Attendees most commonly reported having two children ($M = 1.92$ children, $SD = 1.42$ children). Three-quarters (76.3%, $n = 29$) of attendees reported working outside the home. Of those who worked, 68.9% ($n = 20$) worked at a small business (fewer than fifty employees) and 24% ($n = 7$) worked at a large business (more than fifty employees); two attendees did not provide this information. Attendees' average age was 37.24 years old ($SD = 13.3$ years). Most attendees identified as White (86.8%); attendees also identified as African American (5.3%), Asian (5.3%), and American Indian (2.6%).

RHETORICAL ANALYSIS

Guided by an understanding of the similarities and differences across each community context, we used rhetorical field methods and applied rhetorical criticism to analyze how participants used public discourse at the two public deliberation events. Our analysis highlights how rhetoric *as* rhetorical health citizenship is embodied through the rhetorical forms (Farrell, 1993) of rhetorical agency, public deliberation, and health citizenship. These three aspects of rhetorical health citizenship come together in rhetorical praxis in deliberating health issues of breastfeeding support and substance abuse. First, in the *rhetorical agency* is *material and collective* section, we explore (a) individual agency and (b) collective agency. Second, in the *public deliberation* is *an inclusive space to engage complex public problems* section, we explore characteristics of the public deliberation process including (a) inclusiveness and (b) weighing trade-offs and tensions. Third, in the *health citizenship* is *inclusive through action* section, we explore how health citizenship (a) educates and (b) encourages action.

Rhetorical Agency *Is* Material and Collective

In our case studies, rhetorical agency is expressed as a rhetorical form (Farrell, 1993) in both the community members who attended the public deliberations and the faculty and students who led, developed, and facilitated the events. Our analysis demonstrates two facets of rhetorical agency present in these events. First, rhetorical agency *is* individual, and it often takes the form of materialist agency (Greene, 2004) communicated through personal experience. Second, rhetorical agency *is* collective, because agency is dynamic (Geisler, 2005) as it interacts between people and structures (Foss, 2006).

Personal experience *is* materialist, individual agency. Participants at the public deliberations articulated their agency through a materialist approach (Cooper, 2011; Ewalt, 2016; Greene, 2004) that relied on lived experiences. Participants used personal experiences as motivation to attend. At the Brookings event, participants across six tables expressed personal struggles with combining breastfeeding and work as an impetus for attending. While the issue of substance abuse is challenging to publicly discuss, several tables had participants relay their experiences with abuse and recovery. Eight of the ten tables expressed a personal reason for attending, such as close friends or relatives struggling with substance abuse. Expressing personal connections and lived experiences related to the topic allows participants to illustrate their commitment to the deliberative process and to making a positive change in their communities.

Participants also used personal experience to advocate for structural changes or policy creation. In this way, individuals' agency was dynamic between the individual and various structures (Foss, 2006), such as participants' workplaces or connections with recovery programs. Both public deliberations included participants who used their personal experiences and connections in their communities as rhetorical strategies to situate themselves in discussing actions. In Brookings, participants used material conditions of going through breastfeeding or previously needing to pump at work to talk with others about developing a lactation room or written breastfeeding policy. A participant from Table 1 said: "I am here because I'm a mother too, who has breastfed in Brookings . . . I've been in the position of being a breastfeeding mom, a pumping mom, working and pumping, also being a supervisor to people who are pumping."

The discussion at Table 1 drew upon personal experiences and past struggles of combining breastfeeding and work to advocate for clearer, written breastfeeding policies in local businesses. In Montgomery County, one local organization offered an opportunity for individuals in a recovery facility to attend the public deliberation, and many tables had representatives who were involved in substance abuse recovery programs. Many of these individuals offered examples of how more recovery facilities, including different types, were needed to address the problem of substance abuse in the community (Table K). Participants relied on the rhetorical strategy of using personal, lived experiences to situate their desire to create community change, and specifically structural changes such as written breastfeeding policies or recovery programs.

Collective agency *is* empowerment. Both public deliberations had examples of collective agency, specifically through empowering *others'* rhetorical agency. Collective agency is the interaction between one's own agency and assisting others to realize their own agency (Campbell, 2005). At the Brookings event, three tables discussed enabling women to enact their individual agency in asking for breastfeeding support from their supervisors, to "empower mothers to find their voice" (Participant 2, Table 10), or to learn *how* to talk about their needs for breastfeeding support when they return to work. At the Montgomery County event, tables discussed the need to "empower people who care" (Table C) to enact their agency through various roles. Table I stressed the need for the newspaper to highlight community awareness, later suggesting that a key action would be to "publish statistics" to "enhance community" awareness. Similarly, a participant (Table 6) from the breastfeeding public deliberation commented that improving breastfeeding mothers' individual agency "could have a community-wide benefit." At both, the collective interactions of participants (Campbell, 2005; Hanchey, 2016) engaged rhetorical agency as a form to encourage the empowerment of individual agency as a means to cultivating broader, collective agency in the community.

Collective agency occurs through social networks (Campbell, 2005; Geisler, 2004; Greene, 2004), when community citizens work together. At the Brookings event, participants highlighted two examples of collaborative breastfeeding support in the community: a community mothers' group and a breastfeeding support group. Both groups use collective agency to provide breastfeeding support to local mothers. Four tables mentioned how the mother's group provides a breastfeeding tent at an annual outdoor community festival. Seven tables talked about a weekly community breastfeeding support group and that group's Facebook page as resources for information, support, and relationship-building. By drawing upon past experiences with collective agency, participants positioned the issue of breastfeeding as an individual action that can be powerfully affected by others' agency. In contrast to the (often) negative experiences of personal agency (breastfeeding) clashing with structures (workplaces), these examples illustrate how personal agency (breastfeeding) can positively interact with community structures (support groups) who are enacting collective agency (Foss, 2006).

At the Montgomery County event, participants considered *potential* types of collective agency, noting that collaboration across citizens and interested community groups was necessary for certain approaches to the health issue of substance abuse. Table F noted in the reflection period that any solution would "need all sectors of [the] community [to be] involved." Table G wrote that there needed to be a "community" organized effort "against" substance abuse. At Table A, when discussing prevention efforts, the notes explained that "getting people involved makes people invested." Across tables, participants recognized the necessity of collective agency to address the health issue of substance abuse. Enabling citizens to act occurs best through social networks (Geisler, 2004) and through fostering relationships between community members and community groups. One way to foster such relationships is through public deliberation.

Public Deliberation *Is* an Inclusive Space to Engage Complex Public Problems

Public deliberation is expressed as a rhetorical form (Farrell, 1993) that encourages inclusivity and the expression of marginalized voices in both the planning and execution of the event. Additionally, public deliberation is a rhetorical praxis of collectively working through public problems, weighing trade-offs and tensions of diverse approaches (Asen, 2015; Nabatchi, 2012). Our analysis shows that public deliberation *is* a discursive space for collaboratively addressing public problems. Public deliberation alters the discursive landscape by engaging, rather than minimizing, the complexity of public problems through a process of weighing trade-offs and tensions.

Public deliberation *is* inclusive. As part of planning and creating the public deliberations, both research teams prioritized creating rhetorical spaces that would encourage voices from a variety of publics, including marginalized voices as well as those with power through elected office or agency status. For both public deliberation events, teams of academics trained in public deliberation produced the issue guides that were guided by local voices from focus groups and interviews (Drury, 2015; Kuehl et al., 2014). In Brookings, participants valued that the deliberation guide allowed them to hear from breastfeeding, working mothers who often feel unable to speak out against their employers' practices or policies. For an issue like breastfeeding that "is something that isn't talked about enough" (Table 9), it was important to participants that the deliberation guide and event "foster public conversations about breastfeeding" (Table 8). The process of designing public deliberations on a health issue involves collecting and amplifying the voices of those most significantly affected, bringing their perspectives to the table and inviting a broader public to consider and understand their views.

In Montgomery County, the issue framing encouraged diverse stakeholders to deliberate different perspectives. In addition to the issue guide based on local perspectives, the team also created a short video featuring prominent community leaders sharing their experiences. Shown at the beginning of the event, the video demonstrated that the issue was being defined by the local community—rather than a state or national agency—and worked to suggest that localized experiences would be valued in the conversation (Drury, 2015). After deliberating, many participants noted (in post-event surveys) that they found the inclusiveness to be quite different than any other community effort to address the issue. One participant shared, "In 20+ years of concerns re: addictions and impacts on families, this is the best attendance I have ever seen. Kudos to the organizers for bringing together so many perspectives." Another wrote, "Interesting perspectives from those in recovery; do not have the opportunity to get this view often." Both the design and the enactment of public deliberation in praxis are ways to encourage representation of marginalized voices (Hicks, 2002), which are crucial to having honest, open, public conversations about health issues (Baum et al., 2009).

However, while public deliberation creates a space to discuss and affirm lived, local experiences, it does not dismiss expertise and scientific evidence. Instead, public deliberation works to be inclusive of both perspectives, contextualizing evidence within public experiences (Carman et al., 2018). In Brookings, one reason for holding the public deliberation came from new protections for breastfeeding mothers returning to work, outlined in the Affordable Care Act. Organizers used health and business expertise, particularly *The Business Case for Breastfeeding* (Office on Women's Health, 2014), to offer a researched, fact-based context for the importance of supporting breastfeeding. Similarly, organizers for the Montgomery County event stressed the seriousness of the problem by using county health statistics and testimony from a local addictions counselor. Additionally, some participants at both events were experts in their fields—doctors, nurses, and lactation consultants at the Brookings event, and counselors, educators, and law enforcement at the Montgomery County event. The deliberative processes of framing the issue inclusively and, at the event, encouraging diverse participation encouraged a hybrid, inclusive rhetoric of expertise and lived experience.

Public deliberation *is* working through trade-offs and tensions. Inherent in the design process of public deliberation is recognizing the public concern as a "wicked problem" (Rittel & Webber, 1973, p. 160), a term that signifies a complex, public problem with many stakeholders that is best addressed through a series of actions and management. Efforts to solve such problems often leave citizens feeling frustrated because of their complexity. A key aspect of public deliberation is to encourage citizens to recognize deliberation as a management cycle, acknowledging that every benefit of addressing a "wicked problem" (Rittel & Webber, 1973, p. 160) has a trade-off that must be addressed, minimized, or accepted (Carcasson & Sprain, 2016). Additionally, a deliberative perspective encourages citizens to recognize the *problem* as wicked rather than the *people involved in the issue*. This framing encourages the public to consider various perspectives and parts of the problem rather than focus on differences. Once the public deliberation begins in praxis, community members engage in active consideration of alternatives, often using facilitators to slow the process and encourage participants to work through the difficulties of the complex public problem's trade-offs (Dillard, 2013). In analyzing our deliberative case studies, we observed an important trade-off: focusing on aiding a specific group—breastfeeding mothers or substance abuse addicts or those in recovery—could result in alienating or ignoring other stakeholders.

At the Brookings event, the process encouraged participants to work through how to be inclusive in their solutions. Tables discussed how to minimize a key trade-off: focusing on helping breastfeeding women could exclude others, especially fathers, family members, and those who could not or chose not to breastfeed, for whatever reason. Table 10 noted that it would be important *not* to alienate those who might have to use formula. Table 9 proposed that in order to *not* minimize involvement of all community members, any campaign for breastfeeding support must "show how it is helpful to everybody. . . . to partners, to other children, to business owners, because that's really culture." These lines of discussion recognized that the trade-off of potentially alienating individuals who were not breastfeeding mothers could be minimized through a more inclusive campaign—the inclusive "culture" suggested by the participant. Importantly, the deliberative process made the group slow their reasoning-through of potential actions, resulting in the prioritization of inclusive actions.

At the Montgomery County event, many table notes included questions that acknowledged the tensions of how to begin addressing a complex public problem. One survey noted, "Yes, [it is] a problem that has many levels"; another lamented, "It is a huge problem that needs to be attacked at all the levels to be successful—can be overwhelming." The post-surveys reflected themes from several tables as they wrestled with a temporal trade-off of whether to focus on immediate treatment needs or on prioritizing prevention. Some tables had participants who suggested that, initially, substance abuse begins with a choice and therefore actions should focus on punishment and prevention. Others noted the need to frame addicts as suffering from a disease rather than an individual failure, stressing that the trade-off of treatment was too important to minimize. For example, in the final stage of deliberation, Table D reflected that substance abuse needed to be seen as a disease rather than as an individual failure, which would address the tension of alienating addicts while offering more preventative treatment through education, mental health diagnosis, and general encouragement.

At both events, participants identified tensions within possible actions and then determined ways forward, often suggesting management of trade-offs. This process of collectively wrestling with trade-offs and tensions is critical for public deliberation in praxis. Discussing trade-offs and tensions enhances the public's ability to better understand the complexity of the public problem. These discussions also help a community work toward reasonable management of the issue, ultimately moving the community forward to address the problem (Carcasson & Sprain, 2016).

Health Citizenship *Is* Inclusive through Action

Public deliberation *is* a rhetorical form (Farrell, 1993) that influences the possibilities for health citizenship to emerge for citizens who attended. Inclusion and actions illustrate rhetorical health citizenship *as* a process that involves a negotiation between an individual health citizen and the collective community, including lay and expert knowledge in discussions of actions. At times, health citizenship *is* a process by which health citizens take on various roles; both activist (Zoller, 2005) and advocate (Brown et al., 2004; Zoller, 2005) roles operate within a public deliberation attended by many health citizens who come from a variety of stakeholder perspectives.

Health citizenship *is* inclusive education. At the public deliberations, participants often discussed the importance of education of diverse stakeholders as a means for creating structural changes (e.g., lactation rooms, breastfeeding policies, drug abuse prevention and treatment) that enable individual actions for health citizenship (e.g., combining breastfeeding and work or seeking treatment for substance abuse). By including different stakeholders, participants recognized the agency of health citizens to influence social structures, like workplaces or recovery programs. Thus, participants explicitly noted the social and institutional contexts (Rimal et al., 1997) and social networks (Campbell, 2005) where breastfeeding mothers and those impacted by substance abuse need the most support.

Participants at the Brookings event emphasized that everyone in the community needed to understand the importance of breastfeeding, so that they understand how it affects them (Table 7) and so that breastfeeding mothers are not always expected to initiate actions to increase support (Table 10). Tables discussed the inclusion and education of specific stakeholder groups such as other parents (Table 10), fathers/spouses/partners (Tables 7 and 10), men (Tables 2, 3, and 7), co-workers and other employees (Tables 1, 3, 5, 7, and 10), business leaders (Tables 1 and 2), children and teenagers (Tables 3, 4, 7, and 10), and older generations or grandparents (Table 2). Similarly, at the Montgomery County event, participants stressed the importance of including and educating various stakeholders connected to the community members impacted by substance abuse (Tables A, C, F, and G).

Participants at the Brookings event prioritized actions that expanded the community's understanding and awareness of the issues, reflecting that health citizenship could increase through continued conversations on prevention and treatment. We did not collect specific information about stakeholders at each table, because of the anonymity of the substance abuse deliberation and the contingent nature of participant discussions at the breastfeeding deliberation. For example, some people moved to different tables as a result of condensing tables or came and went due to breastfeeding their babies during the deliberation. However, given the variety of different types of stakeholders explicitly mentioned at the breastfeeding deliberation noted above, and the qualitative comments that emphasized multiple stakeholders at the substance abuse deliberation, we see inclusive education *as* an important component in these discussions about health citizenship across both community contexts.

Health citizenship *is* action. At the Brookings event, discussions generated a wide range of actions regarding health citizenship in the community. Tables discussed putting a lactation room in the new university football stadium (Table 5), creating a billboard to promote and normalize breastfeeding (Tables 5, 6, and 7), creating a speaker series to reach multiple stakeholders (Table 6), and developing a breastfeeding app (Table 10) with locations friendly to breastfeeding. The university football stadium has added a lactation room since the public deliberation. The execution of specific actions from the public deliberation shows the dynamic relationship between the health citizen and the larger system (Rimal et al., 1997), or business community.

One tangible action that developed across nine tables at the Brookings event was having "breastfeeding-friendly businesses" that publicly display a breastfeeding symbol indicating that breastfeeding customers and employees will be accommodated. Six months after the public deliberation, the South Dakota Department of Health (SDDOH) contacted Kuehl and Anderson to discuss collaborating on community breastfeeding support. Stakeholders agreed on a breastfeeding-friendly business initiative, which aligned with two of the prioritized actions from the public deliberation: securing breastfeeding employer support and changing breastfeeding culture. Over 100 Brookings businesses are now "breastfeeding-friendly," meaning they have pledged to provide breastfeeding support to employees and customers (SDDOH, 2017). The initiative has spread to other communities across the state. This action specifically constitutes health advocacy rather than health activism (Zoller, 2005), in that faculty, students, community members, breastfeeding mothers, health-care providers, and business representatives worked together to collaborate within existing structures, using the resources and connections with the city's Chamber of Commerce and the state health department, to initiate this particular health citizenship action.

At the Montgomery County event, rhetorical agency cultivated by the public deliberation developed into health citizenship through integrating the results of the deliberation into the work of the Drug Free Montgomery County Coalition. Spurred by the deliberation process, the coalition brought together concerned citizens, recovering addicts, health workers, individuals based in community organizations, and others to work together to prevent and treat substance abuse. The coalition continued their work on the issue, using the public deliberation report (Drury & Abbott, 2013) to guide their organization's actions, which later included a second, smaller public deliberation event focused around strategic planning and future action. This lengthy process reflects the so-called cycle of deliberative inquiry of how a community can manage "wicked problems" (Rittel & Webber, 1973, p. 160)—in this case, a massive public health problem—in contrast to seeking out a tangible outcome or concrete solution (Carcasson & Sprain, 2016). Similar to the breastfeeding-friendly business initiative, this coalition is an example of health advocacy (Brown et al., 2004), which draws upon the benefits of working with established community structures and organizations in advocating for health citizenship.

CONCLUSION: RHETORIC *AS* RHETORICAL HEALTH CITIZENSHIP

Our analysis conceptualizes rhetoric *as rhetorical health citizenship*, which brings together rhetorical agency, public deliberation, and health citizenship *as* conceptualized in a way that matches our experiences of how rhetoric *is* in praxis in our communities. Similar to Asen's (2004) labeling of discursive citizenship, we define rhetorical health citizenship as the myriad ways to discursively enact health citizenship through collaborative civic practice. Rhetorical health citizenship highlights the importance of citizens coming together to discuss public health issues: in a way that occurs through public deliberation, which requires rhetorical agency of participants before and after a public deliberation and enacts health citizenship or enables health citizenship for others. Given that citizenship is a "mode of public engagement" (Asen, 2004, p. 191), rhetorical health citizenship allows participants at public deliberations to engage with fellow stakeholders invested in a particular health issue in a way that is collaborative yet also contested, especially in discussing trade-offs of a given "wicked problem" (Carcasson & Sprain, 2016; Rittel & Webber, 1973). This conceptualization highlights multiple public practices, performances, or enactments of citizenship by different, often marginalized groups (Bennett, 2009; Cisneros, 2013; Stillion-Southard, 2011).

Rhetorical health citizenship *is* a practice that engages citizens, public officials, and experts in public deliberation to critically examine social structures and generate collaborative solutions that improve public health. Whereas health citizenship focuses on individual health decision-making (Rimal et al., 1997), often between a patient and provider, *rhetorical* health citizenship is the communicative interaction between individuals and structures, or between individuals and the larger community (Farrell, 1993; Foss, 2006). This dynamic is the fulcrum of the communicative process whereby health citizenship and various public actions are enacted in communities through social networks (Geisler, 2004), across institutional contexts (Rimal et al., 1997), and through a community's management of a complex public problem over time (Carcasson & Sprain, 2016). This deliberative perspective encourages a different perspective on engagement, one focused on long-term engagement and management rather than on single solutions. Rhetorical health citizenship therefore *is* a public praxis, embodied in discursive exchanges in small groups and in a community's social networks, that emphasizes shared decision-making.

Rhetorical health citizenship acknowledges the contradictory positions that participants take on as health activists, health advocates, or health citizens, and sometimes all of these, throughout the deliberative process in enacting their rhetorical agency on a community health issue. Yet, many large-scale actions that emerged from these public deliberations fell into the category of health advocacy rather than health activism, which may disappoint some stakeholders. Health activism requires an "oppositional consciousness" (Zoller, 2005, p. 352), rather than the passionate impartiality that is characteristic of public deliberation (Carcasson & Sprain, 2016), and the willingness to work *with* existing structures to enact change that characterizes health advocacy (Brown et al., 2004). For example, at the Brookings event, participants disagreed over the best location for a permanent breastfeeding support space. Taking the position of a health activist (Zoller, 2005), a participant at Table 3 was adamant that it *not* be affiliated with the local hospital. Our field notes indicated that activists felt that affiliating it with the hospital would over-medicalize breastfeeding and de-emphasize the community-building element.

In contrast to the health activists' position, health advocates (Brown et al., 2004) employed at the local hospital wanted a permanent breastfeeding support space in the hospital, in order to provide accurate information and make medical referrals. Ultimately, the hospital currently operates a breastfeeding support space, staffed with nurses who are certified lactation consultants. This health citizenship action is classified as advocacy that works *within* the existing social structures in the community. Although this is an excellent resource in the community, not everyone was pleased with this action. This demonstrates that even though multiple stakeholders are involved in the deliberation process, outcomes from an event might not have unanimous support.

This chapter demonstrates how rhetoric is useful not only for analyzing pressing public problems but also for creating new public spaces to foster collaborative deliberative rhetoric. Our experiences suggest the importance of working authentically and openly with the community to encourage efficacious rhetorical health citizenship: specifically, partnering with relevant community organizations to foster broad engagement in the public deliberation, recording conversations through table notes and, when possible, audio-recordings, to create a public record; and analyzing the event's data into an event report that is then presented to the public (Drury & Abbott, 2013; Drury et al., 2015). Furthermore, this chapter is an example of how, after the event's conclusion, applied rhetorical criticism (Condit & Bates, 2009) can be used to understand the language strategies across deliberative texts while still producing acts of health citizenship and enabling rhetorical agency across many different stakeholders in our communities through our rhetorical fieldwork (McKinnon et al., 2016).

Because we analyzed two case studies across different health issues of breastfeeding support and substance abuse, our conclusions are limited by local community context and issue. The two health issues were selected for public deliberations because community members approached the authors in the different communities to inquire about assistance with public communication about the issues of substance abuse and breastfeeding support. Despite the different health topics, as noted above, the process of public deliberation was similar (Anderson et al., 2017). Both case studies engaged in the same process of creating a research team (with community-based partners), conducting formative research (through focus groups and interviews with community stakeholders), holding the public deliberation events (through community promotion and engaging diverse stakeholders), and hosting a follow-up community meeting (to engage the most active community members in beginning to take action).

Although the two case studies have significant differences in terms of context, we are encouraged by the interplay of concepts important to rhetorics of health and medicine, and therefore call for additional work applying rhetorical health citizenship to other health issues and geographical or cultural contexts. We can envision a number of health-based "wicked problems" (Rittel & Webber, 1973, p. 160) that would benefit from this approach, including hunger, water quality, and green initiatives. Fostering rhetorical health citizenship encourages communities to address public problems through rhetorical agency, public deliberation, and health citizenship. In praxis, rhetorical health citizenship *is* a collective mode of public engagement that improves the physical and civic health of communities.

REFERENCES

Anderson, J., Kuehl, R. A., Mehltretter Drury, S. A., Tschetter, L., Schwaegerl, M., Yoder, J., . . . & Hildreth, M. (2017). Brookings supports breastfeeding: Using public deliberation as a community-engaged approach to dissemination of research. *Translational Behavioral Medicine, 7*(4), 783–792. https://doi.org/10.1007/s13142-017-0480-6

Asen, R. (2004). A discourse theory of citizenship. *Quarterly Journal of Speech, 90*, 189–211. https://doi.org/10.1080/0033563042000227436

Asen, R. (2015). *Democracy, deliberation, and education.* University Park, PA: Pennsylvania State University Press.

Baum, N. M., Jacobson, P. D., & Goold, S. D. (2009). "Listen to the people": Public deliberation about social distancing measures in a pandemic. *American Journal of Bioethics, 9*(11), 4–14. https://doi.org/10.1080/15265160903197531

Bennett, J. A. (2009). *Banning queer blood: Rhetorics of citizenship, contagion, and resistance.* Tuscaloosa, AL: University of Alabama Press.

Brown, P., Zavestoski, S., McCormick, S., Mayer, B., Morello-Frosch, R., & Altman, R. (2004). Embodied health movements: New approaches to social movements in health. *Sociology of Health & Illness, 26*, 50–80. https://doi.org/10.1111/j.1467-9566.2004.00378.x

Campbell, K. K. (2005). Agency: Promiscuous and protean. *Communication and Critical/Cultural Studies, 2*, 1–19. https://doi.org/10.1080/1479142042000332134

Carcasson, M., & Sprain, L. (2016). Beyond problem-solving: Reconceptualizing the work of public deliberation as deliberative inquiry. *Communication Theory, 26*, 41–63. https://doi.org/10.1111/comt.12055

Carman, K. L., Maurer, M., Mallery, C., Wang, G., Garfinkel, S., Richmond, J., . . . Fratto, A. (2014/2018). *Community forum deliberative methods demonstration: Evaluating effectiveness and eliciting public views of use of evidence* (AHRQ Publication No. 14(15)-EHC007-EF). Rockville, MD: Agency for Healthcare Research and Quality. https://doi.org/10.2139/ssrn.3123559

Cisneros, J. D. (2013). *The border crossed us: Rhetorics of borders, citizenship, and Latina/o identity.* Tuscaloosa, AL: University of Alabama Press.

Condit, C. M., & Bates, B. R. (2009). Rhetorical methods of applied communication scholarship. In L. R. Frey & K. N. Cissna (Eds.), *Routledge handbook of applied communication research* (pp. 106–128). New York, NY: Routledge.

Cooper, M. M. (2011). Rhetorical agency as emergent and enacted. *College Composition and Communication, 62*, 420–449. Retrieved from http://www.jstor.org/stable/27917907

Dillard, K. N. (2013). Envisioning the role of facilitation in public deliberation. *Journal of Applied Communication Research, 41*, 217–235. https://doi.org/10.1080/00909882.2013.826813

Drury, S. (2015, August 1). *Community conversation on substance abuse, 2013* [Blog post]. Retrieved from http://blog.wabash.edu/wabashdpd/2015/08/01/final-report-substance-2013/

Drury, S. A. M., & Abbott, J. Y. (2013, December). *Community conversation on substance abuse in Montgomery County: November 6 public deliberation report.* Retrieved from http://blog.wabash.edu/wabashdpd/wp-content/uploads/sites/21/2015/10/Nov6Report_Final.pdf

Drury, S. A. M., Kuehl, R. A., & Anderson, J. (2015). *Report on the community conversation on breastfeeding in Brookings businesses. Communication Studies Publications, 13*. Retrieved from http://openprairie.sdstate.edu/comm-theatre_pubs/13/

Endres, D., Hess, A., Senda-Cook, S., & Middleton, M. K. (2016). *In situ* rhetoric: Intersections between qualitative inquiry, fieldwork, and rhetoric. *Cultural Studies Critical Methodologies, 16*(6), 511–524. https://doi.org/10.1177/1532708616655820

Ewalt, J. P. (2016). The agency of the spatial. *Women's Studies in Communication, 39*, 137–140. https://doi.org/10.1080/07491409.2016.1176788

Farrell, T. B. (1993). *Norms of rhetorical culture*. New Haven, CT: Yale University Press.

Foss, S. K. (2006). Interdisciplinary perspectives on rhetorical criticism: Rhetorical criticism as synecdoche for agency. *Rhetoric Review, 25*, 375–379. https://www.jstor.org/stable/20176742

Geisler, C. (2004). How ought we to understand the concept of rhetorical agency? Report from the ARS. *Rhetoric Society Quarterly, 34*, 9–17. https://doi.org/10.1080/02773940409391286

Geisler, C. (2005). Teaching the post-modern rhetor: Continuing the conversation on rhetorical agency. *Rhetoric Society Quarterly, 35*, 107–113. https://doi.org/10.1080/02773940509391324

Greene, R. W. (2004). Rhetoric and capitalism: Rhetorical agency as communicative labor. *Philosophy and Rhetoric, 37*, 188–206. https://www.jstor.org/stable/40238183

Hanchey, J. N. (2016). Agency beyond agents: Aid campaigns in sub-Saharan Africa and collective representations of agency. *Communication, Culture & Critique, 9*, 11–29. https://doi.org/10.1111/cccr.12130

Hauser, G. A., & Benoit-Barne, C. (2002). Reflections on rhetoric, deliberative democracy, civil society, and trust. *Rhetoric & Public Affairs, 5*(2), 261–275. https://doi.org/10.1353/rap.2002.0029

Hicks, D. (2002). The promise(s) of deliberative democracy. *Rhetoric & Public Affairs, 5*, 223–260. https://doi.org/10.1353/rap.2002.0030

Jansen, T. (2016). Who is talking? Some remarks on nonhuman agency in communication. *Communication Theory, 26*, 255–272. https://doi.org/10.1111/comt.12095

Kuehl, R. A., Anderson, J., Drury, S. A. M., Bachman, C., Hildreth, M., Lamp, J., . . . & Yoder, J. (2014). *Community conversation guide: How can our community support the breastfeeding experience in Brookings Businesses*. Communication Studies Publications, 12. Retrieved from http://openprairie.sdstate.edu/comm-theatre_pubs/12/

McKinnon, S. L., Asen, R., Chavez, K. R., & Howard, R. G. (2016). *text + field: Innovations in rhetorical method*. University Park, PA: Pennsylvania State University Press.

Middleton, M., Hess, A., Endres, D., & Senda-Cook, S. (2015). *Participatory critical rhetoric: Theoretical and methodological foundations for studying rhetoric in situ*. Lanham, MD: Lexington Books.

Miller, C. R., Walsh, L., Wynn, J., Kelly, A. R., Walker, K. C., White, W. J., & Winderman, E. (2016). The great chain of being: Manifesto on the problem of agency in science communication. *POROI: Project on Rhetoric of Inquiry, 12*(1), Article 2. https://doi.org/10.13008/2151-2957.1246

Nabatchi, T. (2012). An introduction to deliberative civic engagement. In T. Nabatchi, J. Gastil, G. M. Weiksner, & M. Leighninger (Eds.), *Democracy in motion: Evaluating the practice and impact of deliberative civic engagement* (pp. 3–18). New York, NY: Oxford University Press.

Office on Women's Health, US Department of Health and Human Services. (2014). *Business case for breastfeeding*. Retrieved from https://www.womenshealth.gov/breastfeeding/business-case-for-breastfeeding.html

Rimal, R. N., Ratzan, S. C., Arntson, P., & Freimuth, V. S. (1997). Reconceptualizing the "patient": Health care promotion as increasing citizens' decision-making competencies. *Health Communication, 9*(1), 61–74. https://doi.org/10.1207/s15327027hc0901_5

Rittel, H. W. J., & Webber, M. M. (1973). Dilemmas in a general theory of planning. *Policy Sciences, 4*, 155–169. https://doi.org/10.1007/BF01405730

South Dakota Department of Health. (2017). *Become a breastfeeding-friendly business.* Retrieved from http://healthysd.gov/category/breastfeeding+workplace/?tag=breastfeeding-friendly-businesses

Stillion-Southard, B. A. (2011). *Militant citizenship: Rhetorical strategies of the National Woman's Party, 1913–1920.* College Station, TX: Texas A&M University Press.

Zoller, H. M. (2005). Health activism: Communication theory and action for social change. *Communication Theory, 15*(4), 341–364. https://doi.org/10.1111/j.1468-2885.2005.tb00339.x

CHAPTER 8

Challenging Racial Disparities in and through Public Health Campaigns

The Advocacy of Social Justice

JENNIFER HELENE MAHER

1. Everyone has the right to a standard of living adequate for the health and well-being of himself and of his family, including food, clothing, housing and medical care and necessary social services, and the right to security in the event of unemployment, sickness, disability, widowhood, old age or other lack of livelihood in circumstances beyond his control.
2. Motherhood and childhood are entitled to special care and assistance. All children, whether born in or out of wedlock, shall enjoy the same social protection.

—Article 25, Universal Declaration of Human Rights

ON DECEMBER 10, 1948, the General Assembly of the United Nations adopted the Universal Declaration of Human Rights, which, according to the opening lines of its preamble, affirmed that "the inherent dignity and of the inalienable rights of all members of the human family is the foundation of freedom, justice and peace in the world." Among the inalienable rights identified in the declaration was access to quality medical care. Since then, progress in global health has led to the elimination of smallpox and the near eradication of polio. And global health initiatives continue to work toward decreasing infection and mortality rates related to diseases like malaria and HIV/AIDS. The effect of these initiatives has resulted in both a decreased infant mortality rate and increased life expectancy. Between the periods 1950–55 and 2010–15, the infant mortality rate, meaning the rate of death among children under one year of age, decreased worldwide from 142 deaths per 1,000 to 36 deaths per 1,000 (Population Division, United Nations, 2015). During the same periods, life expectancy increased globally from 46.81 to 70.47 years. As health policy experts Daniels, Donilon, and Bollyky (2014) summed up, "It is easy to be discouraged about the state of international cooperation today, but global health remains an area in which the world has come together to do significant good."

Despite progress in global health, disparities in care and outcomes continue often as a result of social injustice that, according to Levy and Sidel (2013), "creates conditions that adversely affect the health of individuals and communities" (p. 6). For instance, according to the World Health Organization's 2013 *World Health Statistics,* the life expectancy in Chad was forty-four years; in Japan, seventy-nine years. While the economic disparities between a poor country like Chad and a wealthy country like Japan offer obvious reasons for this difference in life expectancy, other sociocultural factors that can include gender, disability, age, race, ethnicity, or sexual orientation also create disparities in life expectancy and health outcomes; and these disparities are by no means limited to country-to-country comparisons. Disparities related to racism and ethnic prejudice in the US affect attention to and treatment of a whole range of conditions that include, but are by no means limited to, mental health, cancer, and addiction (Chin, Walters, Cook, & Huang, 2013; LaVeist & Isaac, 2013; US Department of Health and Human Services, 2015). While a contributing factor to a shortened life expectancy that, in 2014, was 75.2 years for the non-Hispanic black population and 78.8 years for the non-Hispanic white population (Hamilton et al., 2015), according to the Centers for Disease Control and Prevention (CDC), racial disparities actually begin before birth. For example, in 2012, 13 percent of babies born to non-Hispanic black mothers had low birth weights, in contrast to 7 percent of babies born to non-Hispanic white mothers.

At birth, disparities only continue. In 2013 the mortality rate for non-Hispanic black infants was 11.11 per 1,000 live births; the mortality rate of non-Hispanic white infants during the same period was 5.06 (Matthews, MacDorman, & Thoma, 2015). Even among sudden unexplained infant deaths (SUID), which includes sudden infant death syndrome (SIDS), the rate of death among non-Hispanic white infants (84.4/100,000) more than doubled among non-Hispanic black (171.8) and American Indians / Alaskan Natives (190.5), according to the CDC. In sum, racial and ethnic disparities in health care persist from the womb to the tomb as a form of social injustice.

Martin Luther King Jr. remarked in 1966, "Of all the forms of inequality, injustice in health is the most shocking and the most inhuman because it often results in physical death" (Associated Press). For Dr. King, the answer then, as it is now, was "direct action and creative nonviolence to raise the consciousness of the nation." Imperative to action and consciousness-raising in the pursuit of social justice is the rhetorical activity of advocacy, which the World Health Organization (WHO) has identified as one of three prerequisites for improving health. In the context of advocacy, the rhetoric of health and medicine *as* social justice aims to bring awareness to the causes and effects of racial and ethnic disparities, among other social and economic injustices, in health care and to transform the materializations of these injustices in everyday life in order to bring about health equity. At a broader level, this means revealing what Swartz (2012) described as the ways in which "the systemic manipulations of culture" in the realms of health and medicine have permitted and reproduced not only unequal health-care conditions for marginalized races and ethnicities but also physical abuses that have included forced sterilization and experimentation (Brandt, 1978; Richardson, 2013; Roberts, 1997; Secundy, Dula, & Williams, 2000; Washington, 2006), which together have created distrust of health-care professionals, especially in African American communities (Armstrong, Ravenell, McMurphy, & Putt, 2007; Brandon, Isaac, & LaVeist, 2013; Braunstein et al., 2008; Jacobs et al., 2006).

As complement to the rhetoric of health and medicine *as* social justice, the rhetoric of health and medicine *is* social justice seeks to intervene in ways that seek not only to challenge these conditions through which the "health gap" (Byrd & Clayton, 2002; Marmot, 2015) persists but also to improve the lived experiences of those subject to these disparities. But to do so demands that researchers in the rhetoric of health and medicine identify, challenge, and work to transform the materiality of injustice at the local level (Agboka, 2013; Lawrence, Hausman, & Dannenberg, 2014; Sequist & Schneider, 2006; Zoller & Melonçon, 2013). To illustrate the rhetoric of health and medicine *as/is* social justice, I first discuss the relationship between social justice, health advocacy, and race, and second analyze two public health campaigns that sought to lower infant mortality rates due to SIDS in order to illustrate the importance of locally grounded public health campaigns in addressing racial disparities.

SOCIAL JUSTICE ADVOCACY

What does it mean to advocate for social justice in health and medicine? As a rhetorical endeavor, social justice advocacy deals in what is probable, rather than what is true. As Aristotle (1984c) explained, unlike in matters that "cannot now or in the future be, other than they are," rhetoric is a matter of persuasion, dealing with that which can be otherwise (1356a 24). In a realm defined by empirical evidence, the rhetoric of health and medicine *as* social justice may seem an unnecessary distraction inasmuch as certain principles attesting to the importance of health, as in the Universal Declaration of Human Rights, may suffice. Although such declarations crystallize those fundamental rights that all human beings ought to be entitled to, this kind of essentializing does not readily provide theoretical landscapes or practical pathways by which to help ensure that these rights are materialized in lived experience. Theorizing and applying the rhetoric of health and medicine *as/is* social justice seeks to do just that.

Foregrounding the rhetoric of health and medicine *as* social justice is not without challenges, however. Foege (2013) explained, "Some people argue that 'social justice' is a soft subject, and, therefore, almost unscientific" (xiii). And coupling social justice with rhetoric only compounds the problem for those for whom evidenced-based medicine is the gold standard. But, social injustice is, in fact, readily evident in "hard statistics" (Foege, 2013). Disparities related to racism and ethnic prejudice in the US affect attention to and treatment of conditions including mental health issues (Atdjian & Vega, 2005; Primm et al., 2010; Wells, Klap, Koike, & Sherbourne, 2001), cancer (Bickell et al., 2006; Brawley, 2006; Happe, 2006; Suneja et al., 2014), diabetes (Cowie et al., 1989; Heisler et al., 2003), and diseases of the heart (Ayanian et al., 1993; Schulman et al., 1999). Although improvements have been made in addressing health inequities, they have been at best modest (Benz, Espinosa, Welsh, & Fontes, 2011). More specifically, Hoberman (2012) noted, "The sheer magnitude of the African American health crisis has been documented repeatedly, exhaustively, and—in important ways—fruitlessly" (p. 19). Undoubtedly, a significant reason for the difficulty in improving health with respect to social justice is the confluence of factors that are involved in ways that can be difficult to account for, let alone measure. In light of this, Healthy People 2010, initiated by the US Department of Health and Human Services Office of Disease Prevention and Health Promotion to address racial and ethnic disparities in health care, was revised to account for disparities that Rouse (2016) identified as stemming from other social factors such as income and geography.

However, the challenge of social justice, generally, and in health, specifically, is what makes advocacy all the more salient. As Artz (2012) remarked, "If social justice means securing for humanity the right to all the burdens and benefits of humanity, then working for social justice must also mean we have responsibility to advocate, advance, and secure those rights as democratically, persuasively, and effectively as possible, as soon as possible, in opposition to all existing obstacles" (p. 247). Significant features of social justice advocacy include calling attention to disparities and working to minimize the ways in which those disparities affect people's everyday lives (Jones, 2016; Kreps, 2003, 2005). The Healthy People 2020 initiative states that *health disparities* are present "if a health outcome is seen to a greater or lesser extent between populations." Although not unimportant differences exist among terms like *disparity, inequality,* and *inequity* in health care (Braveman, 2016), social justice is essentially concerned with addressing lack of fairness, stemming from social and economic factors. Whether described in terms of parity, equality, or equity, we might best understand that what is at the heart of these issues in the rhetoric of health and medicine is the pursuit of justice that maximizes the potential for good health for all.

Yet, theories of social justice, including but not limited to health research, are hardly in agreement about what constitutes justice. Without delving into the whole range of these theoretical distinctions and their implications, which would take me too far afield for my aims here (see instead Ruger, 2009, pp. 19–44), I concentrate on two theories that have significantly influenced discussions of health and social justice: Rawls's "justice as fairness" and Aristotle's "human flourishing" (see Daniels, 2008; Ekmekci & Arda, 2015; Majumdar, 1996; Moskop, 1983; Peñaranda, 2015; Peter, 2001; Price, 1985; Rees, 2008; Resnik & Roman, 2007; Ruger, 2004, 2009; Venkatapuram, 2011).

For political theorist Rawls (2001, 2005), equality is one of two essential principles, the other being liberty, that compose fairness in the ideal system of political liberalism. Because a just political system must persist without appeal to religious, philosophical, or moral values, Rawls contended that "justice as fairness" ought to be the elemental foundation upon which what is considered reasonable for a citizenry is built. However, too often, the absence of rights and liberties such as wealth equality and assurance of what he identifies as "basic health care" for all (2005, lvii, 21) results in a system where some experience more freedom and equality and others less. Yet, this does not necessarily mean that health is a "primary good," meaning "the same basic rights, liberties, and opportunities, and the same all-purpose means such as income and wealth" (2005, p. 180). As Rawls explained, justice as fairness "presents itself as a conception of justice that may be shared as a basis of a reasoned, informed, and willing political agreement" (2005, p. 10). Through this conception of justice, a liberal politic is able to generate "overlapping consensus" even among those with not simply competing, but oftentimes, incommensurable moral, philosophical, or religious beliefs. This consensus is made possible by "two principles of justice," which read as follows:

a. Each person has the same indefeasible claim to a fully adequate scheme of equal basic liberties, which scheme is compatible with the same scheme of liberties for all; and

b. Social and economic inequalities are to satisfy two conditions: first, they are to be attached to offices and positions open to all under conditions of fair equality and opportunity; and second, they are to be the greatest benefit of the least-advantaged members of society. (Rawls, 2001, pp. 42–43)

Furthermore, justice as fairness foregrounds the role of a kind of secular morality in a liberal politic. With what Rawls described as "two moral powers," citizens are understood as essentially moral beings who have both "the capacity for a sense of justice and the capacity for a conception of good" (2005, p. 81). Justice as fairness consequently depends upon these moral powers to foster a shared sensibility about what is just and good for citizens.

In Aristotle's conception, justice is a virtue of character, one that is shaped both by education and habit stoked by just laws. Aristotle (1984a) wrote, "We see that all men mean by justice that kind of state which makes people disposed to do what is just and makes them act justly and wish for what is just; and similarly by injustice that state which makes them act unjustly and wish for what is unjust" (1129a9–10). While somewhat ambiguous in this configuration (see Bostock, 2000, pp. 54–58), justice is, in contrast to other virtues such as liberality, courage, and magnanimity, "the greatest of excellences" (Aristotle, 1984a, 1129b28–29) because he "who possesses it can exercise his excellence towards others too and not merely by himself" (Aristotle, 1984a, 1129b32–33). Put another way, "justice . . . is thought to be another's good, because it is related to others; for it does what is advantageous to another" (Aristotle, 1984a, 1130a32–34). But justice in itself is not the ultimate end for Aristotle. Rather, the ultimate end to which all excellences, including the technical and intellectual, are oriented toward, without question, is *eudaimonia,* or "human flourishing." Also defined as *happiness,* but not without problematic connotations, *eudaimonia* as human flourishing signifies the "highest of all goods achievable by action" (Aristotle, 1984a, 1095a15–16). Essential to human flourishing in a way more elemental than most is health, which is why in Aristotle's description of the ideal city-state, even the location must first give consideration to how it fosters health; for, "health—this is a necessity" (Aristotle, 1984b, 1330a36–37).

Differences between Rawls's justice as fairness and Aristotle's human flourishing are many, despite obvious similarities. Most obviously, in health and social justice research, one of the most notable differences is the significance of health. For example, informed by a Rawlsian justice, Daniels (2001) argued, "Our health is affected not simply by the ways with which we can see a doctor—though that surely matters—but also by our social position and the underlying inequality of our society" (p. 21). Consequently, health disparities are a by-product, in many ways, of more insidious and obfuscated injustices. The result of prioritizing health in matters of social justice has therefore resulted in treating the symptom rather than the cause. As Daniels further explained, "Much contemporary discussion about reducing health inequalities by increasing access to medical care misses this point. Of course, we still want that ambulance there, but we should be looking as well to improve social conditions that help to determine the health of societies" (p. 21). But for an Aristotelian-inspired conceptualization like Ruger's, one grounded in readings by Martha Nussbaum's (1992, 2001) and Amartya Sen's (1992, 1999) respective readings of Aristotle's notion of capability, it is the absence of a collective concern for human flourishing that undermines such arguments, as the "Rawlsian project not only did not attempt to define the good life, but was quite skeptical of such an exercise" (Ruger, 2009, p. 36). Ruger (2016) subsequently explained:

> Human flourishing is a morally central aim shared by all persons by virtue of their humanity. Human flourishing captures and incorporates the idea of human capability, what humans are able to do and be and what possibilities they have. Capability includes human agency, an essential human good to be protected and promoted. The ability to direct one's own life, to make one's own choices, is an essential human interest: people flourish by making their own decisions and shaping their own circumstances. Agency includes health agency, the ability to make decisions and choices about one's health. (p. 71)

Whereas health is not a primary good in a Rawlsian conception of social justice, health, in an Aristotelian-inspired understanding of social justice, is an essential good, one upon which all others depend. Because, as Aristotle (1984a) opined, "We deliberate not about ends but about what contributes to ends" (1112b12), only in recognizing health as such an end can deliberations about how to end disparities and maximize health-care quality for all become the focus of health-care social justice.

Despite their respective emphasis on justice, theories such as Rawls's and Aristotle's can leave unrecognized, obfuscate, and even propagate the ways in which work in the name of justice, whether in theory or practice, is not always just and sometimes downright unjust. With Aristotle's defense of the "natural slave" (1984b), this point cannot be made clearer. But, even in a contemporary theorization of justice offered by Rawls, an emphasis on consensus born out of reasonable plurality ignores how justice as fairness is always already compromised by the existence and perpetuation of inequalities that denies to some, to the benefit of others, basic liberties and moral powers. (For more in-depth critiques, see Anderson, 2010; Blum, 2007; Garcia, 1996; Matsuda, 1986; Mills, 2017; Okin, 2005) Consequently, theories of justice in the rhetoric of health and medicine *as* social justice must be complemented, challenged, and even rejected through intersectionality. Defined by Collins and Bilge (2016),

> Intersectionality is a way of understanding and analyzing the complexity in the world, in people, and in human experiences. The events and conditions of social and political life and the self can seldom be understood as shaped by one factor. They are generally shaped by many factors in diverse and mutually influencing ways. When it comes to social inequality, people's lives and the organization of power in a given society are better understood as being shaped not by a single axis of social division, be it race or gender or class, but by many axes that work together and influence each other. Intersectionality as an analytic tool gives people better access to the complexity of the world and of themselves. (p. 2)

In the context of health, intersectionality has helped explain how constructed social categories, such as race, class, and gender, have contributed to health disparities in biomedical research, health-care access, and bioethics (López & Gadsden, 2016; Rogers & Kelly, 2011; Schulz & Mullings, 2006). What can otherwise be overlooked without the rhetoric of health and medicine *as* social justice are the macro-level conditions, what Wall (2008) identified as the "historical legacies and contemporary forces of oppression, domination, and discrimination" that perpetuate healthy inequality. For instance, in a Rawlsian conception of social justice in health, the large-scale social and economic conditions that work across such disparate, national contexts cultivate injustice as a lack of fairness perpetuated through a global, neoliberal politic that negatively affects already socially and economically disadvantaged populations. In an Aristotelian conception, the lack of a committed collective sense that the end of all action must be the human flourishing of all too often serves to accommodate health inequalities, as well as the socioeconomic conditions that perpetuate those inequalities. But without the infusion of intersectionality, invocations of *justice* can mask and perpetuate injustice. Describing the paradox of diversity work, Ahmed (2012) wrote, "Having an institutional aim to make diversity a goal can even be a sign that diversity is *not* an institutional goal" (pp. 22–23). For social justice work to account for, confront, and overcome the same challenge necessitates recognizing and attending to the myriad ways in which *and justice for all* remains a broken promise that can only be fixed by "paying special attention to the needs of those groups that have suffered injustice, and taking action to improve their health" (Wall, 2008, p. 2).

Yet, in many ways, an emphasis on persuasion as praxis (Blundell, 1992; Katz, 1993; Lupton, 1994) in the rhetoric of health and medicine *as* social justice frees us from becoming set too adrift in the abstraction of theory that, while obviously important for conceptualizing social justice and implementing policies, initiatives, and practices that address health disparities, can also make addressing health disparities appear overwhelming, if not futile. But in advocating for social justice in health, the values of justice, morality, and goodness function as a powerful kind of proof that can put these values into action regardless of their ultimate cause. As a result of the WHO's First International Conference on Health Promotion held in November 1986, "advocating," in addition to "enabling" and "mediating," was identified as a prerequisite for promoting better health. As outlined in the Ottawa Charter for Health Promotion that resulted from the conference, "Good health is a major resource for social, economic and personal development and an important dimension of quality of life. Political, economic, social, cultural, environmental, behavioural and biological factors can all favour health or be harmful to it. Health promotion action aims at making these conditions favourable through advocacy for health." The practice of health advocacy, as the WHO would later explain in 1998, is "a combination of individual and social actions designed to gain political commitment, policy support, social acceptance and systems support for a particular health goal or programme." Because rhetoric is not only a craft to be put to use but also an ethical endeavor (Aristotle, 1984c; Katz, 1992), advocacy in the pursuit of social justice can work to cut through these questions of which causes which, in order to make a real difference in the lives of those subject to disparities, whatever the cause or causes. Jones (2016) explained in a broader discussion of social justice that advocates "concerned with the social, economic, and political implications of their work must now consider ways to critique, intervene in, and create communicative practices and texts that positively impact the mediated experiences of individuals" (p. 344). This is the aim when the rhetoric of health and medicine *is* social justice.

SIDS AWARENESS AND PREVENTION

In 1974 the National SIDS Act provided for the first time funding for SIDS programs in each state in the US. In *The "Discovery" of Sudden Infant Death Syndrome*, pediatrician and SIDS awareness advocate Robert Baumiller (1989) recalled efforts made by individuals (including parents and doctors) and organizations such as the American Guild for Infant Survival to draw attention to SIDS as "a major American health problem," one largely unknown to most Americans. Although a number of initiatives such as the Guild's plan to simplify prescribed home infant apnea/cardiac monitoring for high-risk babies was promoted nationwide starting in the late 1970s, SIDS remained largely known only to health-care professionals and those families that had lost a child to SIDS. To illustrate, in the April 1984 issue of the Newport Beach–based lifestyle publication *Orange Coast Magazine,* peppered with ads for "Boudoir Portraiture" and luxury automobiles such as Ferrari and Mercedes, an article entitled "Crib Death: Chasing Down a Thief That Gives No Warning and Leaves No Tracks" described the veil that still shrouded SIDS at the time:

> The morning sun slowly slices through the lacy curtains of a baby's nursery. But each morning 20–30 families in America wake up to become victims of the "silent killer," more commonly known as crib death or SIDS—Sudden Infant Death Syndrome. The cheery and youth-filled room is left quiet, the crib is left still, the family is left shattered. Because death comes so suddenly and silently, and because these innocent babies have had little time to become known outside their own family, the general public is unaware that this dilemma exits. Nor do these infants linger in a handicapped or suffering condition to enlist society's sympathy and help. (Lentz, 1984, pp. 43–44)

Even among such an economically privileged readership, SIDS remained a largely unknown phenomenon.

Defined as "the sudden death of an infant under one year of which, which remains unexplained after a thorough case investigation, including performance of a complete autopsy, examination of the death scene, and review of the clinical history" (Willinger, James, & Catz, 1991, p. 678), infant mortality rates due to SIDS have declined by more than 50 percent since 1988. A significant reason for this decline is the national health campaign Back to Sleep, initiated by partners that included the National Institutes of Child Health and Human Development, the Association of SIDS and Infant Mortality Programs, and the American Academy of Pediatrics (AAP). In 1992 the AAP recommended placing infants on their side (lateral) or back (supine) for sleep rather than on their stomach (prone), later amending this recommendation to back only. To disseminate this recommendation, as well as others subsequently made, the national health campaign Back to Sleep launched in 1994 and used communication outlets and mediums that included health-care professionals, professional journals such as *Pediatrics,* medical settings, and print articles and advertisements such as in parent and infant-caregiver-oriented publications like *Parents Magazine* and its related publications. In 1996, for instance, a "PARENTS' ALERT" in *Parents' Magazine's It Worked For Me! From Thumbsucking to Schoolyard* reiterated information from the Back to Sleep campaign:

Each year more than 6,000 babies in the United States die of sudden infant death syndrome (SIDS). To reduce the number of babies who fall victim to SIDS, the U.S. Public Health Service and the American Academy of Pediatrics (AAP) are urging that healthy babies—even those who can turn over on their own—be put to sleep on their backs or sides. Many parents place their baby face down, believing that if an infant is laid on his back he may choke if he spits up. But research links the prone position to SIDS, the leading cause of death during the first year of life. (Researchers suspect that infants who sleep face down may breathe their own expired air and suffocate particularly if they are placed on a soft surface.) "Keep your baby's crib free of soft pillows, comforters, sheepskins and other soft objects that can trap gas," advises John Kattwinkel, M.D., chairman of the AAP task force on SIDS. "Ideally, your baby should sleep on a standard infant mattress covered by a sheet." For the free brochure "Reducing the Risk of Sudden Infant Death Syndrome: What You Can Do" and a crib sticker that reminds caretakers of the proper sleep position, call 800-505-CRIB. (Murphy, 1997, p. 33)

So successful was the Back to Sleep campaign, renamed in 2012 Safe to Sleep in order to "expand the campaign to emphasize its continued focus on safe sleep environments and back sleeping as ways to reduce the risk of SIDS and other sleep-related causes of infant death" (National Institutes of Health, n.d.), that infant mortality due to SIDS had been almost halved in the US by 2009.

Yet, "one-size-fits-all health promotion, health campaigns, health services or even statistical approaches to health data" have proved problematic (Mays, Ponce, Washington, & Cochran, 2003), with many noting that public health campaigns often fail to reach those populations most in need of the information (Backer, Rogers, & Sopory, 1992; Bennett; Benz, Espinosa, Welsh, & Fontes, 2011; Kreps, 2005; Kwate, 2014; Mays et al., 2003). Despite the significant decrease in SIDS-related deaths nationwide, the national SIDS awareness campaign had significantly less impact in large urban areas with a sizable black population, which is disproportionately affected by SIDS. In 2009, for example, the city of Baltimore had the fourth-worst infant mortality rate in the US, with 12.1 deaths per 1,000 live births; the national rate was 6.9 deaths (Maryland Department of Health and Mental Hygiene, 2010). And the rate for Baltimore's non-Hispanic black population was 14.3 deaths per 1,000 live births; among the non-Hispanic white population, the rate was 7.3. Just as was the case nationally for infants one month to one year of age, the leading cause of death, regardless of race, was SIDS, which is also the leading cause of death in the broader category of SUID that includes deaths due to unknown cause and accidental suffocation and strangulation in bed (CDC, 2019). As is the case nationally, SIDS remained the leading cause of death of among infants one to twelve months old (CDC, 2017). However, unlike nationally, the number of SIDS/SUID cases had routinely increased in Baltimore, with a decade-long high of twenty-seven deaths occurring in 2009. Of these deaths, the rate among Baltimore's black population was more than twice that of its non-Hispanic white population.

Although celebrated as a national health campaign that generated significant success in reducing the number of SIDS-related deaths nationwide, Back to Sleep was less successful in addressing the racial disparities that existed in SID/SUID mortality rates. To address these disparities, the Baltimore City Health Department and its partner organizations, which include the Family League of Baltimore City and the Johns Hopkins Bloomberg School of Public Health, implemented in 2010 the B'More for Healthy Babies initiative, which included a campaign to reduce infant mortality due to SIDS/SUID. Having lost 30 percent of its population from 1970 to 2000, for reasons that include deindustrialization and white flight, Baltimore has a population of 621,849, according to the US Census Bureau (2015). Of this population, 62.0 percent are black, 31.7 percent are white, 4.8 percent are Hispanic or Latino, and 2.8 percent are Asian. Located in the wealthiest state in the country, with a median household income of $74,551 and poverty rate of 9.7 percent, Baltimore, in contrast, has a median household income of $42,241 and a poverty rate of 22.7 percent. The overall poverty rate for the US in the same year was 13.5 percent. Through a confluence of factors that contribute to disparities in Baltimore, including education and neighborhood location, in addition to race and income, no other population experiences health disparities in Baltimore to a greater degree than African Americans, including those less than one year in age.

Using the slogan—SLEEP SAFE. Alone. Back. Crib. NO EXCEPTIONS— the Baltimore campaign to raise awareness among city residents about SIDS and to provide education about ways to reduce the risks has used mass media campaigns, community outreach, door hangers, and even safe sleep prescriptions to spread its message. Because of the importance of tailoring both message and medium to underrepresented groups, a rhetorical strategy that is particularly important in addressing racial disparities in health (Campbell & Quintiliani, 2006; Freimuth & Quinn, 2004; Hawkins et al. 2008), outdoor outlets for the SLEEP SAFE media campaign used not only billboards but also posters placed in bus shelters in recognition of the significant role that mass transits plays in urban communities, especially among the poor and working class.

In addition to radio spots, nonprint mediums included testimonial videos of Baltimore mothers who had lost children to SIDS. These videos play on maternity units in eight Baltimore hospitals, in community centers, and at Women, Infant, & Children sites. In a public service announcement (PSA) video, produced by B'More for Healthy Babies, Mission Films, and the Johns Hopkins Bloomberg School of Public Health Center for Communication Program, Baltimore mothers Ayanna Williams, Dearea Matthews, and Lottie Plumley speak about the loss of their children to SIDS:

AYANNA: I am Ayanna Williams. I have one daughter. She is twelve years old. And I had a younger son. He would have been eleven months old. [Her baby's picture appears on-screen.] His name is Brandon Lawson.

DEAREA: My name is Dearea, and I live in the northern part of Baltimore. I have husband, three children—a four-year-old, his name is Eugene. I have a one-year-old; her name is Saniya. [Her baby's picture appears on-screen.] And I had a baby boy. His name was Charlie.

LOTTIE: My name is Lottie Plumley. My son was born in Baltimore, Maryland on [Crib with picture of her baby appears on-screen.] November 12, 2009. My son's name was William Woodward.

AYANNA: I basically got a phone call from another family member that was living in the house that the ambulance was at the home trying to resuscitate the baby and that they were rushing him to Hopkins. [Picture of their bed appears on-screen.] He was not in his crib. He was in the bed, in our bed.

LOTTIE: When I woke up at 4:30, he was gone. We had found him dead [Lottie and her baby's father sitting on their bed staring at the crib against the wall appear on the screen] in the middle of our bed.

DEAREA: On December 29, Charlie passed away. He turned a month that day. [Charlie's picture appears on-screen.] And that morning, he was in the bed with us. And when I woke up and looked over at him, he just wasn't breathing. [Dearea appears back on-screen.] If I had a chance to go back to December 29, knowing what I know now, I probably would have changed a lot of things.

The video continues with Ayanna, Dearea, and Lottie, as well as other women, sharing statistics related to SIDS, factors that contribute to SIDS death, and measures for preventing SIDS:

SOFIA: I have a seven-month-old baby, and I learned when I went to his doctor for his first appointment that all the babies need to sleep safe. That means alone, no parents, no brothers or sisters, on his back, not on his tummy, and in the crib. That means that in the crib they don't need any bumpers or pillows or blankets, any teddy bears, no exceptions.

DEAREA: For you to be asleep with that baby. I don't think that's a good idea. I don't think that's worth the child's life. Research shows that babies who sleep with a parent are three times more likely to die than babies who sleep alone in a crib. Every month an average of two babies, less than a year old, die in Baltimore city. These are preventable deaths.

HOUSTON: I'm Dr. Avril Melissa Houston. I'm a pediatrician working for the Baltimore City Health Department, and I'm a mother of twins. It is so important that babies are put to bed alone, on their back and in a crib. When we go to sleep at night, we toss, we turn. And the little babies, they're not strong enough to kick back and say, "I'm still here. Don't roll on me." And so that's how a lot of infants end up dying.

LOTTIE: You could possibly roll over the baby. Um, your arm or the brothers or sisters could, you know, put their arms on the windpipe and could suffocate. Or the baby could possibly roll over to the side and not be able to get any air.

Because a multigenerational influence is particularly strong in black, urban areas (Sharkey, 2008), Dearea also directly addresses the importance of parents asserting themselves in order to ensure that their infants are put to sleep according to SIDS prevention guidelines:

DEAREA: I know a lot of times older people do things the way that they did it when they were, you know, raising their children. And you know sometimes kind of have to let them know this is how I want my baby to sleep or you know this is where I want him to sleep. This is what I prefer for him or her. You know. It's your baby. You have to let them know what you want for your baby. You know. At the end, if something was to happen, you have to live with it, not them. You can never replace that child that you lost. Ever. And you'll never ever forget it. Something you have to live with every single day. To wake up and your arms be empty. Or, you know, your home is missing a child. Or, you'll never be able to have grandchildren from that one child. It's something you, you can never change it.

For Dearea, who was also featured in a flyer that was placed throughout the city, the use of Baltimore mothers who had lost babies to SIDS in the SLEEP SAFE campaign was incredibly important. As she explained, "I would have listened if it was a real mother talking" (Cohen, 2010). In telling their stories as Baltimore mothers to Baltimore mothers, this diverse group of women were able to sponsor health literacy in ways not possible with or imagined by the national Back to Sleep campaign.

In addition to hospitals and mother-and-child facilities, SLEEP SAFE videos also played in the waiting room of the Department of Corrections' Central Booking & Intake Center. Given the mass incarceration of black men in the US, in nothing short of what Alexander (2010) identified as a "racial caste system," it is hardly surprising that a disproportionate number of black men are jailed in Baltimore. According to the Justice Policy Institute and Prison Policy Initiative (2015), "While 1 out of 10 Maryland residents is from Baltimore, *one out of three* Maryland residents in state prison is from the city. With an incarceration rate three times that of the State of Maryland and the national average, Baltimore is Maryland's epicenter for the use of incarceration." The recognition of this fact made the Central Booking & Intake Center a necessary site by which to share SLEEP SAFE information.

To address that kind of racial residential segregation that fosters racial and ethical disparities in health care (Caldwell et al., 2017; Williams & Collins, 2001) within the city, door-to-door education also took place in neighborhoods with high infant mortality rates. The neighborhood of Patterson Park is a high-incarceration community, meaning that it is one of the twenty-five Baltimore communities that account for 75 percent of the city's prison inmates (Justice Policy Institute and Prison Policy Initiative, 2015). Predominately poor and black, the northwest edge of the neighborhood is a mere 0.3 miles from the internationally renowned Johns Hopkins Hospital. And in 2013 the campaign more obviously reached out to men with videos featuring Baltimore fathers, who had learned about safe sleep habits. In one PSA, Baltimore father Antoine Dow encouraged men to become "SLEEP SAFE ambassadors because the more that know the more children we can save." To illustrate how such advocacy can work, Dow recounted how he shares information at his neighborhood business, Cutt Styles Unisex Barbershop. "We talk about everything in the shop," Dow explained. "Bad sleep habits are a learned behavior . . . General information you share with someone can save a child's life. Because just one child is too many." Thus, SLEEP SAFE became a campaign not only for SIDS/SUID awareness but for health literacy and advocacy by and for community members.

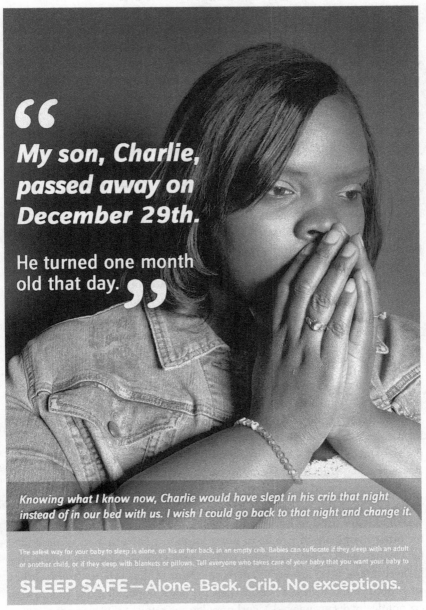

Baltimore Mother Dearea Matthews in Back to Sleep Campaign
Advertisement. Credit: B'More for Healthy Babies.

THE INTERSECTIONAL LENS

Since the start of SLEEP SAFE, instances of SIDS/SUID have dropped in Baltimore from twenty-seven in 2009 to thirteen, which has contributed to a decline in the city's infant mortality rate from 13.5 deaths per 1,000 live births to 8.4 during the same period. Motivated to reduce the rate of SIDS/SUID in Baltimore, this locally grown campaign engaged in advocacy that was tailored to a population that had been otherwise left behind by the national Back to Sleep campaign. As an example of the rhetoric of health and medicine *is* social justice, SLEEP SAFE necessarily cuts through differences between varying theories of justice. After all, such theoretical distinctions, while important, can matter little when lives are at stake. But social justice can certainly be seen to propel the work of SLEEP SAFE in that it recognizes and responds locally to the effect of conditions that materialized a stagnant, or, in some years, higher rate of SIDS/SUID in Baltimore, even while most other parts of the county benefited from a more than 50 percent reduction.

Yet, the SLEEP SAFE campaign must not be confused with speaking directly to the conditions that made Baltimore rates of SIDS/SUID among the non-Hispanic black population disproportionately higher in the first place. Even with SLEEP SAFE and the resulting reduction in infant mortality rates across black and white populations in the city, the SIDS/SIUD percentage among live births remained more than five times that for the non-Hispanic black population (82.5) than the non-Hispanic white population (15.8) during the period 2010–14 (Baltimore City Health Department, 2016). Understanding the conditions that create such disparity necessitates a broader, theoretical understanding of the social injustice that marginalized peoples face beyond local contexts. But, at the same time, attention to the specific ways that disparities and inequalities materialize in specific situations for specific individuals must also be identified and addressed.

An intersectional approach therefore encourages a recognition that, much as Back to Sleep did not speak to many African Americans in urban areas, the specific tactics used in Baltimore's SLEEP SAFE campaign might not work for other marginalized people in other locations. For instance, as described by Tipene-Leach, Abel, Haretuku, and Everard (2000), New Zealand had the highest rate of SIDS among Western countries in the early 1980s. Much like what occurred in Baltimore's non-Hispanic black population, the indigenous, economically disadvantaged Māori population's rate of SIDS was not decreasing at the same rate as that of non-Māori, a fact undoubtedly influenced by government-funded social services in New Zealand. In response to the failed messaging to the Māori people in the otherwise successful 1991 national SIDS prevention campaign, the Māori SIDS Prevention Programme, funded as a national contract with the Public Health Commission, began in 1994 with the appointment of a national coordinator who was also a "Māori woman with a strong background in community development" (Tipene-Leach, Abel, Hare-tuku, & Everard, p. 3). Working with community health providers and indig-enous communities, including Māori families who had lost a child to SIDS, this program "aimed to promote infant wellness by building on their commu-nity's beliefs and behaviours, and by working the SIDS prevention messages into local infant care practices at every opportunity" (p. 4). While a range of issues, including the broadened definition of Māori ethnicity, did not allow for a clear-cut measurement of the SIDS rate in the study, the foreground-ing of Māori culture and its communities encouraged a productive change in practices among parents, medical professionals, and health advocates. Given that, in the US, the rate of SIDS from 2013 to 2015 was twice as high in rural counties than in large urban counties (Ely & Hoyert, 2018, p. 2), the kind of praxis-oriented advocacy demonstrated in both Baltimore City's and New Zea-land's SIDS campaigns offer strategies that can be rhetorically crafted with and to rural communities.

Rhetoric of health and medicine *is* social justice is integral to the goal of improving the lives of those whose lives and health suffer as the result of injustice, in that as praxis it can catalyze transformation in the lives of those who are too often overlooked, ignored, erased by what are successful, even life-saving, health advocacy projects like the national campaign Back to Sleep. What a campaign such as Baltimore's SAFE SLEEP illustrates is how success too often comes at the expense of those who already face inequality and the importance of speaking to and with those populations and individu-als however and wherever they are to ensure, in this case, the most elemental of health needs: the survival of infancy. In this way, the rhetoric of health and medicine *is* social justice becomes the very kind of work that is transformative not only in the lives of individuals but also in our knowledge of the world. As Rogers and Kelly (2011) summarized in their call for intersectionality in the context of biomedical research, "An intersectionality explains the multiple, complex dimensions of inequality and power structures that create roles of domination and subordination under the rubric of race, class, gender, and sexuality. The multiplicative effect of discrimination certainly influences a per-son's health; yet this effect is not typically considered by health researchers" (p. 399). But through a recursivity instantiated in both the *as* and the *is* of the rhetoric of health and medicine *as/is,* social justice advocacy is able to mate-rialize those abstract notions of justice, morality, and goodness not only to reimagine them but also to intervene in the everyday lives of those for whom such notions are too often absent in health care and to continue work toward health equality for all.

REFERENCES

Agboka, G. Y. (2013.) Participatory localization: A social justice approach to navigating unenfranchised/disenfranchised cultural sites. *Technical Communication Quarterly, 22*(1), 28–49.

Ahmed, S. (2012). *On being included: Racism and diversity in institutional life*. Durham, NC: Duke University Press.

Alexander, M. (2010). *The new Jim Crow: Mass incarceration in the age of colorblindness*. New York, NY: New Press.

Anderson, E. (2010). *The imperative of integration*. Princeton, NJ: Princeton University Press.

Anderson, W. (2006). *Colonial pathologies: American tropical medicine, race, and hygiene in the Philippines*. Durham, NC: Duke University Press.

Aristotle. (1984a). *Nicomachean Ethics*. In J. Barnes (Ed.), *The complete works of Aristotle* (Vol. 2, pp. 1729–1867). Princeton, NJ: Princeton University Press.

Aristotle. (1984b). *Politics*. In J. Barnes (Ed.), *The complete works of Aristotle* (Vol. 2, pp. 1986–2129). Princeton, NJ: Princeton University Press.

Aristotle. (1984c). *Rhetoric*. In J. Barnes (Ed.), *The complete works of Aristotle* (Vol. 2, pp. 2152–2269). Princeton, NJ: Princeton University Press.

Armstrong, K., Ravenell, K. L., McMurphy, S., & Putt, M. (2007). Racial/ethnic differences in physician distrust in the United States. *American Journal of Public Health, 97*(7), 1283–1289.

Artz, L. (2012). Conclusion: On the material consequence of defining social justice. In O. Swartz (Ed.), *Social justice and communication scholarship* (pp. 239–248). New York, NY: Routledge.

Associated Press. (1966). King berates medical care given Negroes. *Oskhosh Daily Northwestern*, March 26, p. 22. Retrieved from https://www.newspapers.com/ clip/12049661/ oshkosh-daily-northwestern-32666/

Atdjian, S., & Vega, W. A. (2005). Disparities in mental health treatment in U.S. racial and ethnic minority groups: Implications for psychiatrists. *Psychiatric Services, 56*(12), 1600–1602.

Ayanian J. Z., Udvarhelyi, I. S., Gatsonis, C. A., Pashos, C. L., & Epstein, A. M. (1993). Racial differences in the use of revascularization procedures after coronary angiography. *JAMA, 269*, 2642–2646.

Backer, T. E., Rogers, E. M., & Sopory, P. (1992). *Designing health communication campaigns: What works?* Newbury Park, CA: Sage.

Baltimore City Health Department. (2016). *Profile of maternal and infant characteristics: Baltimore City 2010–2014* [PowerPoint deck]. Retrieved from http://www.healthybabiesbaltimore. com/uploads/files/BirthProfile2010_14_generalpublic_5_7_2016.pdf

Baumiller, R. C. (1989). The discovery of sudden infant death syndrome—Lessons in the practice of political medicine. Seattle, WA: University of Washington Press.

Benz, J. K., Espinosa, O., Welsh, V., & Fontes, A. (2011). Awareness of racial and ethnic health disparities has improved only modestly over a decade. *Health Affairs, 30*(10), 1860–1867.

Bickell, N. A., Wang, J. J., Oluwole, S., Schrag, D., Godfrey, H., Hiotis, K., . . . Guth, A. A. (2006). Missed opportunities: Racial disparities in adjuvant breast cancer treatment. *Journal of Clinical Oncology, 24*(9), 1357–1362.

Blum, L. (2007). Racial virtues. In R. L. Walker & P. J. Ivanhoe (Eds.), *Working virtue: Virtue ethics and contemporary moral problems* (pp. 225–249). New York, NY: Oxford University Press.

Blundell, M. W. (1992). *Ethos* and *dianoia* reconsidered. In A. O. Rorty (Ed.), *Essays on Aristotle's Poetics* (pp. 155–176). Princeton, NJ: Princeton University Press.

B'More for Healthy Babies & the Johns Hopkins Bloomberg School of Public Health Center for Communication Program. (2013). *USA/maternal/child health: Baltimore B'More Babies Safe Sleep Campaign—Safe Sleep PSA for fathers*. Retrieved from https://www.youtube.com/watch?v=F194I4a5CLk

B'More for Healthy Babies, Mission Films, & the Johns Hopkins Bloomberg School of Public Health Center for Communication Program. (2011). *USA/maternal/child health: B'More Babies Safe Sleep Campaign video*. Retrieved from https://www.youtube.com/watch?v=yBBiG6e4xRw

Bostock, D. (2000). *Aristotle's ethics*. Oxford, UK: Oxford University Press.

Brandon, D. T., Isaac, L. A., & LaVeist, T. A. (2013). The legacy of Tuskegee and trust in medical care: Is Tuskegee responsible for race differences in mistrust of medical care? In T. A. LaVeist & L. A. Isaac (Eds.), *Race, ethnicity, and health: A public health reader, 2nd Edition* (pp. 557–568). San Francisco, CA: Jossey-Bass.

Brandt, A. M. (1978). Racism and research: The case of the Tuskegee syphilis study. *Hastings Center Report, 8*(6), 14–24.

Braunstein, J. B., Sherber, N. S., Schulman, S. P., Ding, E. L., & Powe, N. R. (2008). Race, medical researcher distrust, perceived harm, and willingness to participate in cardiovascular trials. *Medicine, 87*(1), 1–9.

Braveman, P. (2016). Health difference, disparity, inequality, or inequity—What difference does it make what we call it? An approach to conceptualizing and measuring health inequalities and health equity. In M. Buchbinder, M. Rivkin-Fish, & R. L. Walker (Eds.), *Understanding health inequalities and justice: New conversation across the disciplines* (pp. 33–63). Chapel Hill, NC: University of North Carolina Press.

Brawley, O. W. (2006). Lung cancer and race: Equal treatment yields equal outcome among equal patients, but there is no equal treatment. *Journal of Clinical Oncology, 24*(3), 332–333.

Byrd, W. M., & Clayton, L. A. (2002). *An American health dilemma: Race, medicine, and health care in the United States, 1900-2000*. New York, NY: Routledge.

Caldwell, J. T., Ford, C. L., Wallace, S. P., Wang, M. C., & Takahashi, L. M. (2017). Racial and ethnic residential segregation and access to health care in rural areas. *Health & Place 43*(1), 104–12.

Campbell, M. K., & Quintiliani, L. M. (2006). Tailored interventions in public health: Where does tailoring fit in interventions to reduce health disparities? *American Behavioral Scientist, 49*(6), 775–793.

Carlisle, S. (2000). Health promotion, advocacy and health inequalities: A conceptual framework. *Public Health & Epidemiology 15*(4), 369–376. Retrieved from http://heapro.oxfordjournals.org/ content/15/4/369.full

Centers for Disease Control and Prevention. (2013). CDC health disparities and inequalities report—United States, 2013. *Morbidity and Mortality Weekly Report, 62*(3). Retrieved from https://www.cdc.gov/mmwr/pdf/other/su6203.pdf

Centers for Disease Control and Prevention. (2017). *Sudden unexpected infant death and sudden infant death syndrome*. Retrieved from https://www.cdc.gov/sids/data.htm

Centers for Disease Control and Prevention. (2019). *Sudden unexpected infant death and sudden infant death syndrome*. Retrieved from https://www.cdc.gov/sids/data.htm

Chapman, E. N., Kaatz, A., & Carnes, M. (2013). Physicians and implicit bias: How doctors may unwittingly perpetuate health care disparities. *Journal of General Internal Medicine 28*(11), 1504–1510.

Chin, M. H., Walters, A. E., Cook, S. C., & Huang, E. (2013). Interventions to reduce racial and ethnic disparities in health care. In T. A. LaVeist & L. A. Isaac (Eds.), *Race, ethnicity, and health* (pp. 761–785). San Francisco, CA: Jossey-Bass.

Cohen, B. E., & Marshall, S. G. (2017). Does public health advocacy seek to redress health inequities? A scoping review. *Health and Social Care in the Community, 25*(2), 309–328.

Cohen, M. (2010). Baltimore to promote safe sleeping practices for babies. *Baltimore Sun,* August 9. Retrieved from http://articles.baltimoresun.com/2010-08-09/health/bs-hs-safe-sleep-campaign-20100809_1_infant-mortality-rate-unsafe-sleeping-practices-sids

Collins, P. H., & Bilge, S. (2016). *Intersectionality.* Malden, MA: Cambridge University Press.

Cowie, C. C., Port, F. K., Wolfe, R. A., Savage, P. J., Moll, P. P., & Hawthorne, V. M. (1989). Disparities in incidence of diabetic end-stage renal disease according to race and type of diabetes. *New England Journal of Medicine, 321,* 1074–1079.

Daniels, M. E. Jr., Donilon, T. E., & Bollyky, T. J. (2014). A new direction for global health. *Project Syndicate,* December 15. Retrieved from https://www.project-syndicate.org/commentary/developing-countries-noncommunicable-disease-increase-by-mitch-daniels-et-al-2014-12

Daniels, N. (2001). Justice, health, and health care. *American Journal of Bioethics, 1*(2), 2–16.

Daniels, N. (2008). *Just health: Meeting health needs fairly.* New York, NY: Cambridge University Press.

Ekmekci, P. E., & Arda, B. (2015). Enhancing John Rawls's theory of justice to cover health and determinants of health. *Acta Bioethica, 21*(2), 227–236.

Ely, D. M., & Hoyert, D. L. (2018). Differences between rural and urban areas in mortality rates for the leading causes of infant death: United States, 2013–2015. U.S. Department of Health and Human Services. Retrieved from https://www.cdc.gov/nchs/data/databriefs/db300/pdf

Enoch, S. (2004). The contagion of difference: Identity, bio-politics and national socialism. *Foucault Studies, 1,* 53–70.

Foege, W. H. (2013). Forward. In B. S. Levy & V. W. Sidel (Eds.), *Social injustice and public health* (2nd ed., pp. xiii–xiv). Oxford, UK: Oxford University Press.

Freimuth, V. S., & Quinn, S. C. (2004). The contributions of health communication to eliminating health disparities. *American Journal of Public Health, 94*(12), 2053–2055.

Frey, L. R., Pearce, W. B., Pollock, M. A., Artz, L., & Murphy, B. A. O. (1996). Looking for justice in all the wrong places: On a communication approach to social justice. *Communication Studies, 47*(1–2), 110–127.

Garcia, J. L. A. (1996). The heart of racism. *Journal of Social Philosophy, 27*(1), 5–45.

Hamilton, B. E., Martin J. A., Osterman, M. J. K., . . . Matthews, T. J. (2015). Births: Final data for 2014. *National vital statistics reports, 64*(12). Hyattsville, MD: National Center for Health Statistics.

Hammer, L. (1997). The dark side to donovanosis: Color, climate, race and racism in American South venereology. *Journal of Medical Humanities, 18*(1), 29–57.

Happe, K. E. (2006). The rhetoric of race in breast cancer research. *Patterns of Prejudice, 40*(4–5), 461–480.

Hasian, M. A. Jr. (1996). *The rhetoric of eugenics in Anglo-American thought.* Athens, GA: University of Georgia Press.

Hawkins, R. P., Kreuter, M., Resnicow, K., Fishbein, M., & Dijkstra, A. (2008). Understanding tailoring in communicating about health. *Health Education Research, 23*(3), 454–466.

Heisler, M., Smith, D. M., Hayward, R. A., Krein, S. L., & Kerr. E. A. (2003). Racial disparities in diabetes care processes, outcomes, and treatment intensity. *Medical Care, 41*(11), 1221–1232.

Hoberman, J. (2012). *Black and blue. The origins and consequences of medical racism.* Berkeley, CA: University of California Press.

Jacobs, E. A., Rolle, I., Ferrans, C. E., Whitaker, E. E., & Warnecke, R. B. (2006). Understanding African Americans' views of the trustworthiness of physicians. *Journal of General Internal Medicine, 21*(6), 642–647.

Jones, N. (2016). The technical communicator as advocate: Integrating a social justice approach in technical communication. *Journal of Technical Writing and Communication, 46*(3), 342–361.

Justice Policy Institute and Prison Policy Initiative. (2015, February). The right investment? Corrections spending in Baltimore City. *Prison Policy Initiative.* Retrieved from https://www.prisonpolicy.org/origin/md/report.html

Katz, S. B. (1992). The ethic of expediency: Classical rhetoric, technology, and the Holocaust. *College English, 54*(3), 255–275.

Katz, S. B. (1993). Aristotle's rhetoric, Hitler's program, and the ideological problem of praxis, power, and professional discourse. *Journal of Business and Technical Communication, 7*(1), 37–62.

Kreps, G. L. (2003). The impact of communication on cancer risk, incidence, morbidity, mortality, and quality of life. *Health Communication, 15*(2), 163–71.

Kreps, G. L. (2005). Disseminating relevant information to underserved audiences: Implications from the Digital Divide Pilot Projects. *Journal of the Medical Library Association, 93*(S1), S68–S78.

Kwate, N. O. A. (2014). "Racism still exists": A public health intervention using racism "countermarketing" outdoor advertising in a black neighborhood. *Journal of Urban Health: Bulletin of the New York Academy of Medicine, 91*(5), 851–872.

LaVeist, T. A., & Isaac, L. A. (Eds.). (2013). *Race, ethnicity, and health: A public health reader* (2nd ed.). San Francisco, CA: Jossey-Bass.

Lawrence, H. Y., Hausman, B. L., & Dannenberg, C. J. (2014). Reframing medicine's publics: The local as public of vaccine refusal. *Journal of Medical Humanities 35*(2), 111–129.

Lentz, C. (April 1984). Crib death: Chasing down a thief that gives no warning and leaves no tracks. *Orange Coast Magazine,* pp. 43–49.

Levy, B. S., & Sidel, V. W. (2013). The nature of social injustice and its impact on public health. In B. S. Levy & V. W. Sidel (Eds.), *Social injustice and public health* (2nd ed., pp. 3–18). New York, NY: Routledge.

López, N., & Gadsden, V. L. (2016). Health inequities, social determinants, and intersectionality. *National Academy of Medicine: Perspectives.* Retrieved from https://nam.edu/wp-content/uploads/2016/12/Health-Inequities-Social-Determinants-and-Intersectionality.pdf

Lupton, D. (1994). Toward the development of critical health communication praxis. *Health Communication, 6*(1), 55–67.

Majumdar, S. K. (1996). Aristotle's ethical theory & modern health care. *Bulletin of the Indian Institute of History of Medicine, 26,* 75–80.

Marmot, M. (2015). *The health gap: The challenge of an unequal world.* New York, NY: Bloomsbury.

Maryland Department of Health and Mental Hygiene. (2010). Maryland vital statistics: Infant mortality in Maryland, 2009. Retried from http://www.healthybabiesbaltimore.com/Uploads/file/Maryland%20State%20IMR%20report%202009.pdf

Matsuda, M. J. (1986). Liberal jurisprudence and abstracted visions of human nature: A feminist critique of Rawls' theory of justice. *New Mexico Law Review, 16*(3), 613–630.

Matthews, T. J., MacDorman, M. F., & Thoma, M. E. (2015). Infant mortality statistics from the 2013 period linked birth/infant data set. *National Vital Statistics Reports, 64*(9). Retrieved from http://www.cdc.gov/nchs/data/nvsr/nvsr64/nvsr64_09.pdf

Mays, V. M., Ponce, N. A., Washington, D. L., & Cochran, S. D. (2003). Classifications of race and ethnicity: Implications for public health. *Annual Review of Public Health, 24,* 83–110.

Mills, C. W. (2017). *Black rights / white wrongs.* New York, NY: Oxford University Press.

Moskop, J. C. (1983). Rawlsian justice and a human right to health care. *The Journal of Medicine & Philosophy, 8*(4), 329–338.

Murphy, A. P. (Ed.). (1997). *It worked for me! From thumb sucking to schoolyard fights, parents reveal their secrets to solving the everyday problems of raising kids.* Emmaus, PA: Rodale.

National Institutes of Health. (n.d.). *Key moments in Safe to Sleep® history: 2004–2013.* Retrieved from https://safetosleep.nichd.nih.gov/safesleepbasics/moments/2004-2013

Nussbuam, M.C. (1992). Human functioning and social justice: In defense of Aristotelian essentialism. *Political Theory, 20*(2), 202–246.

Nussbaum, M.C. (2001). *The fragility of goodness: Luck and ethics in Greek tragedy and philosophy.* New York, NY: Cambridge University Press.

Office of Disease Prevention and Health Promotion. (2014). *Disparities.* Retrieved from https://www.healthypeople.gov/2020/about/foundation-health-measures/ Disparities

Okin, S. M. (2005). "Forty acres and a mule" for women: Rawls and feminism. *Politics, Philosophy & Economics, 4*(2), 233–248.

Oliver, M. N., Wells, K. M., Joy-Gaba, J. A., Hawkins, C. B., & Nosek, B. A. (2014). Do physicians' implicit views of African Americans affect clinical decision making? *Journal of the American Board of Family Medicine, 27*(2), 177–188.

Peñaranda, F. (2015). The individual, social justice, and public health. *Ciencia & Saude Coletiva, 20*(4), 987–996.

Peter, F. (2001). Health equity and social justice. *Journal of Applied Philosophy, 18*(2), 159–170.

Population Division, United Nations. (2015). *The world populations prospects: 2015 revision.* Retrieved from http://www.un.org/en/development/desa/publications/world-population-prospects-2015-revision.html

Price, A. W. (1985). Aristotle's ethics. *Journal of Medical Ethics, 11,* 150–152.

Primm, A. B., Vasquez, M. J., Mays, R. A., Sammons-Posey, D., McKnight-Eily, L. R., Presley-Cantrell, L. R., . . . Perry, G. S. (2010). The role of public health in addressing racial and ethnic disparities in mental health and mental illness. *Preventing Chronic Disease: Public Health Research, Practice, and Policy, 7*(1), 1–7.

Rawls, J. (2001). *Justice as fairness: A restatement.* Cambridge, MA: Harvard University Press.

Rawls, J. (2005). *Political liberalism.* New York, NY: Columbia University Press.

Rees, G. (2008). Equity in medical care: An Aristotelian defense of imperfect rules—and bending them. *AMA Journal of Ethics, 10*(5), 320–323.

Reitmanova, S. (2009). "Disease-breeders" among us: Deconstructing race and ethnicity as risk factors of immigrant health. *Journal of Medical Humanities, 30*(3), 183–190.

Resnik, D. B., &. Roman, J. (2007). Health, justice, and the environment. *Bioethics, 21*(4), 230–241.

Richardson, F. (2013). The eugenics agenda: Deliberative rhetoric and therapeutic discourse of hate. In M. F. Williams (Ed.), *Communicating race, ethnicity, and identity in technical communication* (pp. 7–22). Amityville, NY: Baywood.

Roberts, D. (1997). *Killing the black body: Race, reproduction, and the meaning of liberty.* New York. NY: Vintage Books.

Rogers, J., & Kelly, U. A. (2011). Feminist intersectionality: Bringing social justice to health disparities research. *Nursing Ethics, 18*(3), 397–407.

Rouse C. M. (2016). Racial health disparities and questions of evidence. In M. Buchbinder, M. Rivkin-Fish, & R. L. Walker (Eds.), *Understanding health inequalities and justice: New conversation across the disciplines* (pp. 259–284). Chapel Hill, NC: University of North Carolina Press.

Ruger, J. P. (2004). Health and social justice. *Lancet, 363*(9439), 1075–1080.

Ruger, J. P. (2009). *Health and social justice.* New York, NY: Oxford University Press.

Ruger, J. P. (2016). Global health inequalities and justice. In M. Buchbinder, M. Rivkin-Fish, & R. L. Walker (Eds.), *Understanding health inequalities and justice: New conversation across the disciplines* (pp. 64–87). Chapel Hill, NC: University of North Carolina Press.

Schulman, K., Berlin, J. A., Harless, W., Kerner, J. F , Sistrunk, S., Gersh, B. J., . . . Escarce, J. J. (1999). The effect of race and sex on physicians' recommendations for cardiac catheterization. *New England Journal of Medicine, 340,* 618–626.

Schulz, A. J., & Mullings, L. (Eds.). (2006). *Gender, race, class, and health: Intersectional approaches.* San Francisco, CA: Jossey-Bass.

Secundy, M., Dula, A, & Williams, S. (Eds.). (2000). *Bioethics research concerns and directions for African-Americans.* Tuskegee University National Center for Bioethics in Research and Health Care.

Sen, A. (1992). *Inequality reexamined.* New York, NY: Oxford University Press.

Sen, A. (1999). *Development as freedom.* New York, NY: Random House, Inc.

Sequist, T. D., & Schneider, E. C. (2006). Addressing racial and ethnic disparities in health care: Using federal data to support local programs to eliminate disparities. *Health Services Research, 41*(4 Pt 1), 1451–1468.

Sharkey, P. (2008). The intergenerational transmission of context. *American Journal of Sociology, 113*(4), 931–969.

Suneja, G., Shiels, M. S., Angulo, R., Copeland, G. E., Gonsalves, L., Hakenewerth, A. M., . . . Engels E. A. (2014). Cancer treatment disparities in HIV-infected individuals in the United States. *Journal of Clinical Oncology, 32*(22), 2344–2350.

Suthers, K. (2008). *Evaluating the economic causes and consequences of racial and ethnic health disparities.* Retrieved from https://www.apha.org/~/media/files/pdf/factsheets/corrected_econ_disparities_final2.ashx

Swartz, O. (2012). Reflections of a social justice scholar. In O. Swartz (Ed.), *Social justice and communication scholarship* (pp. 1–20). New York, NY: Routledge.

Tapper, M. (1999). *In the blood: Sickle cell anemia and the politics of race.* Philadelphia, PA: University of Pennsylvania Press.

Tipene-Leach, D., Abel, S., Haretuku, R., & Everard, C. (2000). The Māori SIDS prevention programme: Challenges and implications of Māori health service development. *Social Policy Journal of New Zealand, 14.* Retrieved from https://www.msd.govt.nz/about-msd-and-our-work/publications-resources/journals-and-magazines/social-policy-journal/spj14/maori-sids-prevention-programme.html

US Census Bureau. (2015). *Quickfacts.* Retrieved from https://www.census.gov/quickfacts/table/PST045216/24510,24,00

US Department of Health and Human Services, Agency for Healthcare Research and Quality. (2015). *National healthcare quality and disparities report and 5th anniversary update on the National Quality Strategy.* Rockville, MD: Author.

Venkatapuram, S. (2011). *Health justice: An Argument from the Capabilities Approach.* Cambridge, MA: Polity.

Washington, H. A. (2006). *Medical apartheid: The dark history of medical experimentation on Black Americans from colonial times to the present.* New York, NY: Random House.

Wall, W. (2008). *Inventing the "American Way": The politics of consensus from the New Deal to the Civil Rights movement.* New York, NY: Oxford University Press.

Wells, K., Klap, R., Koike, A., & Sherbourne, C. (2001). Ethnic disparities in unmet need for alcoholism, drug abuse, and mental health care. *American Journal of Psychiatry, 158,* 2027–2032.

Williams, D. R., & Collins, C. (2001). Racial residential segregation: A fundamental cause of racial disparities in health. *Public Health Reports, 116,* 404–416.

Willinger, M., James, L. S., & Catz, C. (1991). Defining the sudden infant death syndrome (SIDS): Deliberations of an expert panel convened by the National Institute of Child Health and Human Development. *Pediatric Pathology, 11*(5), 677–684.

Woolf, S. H., & Aron, L. (Eds.). *U.S. health in international perspective: Shorter lives, poorer health.* Washington, DC: National Academies Press.

World Health Organization. (1998). *Health promotion glossary.* Geneva, Switzerland: Author. Retrieved from https://www.who.int/healthpromotion/about/HPR%20Glossary%201998.pdf

World Health Organization. (2008). *Closing the gap in a generation: Health equity through action on the social determinants of health.* Geneva, Switzerland: Author. Retrieved from http://www.who.int/social_ determinants/thecommission/finalreport/en/index.html

World Health Organization. (2015). *World health statistics 2015.* Geneva, Switzerland: Author. Retrieved from http://www.who.int/gho/publications/world_health_statistics/2015/en/

Zoller, H., & Melonçon, L. (2013). The good neighbor campaign as a communication intervention to reduce environmental health disparities. In M. J. Dutta & G. L. Kreps (Eds.), *Reducing health disparities: Communication interventions* (pp. 436–456). New York, NY: Peter Lang.

CHAPTER 9

Decolonizing Medical Discourse through Promotora Practices in Community Health

AMY C. HICKMAN

WHILE ADDRESSING a pervasive Euro-American centrism in rhetorical studies of science, Celeste Condit (2013) encouraged scholars to engage internationalized contexts—both to challenge universalizing tendencies of Western rhetorical orientations and to grow their relevance to broader academic and political concerns. Condit argued that a Eurocentric orientation in science studies leads to a critical myopia that constrains transformative action. Condit contended further that such an orientation leads rhetoricians of health and medicine (RHM) to cast science as the enemy rather than expose the political forces that use (and constrain) scientific authority to support institutional power and organizational goals.

This chapter responds to Condit's (2013) call by examining the rhetorics of public health through the standpoints and practices of Margarita,[1] a community health worker (CHW) active in her Latinx-dominant community. Within the field of health promotion, CHWs work in "neighborhoods, homes, schools, faith and community-based organizations, health departments, clinics and hospitals throughout the United States" to promote health and well-being within their own communities (Rosenthal et al., 2010, p. 1338). CHWs bring a wealth of everyday knowledge about their communities to their work,

---

1. Margarita is a pseudonym chosen by this community health worker to be used in written and spoken references to this project. All proper nouns used in this work are pseudonyms.

and because they are known and trusted within the communities they serve, they have been shown to improve health-care access and outcomes (Findley et al., 2012). As CHWs locate their practice at the intersection of community, medical discourses, and public health policies, rhetorical study of their practices affords a deeper understanding of the colonizing effects of biomedical discourse on public health interventions.

Keeping Condit's (2013) critique in mind, rhetorical study of CHW practices can also expose political ideologies that often inflect public health policy. Biomedicine is a powerful discourse that circulates broadly across social, cultural, political, and economic spheres (Clarke, Mamo, Fishman, Shim, & Fosket, 2003), while CHWs are commonly understood to act as a "cultural bridge" between expert and everyday understandings of health and disease (Findley et al., 2012, p. 1983). Through critical rhetorical analysis of Margarita's pedagogical practices and the texts that inform those practices, I show that CHWs do much more than bridge cultures and discourses; they actively decolonize public health messaging by reconfiguring health citizenship at the site of popular nutrition education. As a medical rhetor, I underscore RHM's commitment to critically interrogate ideological systems at play in medical discourse and practice. Therefore, this case study also demonstrates how RHM is centrally concerned with relations of power in public health. Therefore, RHM, guided by cultural studies as a framework, can participate in decolonial projects by strategically delinking public health messaging from the colonizing effects of biomedical discourse.

This chapter situates RHM within feminist decolonial theory (Sandoval, 2000; Smith, 1999). Tuck and Yang (2012) argued that decolonization is inherently "unsettling" and not just a synonym for, or extension of critical theory (p. 7). Tuck and Yang (2012) offered a crucial reminder that in the context of settler colonialism "settlers make Indigenous land their new home and source of capital and . . . the disruption of the Indigenous relationships to land represents a profound epistemic, ontological and cosmological violence" (p. 5). This chapter argues that medical discourse can operate as a totalizing settler discourse that supplants and dislocates Indigenous and everyday knowledges about health and the body. Accepting the reality of coloniality, the concept of decoloniality was developed by Walter Mignolo (2007) as a "delinking that leads to [a] de-colonial epistemic shift and brings to the foreground other epistemologies, other principles of knowledge and understanding and, consequently, other economies, other politics, other ethics" (p. 453). In response, this chapter examines health-promotion practices through feminist decolonial theory to illuminate how everyday practices strategically use *and* resist public health messaging while also generating new understandings of health in marginalized community contexts.

DIFFERENTIAL CONSCIOUSNESS AND
POWER IN MEDICAL CONTEXTS

Chela Sandoval articulated differential consciousness, in part, through Gloria Anzaldúa's (1987) "*la conciencia de la mestiza*" and Jacque Derrida's (1973) "*différance*" to trace the "process, turn, trope, movement, or identification that contains the means to shatter any economy of difference—any order" (Sandoval, 2000, p. 147). Sandoval (2000) continued to explain that by using tools inherent in subordinated identifications, differential consciousness makes use of the silenced or "deferred" ways of knowing to create new technologies for "decolonizing the imagination" (p. 68). Drawing on Anzaldúa's work (1987), Sandoval (2004) wrote that differential consciousess is an "activity of weaving between and among" oppositional ideologies [found in the social movements of third world feminisms] to create a "new space or mode of oppositional consciousness" (p. 202).

Margarita's praxis in public health contexts makes visible this new hybrid space of oppositional conscious. Everyday ways of knowing about health and disease often become hidden, silenced, or subordinated as Western biomedical ideologies render these epistemologies and practices unimportant and unproductive. González, Moll, and Amanti's (2005) research presented in their landmark book, *Funds of Knowledge: Theorizing Practices in Households, Communities, and Classrooms,* informs my understanding of what constitutes everyday ways of knowing as they theorize how "language practices and [everyday] activities" produce knowledges that are historically contingent, fluid, and located within relations of power (p. 25). This case study involves an analysis of Margarita's teaching practices as a "set of processes, procedures and technologies" that both extend and subvert popular nutrition curricula to produce positive change within her community (Sandoval, 2000, p. 68).

Sandoval (2000) understands differential consciousness as "multidimensional" forms of power (pp. 75–76). Multidimensionality surfaces when everyday knowledges intersect with dominant, expertise-based organizations of power. Sandoval (2000) theorized a differential consciousness at work in communities whose practices and knowledges "combine flat [modalities] with deep" modalities of power "in ways that make journeys, paths, fields and networks of differential consciousness representable" (p. 76). For example, medical expertise can be described as a deep modality of power, as there exists a strong hierarchy of knowledge that is professionalized. In contrast, everyday health knowledges are understood to be a flat modality; one that is superficial and not formally but widely distributed. When medical expertise merges with everyday knowledges, power is refracted through multiple levels. This refraction of power contrasts with what Sandoval (2000) called the "historical vertical orientation" of power traveling downward from expert to novice (p. 72). Because CHWs are positioned at the nexus of medical expertise and everyday ways of knowing, they are often active in the work of knowledge translation and advocacy for marginalized communities of color. By necessity, they are adept at shifting between the deep and hierarchical expert and everyday (flattened) discourses. At the juncture of medical expertise and everyday ways of knowing about health and the body, CHWs combine flat and deep knowledges "from below" (Harding, 2008), thus engaging tensions that rupture to create and make visible new spaces for transformation and change.

The application of Sandoval's (2000) theory of differential consciousness to medical contexts places RHM within the purview of cultural studies. For example, in the West, medicine has evolved into a powerful and profitable discourse that shapes everyday understandings about the body, health, and disease. Scholars have noted the curious paradox that while bodies are increasingly medicalized, chronic disease is often framed as a direct result of personal and individual lifestyle choice (Derkatch, 2011; Derkatch & Spoel, 2017; Spoel, Harris, & Henwood, 2012). However the social and political determinants of health are often positioned well outside the parameters of biomedical expertise and practice (Clarke, Mamo, Fishman, Shim, & Fosket, 2003; DeVoe et al., 2016). Yet as an expert discourse and practice, biomedicine continues to guide public health policy and interventions that address chronic disease prevention, treatment, and management.

Clarke et al. (2003) traced the development of biomedicalization of bodies through stratified and pervasive economic and technoscientific processes. However, Martins (2008) complicated biomedicalization of the diabetic body through rhetorically analyzing the discourse of compliance in diabetes management through habits of embodiment. Because chronic illness is biomedically framed, public health interventions often emphasize individualized behavioral change and pay less attention to lived experiences of community members or to how the social, cultural, political, and economic determinants of health impact health behaviors (Farmer & Sen, 2005 Clarke et al., 2003). In response, I apply decolonial frameworks to medical rhetorical analysis of one CHW's teaching practices and the curricula that inform them. In so doing, this chapter demonstrates how RHM is operative as a critical field of praxis active in exposing colonizing, neoliberal subtexts in public health discourse and practice. Discourse is understood here as language (spoken and written) that shapes and is shaped by social practices and contexts (Wodak & Meyer, 2009). In this sense, discourse indexes a set of "materialities and practices that hang together in a specific, historically and culturally situated way" (Mol, 2008, p. 8). In Latinx community contexts, CHWs are often called *promoto-*

ras de salud. Promotoras are community members who lead through their experience-based expertise to flatten traditional, expert models of health education and care (Balcazar et al. 2011; Pérez & Martinez, 2008).

Feminist critical scholars have contributed insightful work in critiquing the positivist bias within the sciences, yet they have also questioned the purposes for which research is undertaken (Condit, 2013; Haraway, 1988; Harding, 2008; Hartsock, 2004; Hekman, 1997; Segal, 2015). To address these ongoing and pressing issues, rhetorical scholarship in health and medicine deepens understandings of how medical discourse is embedded in relations of power (Condit, 2013; Segal, 2005; Derkatch & Spoel, 2017). RHM is thus well positioned to engage in participatory research that interrogates the cultural, social, and decolonial aspects of power in medical and health discourses. Through feminist participatory projects, RHM can effect transformative research within academic and community contexts.

RESEARCH CONTEXTS AND METHODS

This chapter emerges from a three-year participatory project where I partnered with Margarita, an experienced promotora, to explore community health workers' practices at clinic and community sites.[2] Our inquiry took shape around issues of language and power in public health.[3] Together we asked, what are the effects of Margarita's language practices for clinic patients and community members? Over time, through my observations and conversational interviews with Margarita, I began to see that her rhetorical practices engaged unequal relations of power inherent in expert medical discourse. This realization led to choosing a critical discourse studies approach to analyzing state and privately sponsored public health media, including nutrition teaching scripts, resources, and a website that together constituted the official content of Margarita's teaching practice. I then compared the results of this analysis with my observations and rhetorical analysis of Margarita's actual teaching practices and work stories, which were captured on recordings, translated and transcribed for this purpose.

Our research was located at an urban health clinic in southeast Arizona, where Margarita supported patients and community members that she met

---

2. All research activities were reviewed yearly by the University of Arizona's Institutional Review Board and met the ethical standards set by the University of Arizona's Human Subjects Protection Program.

3. As of this writing, Margarita has retired from her work as a promotora. Consequently, I refer to her activities in the past tense. However, in my analysis of the effects of her practices, I use the present and present perfect tenses to indicate ongoing action.

on her rounds through the clinic. At regular intervals, Margarita engaged in more formal nutrition education sessions and demonstrations. Supported by grants, her work extended beyond the clinic, as she also led nutrition demonstrations and educational sessions at local community centers as well as subsidized housing for low-income populations living with mental and/or physical disability. Margarita also worked in schools with both children and teachers. Because of the clinic's outreach to the low-income populations, and its location in a highly diverse area in South Tucson, Margarita's audiences were drawn from communities experiencing poverty, as well as multiple social and political marginalizations. Margarita led the nutrition demonstrations in both Spanish and English, to accommodate the large number of Spanish speakers in the communities she served.

DEFINING KEY TERMS

Relational praxis is a feminist construction with a long and complex history. It has been helpful to this project in its development in standpoint theory (Harding, 2008; Hekman, 1997) and as an epistemic tool (Fox Keller, 1985; Jaggar, 1989). My use of the term is inclusive of everyday, embodied practices of empathy, caregiving, listening, and sharing. However, at the foundational level, when I use the term *relational praxis* I mean everyday practices that emerge from and in relation to others. Relational praxis is a rhetorical strategy but one typically undervalued in medical contexts, where the interaction between community member and physician takes place in clinical settings within a short time frame. Margarita used relational praxis as a "deferred way of knowing" in her work as promotora.

Chicana feminist or *mujerista* **pedagogies** are defined by Elenes, Gonzalez, Delgado Bernal, and Villenas (2001) as teaching and learning practices that critically engage dominant ideologies and discourses "to create political and cultural projects [that] transform existing social inequalities and injustices" (p. 595). In this case study, I found that promotoras use mujerista pedagogies to resist popular notions that Latinx food choices and practices can lead to chronic illness. Such understandings emphasize traditional Latinx cultural food practices and genetic predispositions as causal factors to developing type 2 diabetes (Williams, Lavizzo-Mourey, & Warren, 1994). Margarita responded by recentering Latinx food practices as healthy food practices, as the following analysis shows.

RHETORICS OF HEALTH CITIZENSHIP IN
PUBLIC HEALTH MESSAGING

Public health education campaigns use a combination of behavior change and education strategies to encourage adherence to nutritional guidelines. Naidoo and Wills (2015) wrote in *Foundations for Health Promotion* that the behavior change model "is popular because it views health as the property of individuals" (p. 70). This health as an individual property approach constructs the consumer-subject's "civic-moral imperative of healthy living" especially for populations already marked by the diagnosis of—or at higher risk for—chronic disease (Spoel et al., 2012, p. 620; Derkatch & Spoel, 2017). For example, Arizona Nutrition Network (AZNN) invokes a civic-moral imperative through its slogan "Be a Champion for Change!" (Champions for Change—Arizona Nutrition Network, 2016). Implicit in the slogan is the hero's call to encourage parents to make healthy food choices. It is often uncritically implied that healthy food choices will ensure a positive change in their family's health's status.

At the clinic site, public health curricula and pedagogical practices employed this neoliberal message of self-management. For example, promotoras were funded to conduct nutrition demonstrations in the clinic waiting areas and in low-income housing developments. To demonstrate nutrition concepts, Margarita engaged her audiences through a brief oral questionnaire regarding the topic of the day, such as the importance of low-fat cooking, or the multiple benefits of cooking a vegetable-rich meal. Equipped with a small mobile kitchen unit, Margarita then prepared a simple recipe to demonstrate healthy food preparation and offered the food to those in attendance after the demonstration was finished. This was a teaching by modeling approach designed to persuade individuals to make positive improvements to their cooking practices. Roughly twenty-five to eighty people participated in these nutrition demonstrations, either in the clinic waiting room or in public community centers.

A teaching script provided the structure of each demonstration. These scripts were approved by AZNN, a state- and privately funded agency that financially supported Margarita's activities at clinic and community sites. At the end of each completed module, Margarita tested the knowledge of her audience through an oral question-and-answer format and recorded the answers of the group. In this way, AZNN shaped the content and measured the uptake of Margarita's teaching. Module titles such as *Getting Ready for Change, Personal Steps to Improved Nutrition, Smart Choices for a Healthy*

Weight, and *Focus on the Family: Inspiring Healthy Food Habits* underscore how interventions mirror biomedical understandings of chronic illness as rooted in the individualized body and how health is linked only to specific lifestyle choices.

Although Margarita's work was funded by AZNN, her style of leading these demonstrations was inflected by relational praxis. Rather than uncritically applying the script, Margarita would converse with her audience as she cooked, telling personal stories about the food she was cooking while demonstrating and pointing out low-fat cooking techniques. As I observed Margarita's practice, it was evident that "food demonstrations were not just a way to disseminate nutrition information, they were also an offering. Food is way to connect to the community in a way that is vital but optional. One can refuse the food" (field notes, March 15, 2010).

Margarita explained to me the importance of relational praxis when she described her practice as "sharing not teaching, allowing others to care for you, [so that community members are] not just . . . recipients of care" (field notes, October 21, 2010). These bidirectional relational practices were critical to interrogating the power differentials embedded in the caregiving/receiving contexts. Another example of relational practice was when Margarita noted that at one community site, members were not very enthusiastic about the class. She decided to incorporate movement with the lesson material on nutrition and found that the attitude of community members improved with movement and dance. This practice then became a routine for her and eventually was incorporated into the curriculum at the state level (personal communication, October 28, 2010).Through Margarita's relational praxis, the community critically informed the policy and curriculum of nutrition interventions.

The following analysis demonstrates Margarita's use of differential consciousness through alternating between dominant expert nutrition practices and everyday ways of knowing to decolonize the often disempowering effects of public health messaging. Although Margarita was constrained to employ a curriculum steeped in neoliberal discourse, her relational practices recentered everyday ways of knowing, revalued Latinx cooking practices, and explicitly named the connections between place and disease. As audience and rhetor co-produce rhetorical action, caregivers and care-receivers both inform and transform care practices. In what follows, I offer an analysis of one teaching module, *Getting Ready for Change.* This module was given to Margarita as the teaching content for her nutrition education classes. I then compare the analysis of teaching scripts with actual promotora teaching practices.

CRITICAL ANALYSIS OF TEACHING MODULES
AND MARGARITA'S TEACHING PRACTICE

As the title suggests, the module *Getting Ready for Change* addresses behavioral change in basic nutrition and exercise habits. The module makes three claims: First, health information is good and useful, but change happens only through an individual's decision to change; therefore, personal readiness is important. Second, change happens when an individual learns concrete ways to practice new behaviors. Third, change happens when an individual can overcome obstacles to change. Implicit in this strategy is the understanding that if healthy food choices lead to healthier bodies, unhealthy food choices lead to illness. For example, in the introduction to the module, the script reads, "This series of classes is all about you. You know your lifestyle and food habits better than anyone else, and you are the one who can put healthy changes into action, one step at a time" (Detailed Outline Personal Steps to Improved Nutrition, Getting Ready for Change p. 1). According to this logic, the individual is held solely responsible for her (non)participation in good health citizenship. This logic of choosing well is suspended from and untouched by political, economic, historical, cultural, and environmental contexts. For example, readers are encouraged to leave notes for themselves, to develop a food journal or calendar, to create an internal/external rewards system for positive behavior, to build a social support system, and to tap into a team of medical providers to support and guide their progress. These actions are markers for self-management of health: personal uptake of health information, making "appropriate" food choices, surveillance and accountability, and adequate follow-up measures. There is little emphasis on critically engaging food systems that make heavily discounted, highly processed, high-sugar and high-fat foods widely available (Nestle, 2013). In addition, by relying on a behavioral approach to support positive change, this teaching module ignores the social contexts of food practices including issues of accessibility, affordability, and cultural factors at play in choosing, preparing and consuming food.

The curriculum also identifies key obstacles to change. Fatalism, whether constructed as God's will or as genetic destiny, can immobilize a person's desire for change in nutrition habits. To counteract fatalism, the concept of personal control is invoked in these instances. For example, "choosing food wisely and getting adequate exercise" results in feeling better, having more energy, and improving mood and stress reduction. A causal relationship is established as a teaching strategy to suggest that an individual subject has the control (independence or autonomy) to eat well, and that if they do not choose food wisely, their personal health and well-being is at risk. The responsibility for health and illness thus rests not with fate or destiny but with the individual alone. The broader social determinants of health such as poverty, structural forms of racism and political dispossession, and other forms of precarity are also unconsidered. To put it more bluntly, health and well-being is a lifestyle choice. This relationship is exemplified through the introduction to the Personal Steps to Improved Nutrition, when the promotora is encouraged to show a poster of Champions for Change. The script reads here: "The smiling face belongs to Champions for Change—individuals just like us who have been successful in making small changes in their eating habits." According to this logic, if you are not willing to make changes, you are not "successful," especially compared with others, at promoting positive change. While the curriculum emphasizes personal autonomy and readiness for change, motivation for change emerges from the murky arenas of guilt and fear.

Margarita's actual teaching praxis upended the neoliberalism of AZNN's public health messaging and curriculum. In one class, Margarita asked whether the attendees expected to benefit from the class. She encouraged attendees to describe why they feel they would benefit or not benefit from the information. One attendee responded, "One of the reasons why I think [the class] won't [be a benefit] is that . . . you're going to teach how to eat correctly, how to evaluate the best foods . . . I never follow up on [this advice] . . . even though I know it's good for me." Margarita answered, "Then I shouldn't try to change you . . . [laughter] . . . but we need to have the desire, the intention [to change] (nutrition lecture, May 19, 2011, recorded and transcribed)." In this interaction, Margarita resists messaging that can lead to blaming individuals for not adhering to nutritional advice on healthy eating. Rather, she playfully and reflectively invites participants to consider a desire to change their nutrition habits.

While Margarita works within the AZNN curricula regarding behavioral change, she also identifies the social, political, and economic realities that face newly immigrated community members. Margarita explains, "We have to battle for these changes. For us Hispanic women, who are getting used to life in this country, it is even harder for us, but we should get the best from this country, not the worst . . . people here are very intelligent, but they also have their things that aren't so good, like fast food. This isn't something we should adopt" (nutrition lecture, May 19, 2011). In this segment, Margarita does not invoke fear or shame associated with poor eating habits but clearly associates fast food with American culture and implicitly dissociates Latinx culture from fast food, as developed later in this chapter. In this way, Margarita's teaching praxis decolonizes public health messaging.

To promote healthy eating habits, promotoras in this setting were tasked with following the USDA guidelines in the MyPlate scheme. This scheme was printed on a plastic plate and provided as a teaching tool to help visualize portion sizes of vegetables, meat/protein, and carbohydrates. AZNN provided these plates to be given to community members as a gift along with handouts to identify meats, grains, fruits and vegetables, and dairy items to be incorporated in their diet. To use the information on MyPlate, community members must be able to compare what they currently eat, and their portion sizes, with the types and amounts foods represented in the scheme. However, the food depicted on the resource pages for MyPlate reflects an American diet which in effect privileges Western food preferences, such as oatmeal, bread, brown rice, and chicken drumsticks. In the literature supporting the MyPlate teaching tool, there are no traditional Mexican foods pictured (e.g., hominy-based dishes such as pozole) that reflect the cultural identity of community members. Therefore, in this context, eating healthy means eating food that community members might not recognize or enjoy. This is an inherently disempowering intervention. In addition, from a health literacies perspective, these strategies assume an ability to read and to understand the differences between saturated fat, unsaturated fat, and trans-fatty acids, and to identify the amount of fat allowable for one's age and height. From an embodied standpoint, these strategies also assume an ability to shop and prepare food independently. These strategies are most familiar to those who are able and willing to consult a website or nutrition expert and to assume an individualized meal plan.

However, in observing Margarita's health promotion practices in community settings, I noted that those living with disability in assisted living settings often depend on others to buy food for them. Participants living at Pima Village, a subsidized housing complex for low-income residents living with disability, often do not travel independently and may have lower levels of functional literacy needed to fit within the paradigm of "good" chronic illness management and prevention. In this context, Margarita would sit in the lobby of Pima Village with a few AZNN brochures on the table beside her and listen to community members as they approached her to chat about their lives. I observed Margarita as she engaged in relational praxis in these sessions by listening to people first, and then telling stories about her own experiences with illness, what was difficult for her, and what she learned from her experiences. At our closing interview, Margarita noted that at the beginning of her work with those living at Pima Village, "nobody wanted to talk to each other, nobody wanted to make friends with anyone" (Margarita, closing Interview, June 27, 2013). Through the years of modeling and encouraging relational praxis, and by asking community members to "check up after each other," Margarita's work led to developing a more positive community where residents were noted to know each other's names, and to make space for one another at meetings (Margarita, closing Interview, June 27, 2013). Through relational praxis, residents began to build social capital by caring for one another and building networks of support.

DECOLONIZING PUBLIC HEALTH

Margarita's shifting and multiple positionalities as community leader, school volunteer, church volunteer, and promotora worked to engender the trust of many who lived on the political and economic margins. However, Margarita usually aligned herself as an everyday expert despite the fact that she holds a master's degree in social work. Margarita's positioning in this instance is a decolonial pedagogical strategy because Margarita makes use of Western-based knowledges—but not the power that is often associated with such knowledges. At the time, though, Margarita's choice of positioning puzzled me. As rhetors, teachers often refer to their experience or expertise in order to build trust with their audiences. Yet Margarita indicates that while her degree was useful to her in her work, newly immigrated community members might fear approaching her because of her formal expertise. To relate positively to these community members, Margarita identified as a community leader, rather than as a social worker, to develop a relationship of trust that is foundational to health promotion (Pérez & Martinez, 2008).

This positionality was tested when Margarita was asked by the principal of an elementary school to provide a cooking demonstration for the teachers at the school where Margarita volunteered. In this work story,[4] Margarita relates what she learned from the principle of the school:

> I found out why they were so resistant. First, the class was mandatory, and secondly after I left, the principal spoke with the group and asked them why they were so rude. I found out later that it was because they see me around St. Lukes all the time, and with Fr. Ricardo, and with the children, always with the children, and in the parish as well. They see me a community member that is older, without skills, without education, and they ask, "Why is

---

4. It was not always possible or appropriate for me to attend all of Margarita's nutrition classes. To fill in the gaps when I could not observe Margarita in action, we met weekly and Margarita would tell me of her experiences. I taped these work stories and analyzed them using Catherine Kohler Riessman's (2008) dialogic/performative narrative analysis. For purposes of clarity, I omit all conversational interjections in the following excerpts.

she teaching us? We have a degree in education; some of us have Masters Degrees!" (Field Notes, May 13, 2011)

It seems that Margarita's commitment to identifying with everyday expertise in the presence of this professional audience privileges everyday ways of knowing as central to health; in other words, healthy living is accessible to everyone regardless of their educational status. However in this instance, this choice undercut her ethos with her audience, which led to resistance. Yet, reflecting together on Margarita's positionality led to further insight into how professionalized community members might be shaped by biomedical understandings of disease and their treatment rather than valuing everyday eating practices as preventive and powerful.

Velez-Ibanez and Greenberg (2009) note in their book chapter "Formation and Transformation of Funds of Knowledge" that second- and third-generation Latinxs who complete higher education in the US often experience a shift away from community ways of knowing and place higher priority on academic and professional expertise. As Margarita further reflects on her experience, this shift becomes evident as she recounts the teacher's resistance to preventive nutrition. Margarita connects the resistance of the students to their social and economic context: "They . . . think that they have means, the economical—economical means, and the knowledge to go into the web and find something that they can eat or something they can take—to lower their cholesterol"(conversational interview, March 25, 2011). In other words, the teachers no longer feel the need to depend on community knowledges passed down from generation to generation to thrive and prevent disease; rather, professional audiences reflect popular understanding of biomedicine as cure even in the context of chronic disease.

In her account of interacting with this group of educators, Margarita's approach aligns with decolonizing frameworks. Margarita specifically recenters everyday ways of knowing as funds of knowledge that this community may have devalued as they live and work in the US. As first-generation Latinx families participate in the US economy, nutrition practices that were once rooted in family knowledges passed down from mother to child are increasingly influenced by the US food industry and by public nutrition campaigns.[5] Rather than adopting convenience foods, Margarita encourages her audience to "use your minds . . . use your knowledge . . . from your background" (transcript 1.0, lines 148–150). As promotora, Margarita uses mujerista pedagogies

---

5. For more on this, see how Velez-Ibanez & Greenberg (2009) traced the formation and transformations of traditional funds of knowledge as families moved and settled north across the Mexico–US border.

to place "cultural knowledge and language at the forefront in order to better understand lessons from the home space and local communities" (Delgado Bernal, 2006, p. 114).

As second- and third-generation Latinxs, the teachers responded to Margarita's teaching regarding their parents and grandparent's relationship to food by saying that "life is different now" (personal communication, telephone, November 4, 2014). In the context of busy family and work lives, a new economy of values emerges around convenience foods for families who don't have the time for slower, more traditional cooking practices. In response, Margarita offers simple recipes that use minimally processed foods as an alternative to reliance on prepared foods and fast-food restaurants.

The interview excerpt below reinforces how Margarita's positionality as everyday expert links to a critical awareness of food consumption practices, particularly within the context of medical economies. In this work story, Margarita ponders one educator's response to managing cholesterol through diet:

> I started asking [the] question . . . do you think you can put some of these into practice? That is when I got the answer that "I don't think I can live without 2 pounds of beef a day." . . . and ah, and I thought well maybe not two pounds, but maybe one and three quarters—slightly and slowly go down. And this is really ohh to prevent . . . your cholesterol from rising. [Student response:] "Well, I'll take medication for my cholesterol." . . . but of course I said you can fix that with the pill, I said . . . there are quite a few of those—but did you know that they are expensive—you can afford them—but can you are afford the damage on your kidneys, on your liver? Liver function tests, kidney function tests are expensive. And more than expensive, because sometimes you have the money, but do you have the time to waste on going to the lab back and forth, back and forth, back and forth all the time . . . it's because if you're so busy that you don't have time to go to the doctor, not always [is] a doctor . . . going to be able to accommodate you—at 4 o'clock in the afternoon and that's when you can go to the doctor. And she said "well, that's true." And I said, you can avoid spending money—cholesterol pills, lab, doctors by eating healthy—fruits and vegetables. (Transcript 1.0, lines 184–205)

Margarita recenters everyday nutrition practices as a form of power. Her persuasive strategy is to delink from popular understandings of medicine as a *controlling discourse* with the power to detect, diagnose, and treat disease through a critical pedagogy that exposes the often real cost of medical care in terms of time, money, and possible side effects of medication. Margarita is not advocating avoiding medical care when one actually needs it. Her focus here is to empower community members to pursue prevention first. She explains:

> The problem is that they feel that if they go to the doctor and get a pill—that is all they can do to fix their blood pressure. They need to know and feel that they have the power to help their blood pressure too . . . The main thing is the power. (Field notes, November 9, 2012)

This audience of educators did eventually respond positively to Margarita's message, assisted by the principal, who clarified the importance of Margarita's work at the school as well as her tertiary credentials.

STORYTELLING, CLAIMING, ENVISIONING

Margarita's teaching practices decolonize public health's central focus on personal behavioral change through storytelling and reclaiming histories. Such histories inform communities of what Indigenous life was like before colonization. Decolonial theorist Linda Tuhiwai Smith (1999) called for research and action that uses storytelling and reclaiming to create spaces where community members envision a more just future and initiate change. The excerpts below are taken from a nutrition lecture that Margarita gave at local church to eighteen community members. This nutrition talk was given entirely in Spanish, and no cooking demonstration was given. Margarita introduces herself and situates her work as promotora within the context of an earlier career in social work. Margarita begins with her typical format by reviewing nutrients commonly found in vegetables and fruits, and the importance of including a variety of colors in choosing vegetables to eat.

While this content may seem straightforward, this lecture runs more like a conversation. Audience members interrupt Margarita at regular intervals with personal questions about the material. In addition to the dialogic nature of the class, Margarita continues by sharing stories of her previous family life in Mexico. She also shares the very personal story of caring for her husband, who had survived a heart transplant but who had recently died from complications of diabetes. The personal level of sharing coupled with the conversational style of the lecture suggests a pronounced level of intimacy, alignment, and solidarity that indexes a logic of care through relational praxis. Margarita's vulnerability signals a creative interdependency where she sustains others, while she is sustained by the support she receives from those she cares for.

Margarita uses storytelling as a pedagogical strategy to inform and reconnect students to their history as another key strategy to support community agency. For example, in response to an audience member's query "How did people do before?" Margarita tells a story about her parents' lives in Mexico and relates that her great-grandfather "died at 115 years of age . . . they lived a long time, but also in those times, they died in a lot of pain. They don't know exactly what killed him" (transcript 3.0, lines 3, 5, 6). She then remembers life prior to the advent of industrialized food production and big box stores: "People didn't have cars, they weren't even invented, they walked, [and] they went on horseback. They cut their vegetables from their gardens—without chemicals. They cared for their animals" (transcript 3.0, lines 7–9).

Margarita suggests that her grandfather was healthy and long-lived because of his necessarily active lifestyle and the ready availability of fresh fruits and vegetables. Yet Margarita moves beyond issues of lifestyle as she continues, "There wasn't a hamburger stand on every corner. People made their breakfast, lunch and dinner and they sat down to eat. People worked in the field, packed their lunch, something healthy, without chemicals" (transcript 3.0, lines 14–16).

Margarita implies that the ubiquity of fast-food restaurants (in the US) supplants healthful traditional food practices and dilutes food quality with chemicals. In contrast, Margarita ends her lecture by claiming that the Latinx food culture is fundamentally healthful and not pathogenic:

> Among many people, they say that Mexican food is just full of fat. Mexican food, if it's made here, is full of lard. Our real food isn't like that, the food of our people, it is healthy food. We need to get back to our roots, tell our kids who they are, where they come from, they shouldn't get mixed up in the lifestyle here, they can learn new things here, but they have to remember that their roots are Mexican. That is very important. (Transcript 3.0, lines 49–53)

Note that Margarita is not rejecting medical expertise but shifts between nutritional expertise and everyday ways of knowing. In her nutrition demonstrations, she models low-fat cooking, with an emphasis on fruits and vegetables. She explains the importance of micronutrients, and how to incorporate more of these into an everyday diet to protect the body from disease. What she rejects is the settler mentality that positions Western food practices as healthier choices that in effect replace traditional Mexican food practices. Further, Margarita highlights and resists the proliferation of fast-food restaurants that exist not to nourish but to make a profit. This perspective resists pathologizing Latinx food practices while opening to agencies rooted in reclaimed histories that "rise above present day situations" and that allow others to "dream a new dream and set a new vision" (Smith, 1999, p. 152).

CONCLUSION

Promotora practices decolonize public health messaging by making use of medical expertise while rejecting the colonizing effects of biomedical discourse. Whereas promotoras are constrained by often racialized public health policies, their relational practices interrupt these powerful discourses. By engaging medical discourse on their own terms, so to speak, promotoras do not merely bridge or translate medical discourse for everyday consumption; rather, their practices can strategically appropriate medical discourse—decolonize it—to build healthier communities, especially for those living in conditions of political and economic precarity. Margarita demonstrates a decolonial response to public health through specific rhetorical strategies that liberate, rather than constrain, community members. From this situated case study, Margarita's teaching practices show how mujerista pedagogies decolonize neoliberal public health messaging through relational praxis, storytelling, re/membering histories, and revaluing everyday practices. Margarita's teaching practices resist calling forth the responsible (and blameworthy) consumer-subject, as mujerista pedagogies allow new health knowledges to form that subvert oppressive health management and biomedical discourses. Finally, creative interdependencies form through relational practices that speak back to neoliberal ideals of autonomy and sustain bidirectional caring relationships. Taken together, relational praxis, mujerista pedagogies, and the reclaiming of history and storytelling constitute decolonizing rhetorical strategies that hold the potential for delinking public health messaging from the colonizing effects of medical discourse. This study demonstrates how RHM makes visible transformative rhetorical action in clinical and everyday community contexts as it is guided by feminist decolonial frameworks. As a result, RHM, as it is *situated* within the field of cultural studies, demonstrates rhetorical action central to transformative change.

REFERENCES

Adelman, L. (Prod.) (2008). *Unnatural causes: Is inequality making us sick?* California Newsreel and Vital Pictures Inc.

Anzaldúa, G. (2015). La prieta. In C. Moraga & G. Anzaldúa (Eds.), *This bridge called my back* (p. 198). Watertown, MA: Persephone. Retrieved from https://archive.org/stream/in.ernet. dli.2015.182997/2015.182997.This-Bridge-Called-My-Back_djvu.txt

Anzaldúa, G. 1987). *Borderlands la frontera: The new mestiza*. San Francisco, CA: Aunt Lute Books.

Balcazar, H., Rosenthal, E. L., Brownstein, J. N., Rush, C. H., Matos, S., & Hernandez, L. (2011). Community health workers can be a public health force for change in the United States: Three actions for a new paradigm. *American Journal of Public Health, 101*(12), 2199–2203. https://doi.org/10.2105/ajph.2011.300386

Brown, W. (2006). American nightmare: Neoliberalism, neoconservatism, and de-democratization. *Political Theory, 34*(6), 690–714. https://doi.org/10.1177/0090591706293016

Champions for change—Arizona nutrition network. (2016). Retrieved December 31, 2016, from https://www.eatwellbewell.org/

Clarke, A. E., Mamo, L., Fishman, J. R., Shim, J. K., & Fosket, J. R. (2003). Biomedicalization: Technoscientific transformations of health, illness, and U.S. biomedicine. *American Sociological Review, 68*(2), 161–194. https://doi.org/10.2307/1519765

Condit, C. M. (2013). "Mind the gaps": Hidden purposes and missing internationalism in scholarship on the rhetoric of science and technology in public discourse. *Poroi, 9*(1), 1–9. https://doi.org/10.13008/2151-2957.1150

Delgado Bernal, D. (2006). Learning and living pedagogies of the home: The mestiza consciousness of Chicana students. In D. Delgado Bernal, C. A. Elenes, F. E. Godinez, & S. Villenas (Eds.), *Chicana/Latina education in everyday life* (pp. 113–132). Albany, NY: State University of New York Press.

Derkatch, C. (2011). Does biomedicine control for rhetoric? Configuring practitioner-patient interaction. In J. Leach & D. Dysart-Gale (Eds.), *Rhetorical question of health and medicine* (pp. 129–153). Lanham, MD: Lexington Books.

Derkatch, C., & Spoel, P. (2017). Public health promotion of "local food": Constituti'ng the self-governing citizen-consumer. *Health, 21*(2), 154–170. https://doi.org/10.1177/1363459315590247

Derrida, J. (1973). *Différence* (D. Allison, Trans.). In N. Garver (Ed.), *Speech and phenomena and other essays on husserl's theory of signs* (pp. 129–160). Evanston, IL: Northwestern University Press.

DeVoe, J. E., Bazemore, A. W., Cottrell, E. K., Likumahuwa-Ackman, S., Grandmont, J., Spach, N., & Gold, R. (2016). Perspectives in primary care: A conceptual framework and path for integrating social determinants of health into primary care practice. *The Annals of Family Medicine, 14*(2), 104–108. https://doi.org/10.1370/afm.1903

Elenes, C. A., Gonzalez, F. E., Delgado Bernal, D., & Villenas, S. (2001). Introduction: Chicana/Mexicana feminist pedagogies: *Consejos, respeto, y educación* in everyday life. *International Journal of Qualitative Studies in Education, 14*(5), 595–602. https://doi.org/10.1080/09518390110059900

Farmer, P., & Sen, A. K. (2005). *Pathologies of power: Health, human rights, and the new war on the poor* (2nd ed.). Berkeley, CA: University of California Press.

Findley, S. E., Matos, S., Hicks, A. L., Campbell, A., Moore, A., & Diaz, D. (2012). Building a consensus on community health workers' scope of practice: Lessons from New York. *American Journal of Public Health, 102*(10), 1981–1987. https://doi.org/10.2105/ajph.2011.300566

Fox Keller, E. (1995). *Reflections on gender and science*. New Haven, CT: Yale University Press.

González, N. E., Moll, L. C., & Amanti, C. (Eds.). (2005). *Funds of knowledge: Theorizing practices in households, communities, and classrooms*. Mahwah, NJ: Lawrence Erlbaum.

Haraway, D. (1988). Situated knowledges: The science question in feminism and the privilege of partial perspective. *Feminist Studies, 14*(3), 575–599. https://doi.org/10.2307/3178066

Harding, S. (2003). *The feminist standpoint theory reader: Intellectual and political controversies.* New York, NY: Routledge.

Harding, S. (2008). *Sciences from below: Feminisms, postcolonialities, and modernities.* Durham, NC: Duke University Press.

Hartsock, N. (2004). The feminist standpoint: Developing ground for a specifically feminist historical materialism. In S. Harding (Ed.), *The feminist standpoint theory reader: Intellectual and political controversies* (pp. 35–53). New York, NY: Routledge.

Hekman, S. (1997). Truth and method: Feminist standpoint theory revisited. *Signs: Journal of Women in Culture and Society, 22*(2), 341–365. https://doi.org/10.1086/495159

Hickman, A. C. (2016). *Promotoras and the rhetorical economies of public health: Deterritorializations of medical discourse* (Doctoral dissertation). Retrieved from ProQuest (Order No. 10110993).

Jaggar, A. (1989). Love and knowledge: Emotion in feminist epistemology. *Inquiry, 32*(2), 151–176. https://doi.org/10.1080/00201748908602185

Martins, D.S.(2008). Diabetes management, the complexities of embodiement, and rhetorical analysis. In B. Heifferon & S. C. Brown (Eds), *Rhetoric of healthcare: Essays toward a new disciplinary inquiry* (pp. 75–90). Creskill, NJ: Hampton Press.

Mol, A. (2008). *The logic of care: Health and the problem of patient choice.* New York, NY: Taylor and Francis.

Mignolo, W. D. (2007). Delinking: The rhetoric of modernity, the logic of coloniality and the grammar of de-coloniality. *Cultural Studies, 21*(2–3), 449–514. https://doi.org/10.1080/09502380601162647

Naidoo, J., &Wills, J. (2015). *Foundations for health promotion* (3rd ed.). Edinburgh, Scotland: Baillié Tindale Elsevier.

Nestle, M. (2013). *Food politics: How the food industry influences nutrition and health* (10th ed.). Berkeley, CA: University of California Press.

Nestle, M., & Jacobson, M. (2000). Halting the obesity epidemic: A public health policy approach. *Public Health Reports, 115*(1), 12–24. https://doi.org/10.1093/phr/115.1.12

Pérez, L. M., & Martinez, J. (2008). Community health workers: Social justice and policy advocates for community health and well-being. *American Journal of Public Health, 98*(1), 11–14. https://doi.org/10.2105/ajph.2006.100842

Riessman, C. K. (2008). *Narrative methods for the human sciences.* Thousand Oaks, CA: Sage.

Rosenthal, E. L., Brownstein, J. N., Rush, C. H., Hirsch, G. R., Willaert, A. M., Scott, J. R., . . . Fox, D. J. (2010). Community health workers: Part of the solution. *Health Affairs, 29*(7), 1338–1442. https://doi.org/10.1377/hlthaff.2010.0081

Sandoval, C. (2000). *Methodology of the oppressed.* Minneapolis, MN: University of Minnesota Press.

Sandoval, C. (2004). US third world feminisms: Theory and method of differential consciousness. In S. Harding (Ed.), *The feminist standpoint reader: Intellectual and political controversies* (pp. 202–203). New York, NY: Routledge.

Segal, J. Z. (2005). *Health and the rhetoric of medicine.* New York, NY: Southern Illinois University Press.

Segal, J. Z. (2015). The rhetoric of female sexual dysfunction: Faux feminism and the FDA. *Canadian Medical Association Journal, 187*(12), 915–916. https://doi.org/10.1503/cmaj.150363

Smith, L. T. (1999). *Decolonizing methodologies: Research and indigenous peoples* (1st ed.). London, UK: Zed.

Spoel, P., Harris, R., & Henwood, F. (2012). The moralization of healthy living: Burke's rhetoric of rebirth and older adults' accounts of healthy eating. *Health: An Interdisciplinary Journal for the Social Study of Health, Illness and Medicine, 16*(6), 619–635. https://doi.org/10.1177/1363459312441009

Tuck, E., & Yang, K. W. (2012). Decolonization is not a metaphor. *Decolonization: Indigeneity, Education and Society, 1*(1), 1–40.

Velez-Ibanez, C., & Greenberg, J. (2009). Formation and transformation of funds of knowledge. In N. González, L. C. Moll, & C. Amanti (Eds.), *Funds of knowledge: Theorizing practices in households, communities, and classrooms* (pp. 47–69). New York, NY: Taylor and Francis e-Library.

Williams, D. R., Lavizzo-Mourey, R., & Warren, R. C. (1994). The concept of race and health status in America. *Public Health Reports, 109*(1), 26–41.

Wodak, R., & Meyer, M. (Eds.). (2009). Critical discourse analysis: History, agenda, theory and methodology. In R. Wodak & M. Meyer (Eds.), *Methods of critical discourse analysis* (pp. 1–33). Los Angeles, CA: Sage.

TO HEALTH CITIZENSHIP AND ADVOCACY

On Seeing Health Rhetorics as Deliberation, Power, and Resistance

LISA B. KERÄNEN

FROM PUBLIC DEBATES about the causes of illness in ancient societies to contemporary discussions about reproductive justice, health-care equity, and genomic medicine, people have long rallied around the prominent health issues of their era. Such active public involvement with medical and health matters falls under the banner of *health citizenship*, which Rimal, Ratzan, Arnston, and Freimuth (1997) defined more than two decades ago as the "individual and collective group decision-making processes that are intimately connected with individuals' well-being" (p. 70). The chapters in this section address this process of people coming together to deliberate about health and medical matters, advocating on behalf of themselves and others to create more favorable conditions for health and health-care policy, treatment, research, and practice. While the concept of health citizenship signifies an intensifying interpenetration of health and biological matters with both public and private life, the idea and practice of public policy deliberation is as old as the formal study of rhetoric itself and embodies the Isocratean notion of *synercheste,* of "coming together deliberatively" (Mitchell & McTigue, 2012, p. 92; see also Haskins, 2007; Isocrates, 1929), in this case to consider thought and activity in the realm of health and medicine.

The chapters in this section implicitly take up this Isocratean tradition of *synercheste,* the practice of using discourse to arrive at knowledge and determine action. As Gordon Mitchell and Kathleen McTigue (2012) explained, Isocrates used the concept of *synercheste* "to express interlocking senses" of inquiry, deliberation, and alliance formation (p. 83). Each of the three chapters in this section exemplifies, extends, and, on occasion, challenges the interrelated notions of health citizenship, health advocacy, and health activism. While analyzing several examples of how rhetoric functions *as* health citizenship in situ, these three chapters advance the conceptual work of rhetoric to consider how rhetoric *is*, in turn, a collective mode of public engagement, a means of enacting health-care social justice advocacy, a methodology of interpretation, and a relational praxis. Before addressing the conceptual, methodological, and practical affordances of the health citizenship and advocacy work in this section of the volume, we must first reflect, albeit momentarily, on the limitations of prevailing conceptions of citizenship.

While the dominant conception of *health,* from the Old English term *haelo* or *wholeness* (Jago, 1975) broadly references a person's mental, biological, and social condition and has evolved over time, the notion of *citizenship* conveys an even more vexed and exclusionary lineage, a full accounting of which exceeds the confines of this response (see Chávez, 2015). Noting that rhetoricians have long played "fast and loose" (Chávez, 2015, p. 164) with the idea of citizenship, Chávez (2015) traced the use of the term as a category of legal recognition in relation to the nation-state as a dominant feature of rhetoric studies. Instead, she called for challenging the idea of citizenship by including "non-normative, non-citizen, non-Western perspectives and ways of knowing and being" (p. 164). The limits and problems of conceiving of citizenship as a legal category of belonging in relation to nation-states become clear when we examine "what it obscures and implies about whose rhetorical practices are worthy of engagement, whose rhetorical practices can serve as the material basis for our rhetorical theory, and what modes of rhetorical practice as well as rhetorical theory and criticism matter" (Chávez, 2015, p. 164). Considering the possibilities for more capacious notions of citizenship as engagement and seeking to avoid its marginalizing tendencies, rhetoricians of health and medicine as a collective need to do more work unpacking, critiquing, and reformulating the idea of the "citizen" that underlies most of our models of health citizenship. Although much work remains, we can turn to examine how the chapters in this section extend our understanding of how people think and act regarding matters of health and medicine.

HEALTH CITIZENSHIP AS DELIBERATIVE DEMOCRACY AND/OR AS TECHNIQUE OF POWER

The chapters in this section implicitly invoke two interrelated senses of health citizenship that each foreground a different lineage of the rhetorical tradition and a different sense of the capacities of rhetoric. The first sense emerges from a deliberative democracy perspective and positions health citizenship as a democratically desirable process in which citizens use discourse to enact agency over the conditions of their individual health and the overall health-care systems in which they are embedded. This sense of health citizenship as deliberative democracy resonates with some of the earliest appearances of the term in twentieth-century English-language books when health citizenship often meant civic attention to health and medical matters. For instance, *The Report of the President's Committee on Health Education* (1973) noted that "developing health education programs—where virtually none exist now—in schools, offices, factories and homes; forming active neighborhood groups; involving people in the health care process—all are vital parts of good health citizenship" (p. 17). Here, the idea of health citizenship maps onto the ideal of civic engagement and deliberation. Consistent with the position articulated by Rimal et al. (1997), the traditionally passive role of "patient" is recast into that of "an active citizen who is involved in individual and collective health decision making" (Rimal et al., 1997, p. 70). This process relies on rhetoric as a means of knowing and persuading about future courses of action related to health and medical matters.

This first sense of health citizenship appears most strongly in the chapter by Rebecca Kuehl, Sara Drury, and Jenn Anderson, which merges core rhetorical tenets with the deliberative model of health citizenship to advance the notion of *rhetorical health citizenship*, which suggests that "health citizens enacting rhetorical health citizenship make myriad rhetorical choices that my be classified as activism, advocacy, or both" (p. 164, this volume). Here, citizens deliberate, discuss, challenge, and engage one another about health matters in order to prompt changes that they hope will improve the health and well-being of an expanded scope of people. In this view of health citizenship, health citizens are active agents whose discursive actions reshape health policies and practice. Kuehl, Drury, and Anderson showcase this process at work in their multi-method exploration of the two public deliberations they hosted, one about substance abuse in Indiana and one about breastfeeding support in South Dakota. They conclude that "foster-ing rhetorical health citizenship encourages communities to address public problems through rhetorical agency, public deliberation, and health citizen-ship" (p. 178, this volume). "In praxis," they write, "rhetorical health citizen-ship *is* a collective mode of public engagement that improves the physical and civic health of communities" (p. 179, this volume). By foregrounding rhetoric as democratic deliberation, Kuehl and her co-authors punctuate how community dialogue can be both an intervention into public life and a site for deliberative inquiry (Carcasson & Sprain, 2016).

Jennifer Maher offers a similar take on health citizenship when she addresses health-care advocacy from a social justice perspective. Analyzing two public health campaigns about sudden infant death syndrome (SIDS) that were created with and for African American communities that face disproportionately high rates of SIDS, Maher approvingly quotes Lee Artz (2012) that "if social justice means securing for humanity the right to all the burdens and benefits of humanity, then working for social justice must also mean we have responsibility to advocate, advance, and secure those rights as democratically, persuasively, and effectively as possible, as soon as possible, in opposition to all existing obstacles" (p. 247, as cited in Maher, p. 185, this volume). As she analyzes the workings of two local SIDS campaigns, Maher emphasizes how rhetoric as advocacy can "bring awareness" to health-care injustices and work to change the underlying material conditions that create health disparities and inequities. In line with Zoller's (2005, p. 341) definition of health activism as "efforts, often grassroots, to change norms, social structures, policies, and power relationships in the health arena," Maher shows the power of local narratives to raise consciousness about disparities and injustice.

If the sense of health citizenship in Kuehl, Drury, and Anderson's and in Maher's social justice advocacy positions health citizenship as an agentic, societally productive, and democratic(ally useful) practice, the next and not entirely mutually exclusive sense of health citizenship is at once more skeptical and Foucauldian. This second sense regards health citizenship as a technique of power and reflects the recognition that contemporary subjectivities formed around health and wellness constitute citizens as agents who are responsible for securing their own health and well-being. Drawing on the work of Dorothy Porter (2011), Spoel (2014) reminded us that the rise of what would later be termed health citizenship in the West occurred in eighteenth-century France, when "health became an obligation of the social contract held between the democratic state and its citizens" (n.p.). States thus had a duty to protect the health of the citizenry while citizens had a duty to try to remain healthy for the good of the nation (and, as Foucault would emphasize, for the growth of capitalism). Rose and Novas's (2005) treatment of the Foucauldian concept of *biological citizenship,* which Rabinow and Rose (2006) observed has been rising since World War II, similarly prompts "new kinds of patients' groups and individuals, who increasingly define their citizenship in terms of their rights (and obligations) to life, health and cure" (p. 203). This sense of health citizenship is accompanied by growing bioeconomies (or vital economies) that profit from the creation, curation, cultivation, and flow of biological materials and processes, and rhetoricians of health and medicine would do well to attend more fully to how biological matter is being created, commercialized, and mobilized around the world.

Health citizenship in this Foucauldian sense, as used by Colleen Derkatch and Philippa Spoel in the opening chapter of this volume and in Spoel's (2014) earlier work with the concept, is one that was "developed by scholars in critical health studies to explore how public health systems and policies both presume and encourage particular kinds of citizen rights and obligations in relation to health care" (n.p.). As a form of what Foucault called "knowledge/ power," this sense of health citizenship encourages attention to "how sociopolitical and economic structures of health care influence local or individual experiences, practices, and understandings of health" (Spoel, 2014, n.p.) Many studies of health citizenship in this second sense position themselves against the dominant neoliberal logic of the patient as a consumer of medical and health-care choices.

A middle-of-the-way approach to health citizenship that bears traces of both the senses appears when Amy Hickman merges the results of three years of participatory observation with a community health worker with Chela Sandoval's (2000) concept of *differential consciousness*. In so doing, Hickman illustrates how a *promotoras de salud* used Chicana feminist or *mujerista pedagogies* to reconfigure the racialized subtexts in public health messaging by strategically appropriating dominant medical discourses to promote more healthy—and therefore more resilient—Latinx communities. Hickman straddles the democratic and critical senses of health citizenship both in her focus on the agentic discursive dimensions of health citizenship and in her attention to power dynamics, relational knowledge, and forms of resistance. As such, she positions mujerista pedagogies as a form of resistance to dominant biomedical knowledge, as when, for instance, the promotora recast healthy eating practices in terms of Mexican culture by deploying generational storytelling, harking back to grandparents adopting "healthy" eating practices before the advent of industrialized fast food. Here, issues of difference and power in marginalized communities come to the fore in a community of color in ways that disrupt dominant food practices.

METHODOLOGICAL AND PRACTICAL WORK: THE RHETORIC OF HEALTH AND MEDICINE AS INTERPRETIVE, RELATIONAL, AND TRANSFORMATIVE

Even as they navigate the tension between regarding health-care citizenship as a positive force of agentic democratic deliberation or as a subject-forming

regime of power/knowledge, the essays in this section foreground the heu-
ristic capacities of rhetoric for analyzing and generating health-care rhetoric
and practice. Blending rhetorical field methods with textual analysis and providing road maps for new avenues of study, the chapters in this section have
carved paths for rhetoricians who want to extend the inquiries into and practices of health advocacy. Like Kuehl, Drury, and Anderson, scholars in this
area can draw from deliberative democracy and publics theory to analyze the
dynamics, meanings, and implications of health and medical exchanges. Like
Hickman, they can draw from feminist Chicana theory to develop insights
about how health-care promotion works, and they can merge rhetorical concepts with those from feminist and cultural studies to extend rhetorical theorizing. Like Maher, they can conduct their analyses as a practice of social
justice.

As they work through cases of rhetoric as a means of enacting health
citizenship in situ, the chapters in this section advance the conceptual work
of rhetoric to consider how rhetoric is a methodology of interpretation, a
relational praxis, a collective mode of public engagement, and a means for
promoting social justice around health-care policy and practice. Each of the
chapters extends our understanding of the conceptual/theoretical, methodological, and practical aspects of rhetoric, and each offers examples of rhetoricians of health and medicine collaborating with local citizens and health
workers to produce further health rhetorics. In short, this section reveals rhetoricians of health and medicine enacting their own health citizenship, and
their example encourages the movement of scholarly work from the vita con-
templativa toward the vita activa, focusing on how people can, do, and perhaps *should* enact the various health identities available to them and engage
with the broader health systems and discourses of which they are a part. Here,
viewing academic work as embodied resistance that works to make health-
care structure more equitable represents a robust form of health citizenship.

As rhetorical scholars increasingly collaborate with community groups
and view themselves as embodied sites of resistance who work with marginalized communities, questions of ethical engagement, power differences,
and agency come into sharp focus. How do scholars maintain trust, promote
transparency, and ensure accountability while balancing power and ensuring
continuity of the structures they are building? How do they cultivate a culture of respect, inclusion, and equity, while adhering to the strictures of the
academy? While community-based, participatory rhetorical research is often
seen as more ethical than other approaches, ethical concerns abound from
respecting indigenous forms of knowing to maintaining equal partnership in
all aspects of the research to anticipating future consequences of the partner-

ship for all involved. Humility and listening are a good start but represent only the beginning ethical requirements for such engagement.

Additionally, rhetoricians of health and medicine have more work to do to expand the scope of their focus and collaboration. The health advocacy rhetorics explored in this section take an important cue from scholars like Dutta (2008), Zoller and Dutta (2009), and Condit (2013) in not focusing exclusively on white rhetorics of health. If we look at work in the rhetoric of health and medicine as a whole, however, much room exists to expand our work in ways that center race and other aspects of intersectional identities. As a collective, rhetoricians of health and medicine—and I here readily acknowledge my own failings—certainly need to engage more intentionally with the growing social movement in communication studies that seeks to create a more inclusive field (interested readers can examine the summer 2019 archives of CRTNET, the Communication Research and Theory Network of the National Communication Association, or the Facebook group "Communication Scholars for Transformation" for details). In particular, our subfield—both when attending to health citizenships and well beyond—desperately needs to interrogate more fully, explicitly, and meaningfully the absences, silences, suppressions, and marginalizations of our own membership and scholarship and counter the whiteness that has characterized the communication field in general and our subfield in particular (see, for example, Báez & Ore, 2018; Flores 2016). Attention to race is imperative. As Lisa Flores (2016) asked:

> How could we theorize voice or vernacular *without* attention to race? What would it mean to consider representation and *not* theorize the raced bodies on display? Could we consider theories of citizenship or belonging that ignored race? We do not all need to be race scholars. But we must all be cognizant of race. (pp. xx)

For a subfield that traffics heavily in embodiment, rhetoricians of health and medicine have special obligations to recognize race and adopt explicitly anti-racist research agendas, as a small but growing number of scholars among us have done (see, for example, Dutta, 2008; Happe, 2013). But along with more explicitly centering race in their work, rhetoricians of health and medicine can do more to engage a wider range of constructs, including but not limited to sexuality, gender, social class, nationality, ethnicity, ability, and religion to expose and counter historical inequities and absences of scholarly focus and intervention, as the essays in this section begin to do. Rhetoricians of health and medicine should also draw from a broader set of works addressing difference and power, colonization, and transnational geographies in their work in the future. Admittedly, centering race and other matters of identity is not without its risks and dilemmas, and scholars working in this area need to do so with the utmost ethical care, ensuring that they avoid the "problem of speaking" for others that Linda Alcoff (1991, p. 5) famously wrote about and the tendency to reinscribe conditions of colonization and domination (Colpean & Dingo, 2018). Truly collaborative projects that focus on listening can do this.

In addition to a focus on race and intersectional identities, Condit's (2013) critique of rhetoric of science, technology, and medicine scholarship pointed out the North American focus of so much of this work. Health rhetorics increasingly occur in a world that is simultaneously expanding its global consciousness alongside a parallel reassertion of locality and nationalism. In order to balance the competing differences of multiculturalism with the homogenizing, flattening forces of globalization, rhetoricians of health and medicine will need to grapple with the synergies and tensions between global, national, and local health citizenship. Several questions to drive future work in the area include these:

- What are the preconditions for productive dialogues about health-related matters in diverse global societies? What roles can rhetoricians play in fostering and studying such dialogues? This move toward deliberative inquiry in rhetoric studies complements community-based health rhetoric scholarship and practice but more work is needed to explore and foster productive encounters among cultural, local, and national discourses around the globe.
- Following Condit's (2013) call for more international work in the rhetoric of science, technology, and medicine, what does *global* health citizenship look like, and how does it interrelate to nationally and locally focused forms of health citizenship? Do different forms of health citizenship attach to different regimes of governance? That is, is health citizenship enacted differently in authoritarian, socialist, and democratic nation-states? And how does the notion of universal health citizenship that permeates United Nations and World Health Organization discourses function, and how is this notion deployed across contexts, rhetorics, and cultures, and with what consequence?
- How can rhetoricians of health and medicine center race in their work and produce scholarship that counters the tacit whiteness of our field? Relatedly, what are the underlying assumptions of citizenship in prevailing notions of health citizenship, and whose voices do they exclude? How can rhetoricians of health and medicine work toward globally inclusive concepts, practices, and research concerning health citizenship? What are the ethical requirements of and equitable models for such engagement?

- Finally, more work can be done to articulate the roles that rhetoricians can play when engaging in health citizenship themselves. What are and should be the goals of rhetorical analysis of health citizenship and advocacy? How can rhetoricians as practitioners engage ethically and equitably with other communities, and what structures are needed to do so?

These questions, foci, and methods represent the beginning of a broader conversation to which our three chapters contribute thoughtfully. My hope is that this work stimulates a needed reconsideration of the concept of health citizenship; an elaboration of the methods by which rhetoricians of health and medicine can identify, track, and create interventions for rhetorics of health citizenship around the globe; an expansion of our methods, foci, and perspectives to more fully engage matters of race, nationality, identity, and intersectional biological belonging; and the creation of embodied practices of resistance that transform health structures across local, regional, and global settings.

REFERENCES

Alcoff, L. (1991). The problem of speaking for others. *Cultural Critique, 20,* 5–32.

Báez, K. L., & Ore, E. (2018). The moral imperative of race for rhetorical studies: On civility and walking-in-white in academe. *Communication and Critical/Cultural Studies, 15*(4), 331–336.

Campbell, K. K. (2005). Agency: Promiscuous and protean. *Communication and Critical/Cultural Studies, 2,* 1–19.

Carcasson, M., & Sprain, L. (2016). Beyond problem solving: Reconceptualizing the work of public deliberation as deliberative inquiry. *Communication Theory, 26,* 41–63.

Chávez, K. R. (2011). Counter-public enclaves and understanding the function of rhetoric in social movement coalition-building. *Communication Quarterly, 59,* 1–18.

Chávez, K. R. (2015). Beyond inclusion: Rethinking rhetoric's historical narrative. *Quarterly Journal of Speech, 101*(1), 162–172.

Colpean, M., & Dingo, R. (2018) Beyond drive-by race scholarship: The importance of engaging geopolitical contexts. *Communication and Critical/Cultural Studies, 15*(4), 306–311.

Dutta, M. J. (2008). *Communicating health: A culture-centered approach.* London: Polity.

Endres, D., Hess, A., Senda-Cook, S., & Middleton, M. K. (2016). *In situ* rhetoric: Intersections between qualitative inquiry, fieldwork, and rhetoric. *Cultural Studies, Critical Methodologies, 16*(6), 511–524. https://doi.org/10.1177%2F1532708616655820

Endres, D., Sprain, L. M., & Peterson, T. R., (2009). *Social movement to address climate change: Local steps for global action.* New York, NY: Cambria.

Flores, L. (2016). Between abundance and marginalization: The imperative of racial rhetorical criticism. *Review of Communication, 16*(1): 4–24.

Foss, S. K. (2006). Interdisciplinary perspectives on rhetorical criticism: Rhetorical criticism as synecdoche for agency. *Rhetoric Review, 25,* 375–379.

Frey, L. W., & Palmer, D. (Eds.). (2014). *Teaching communication activism: Communication education for social justice.* New York, NY: Hampton.

Happe, K. (2013). *The material gene: Gender, race, and heredity after the Human Genome Project*. New York, NY: New York University Press.

Haskins, E. V. (2007). *Logos and power in Isocrates and Aristotle*. Columbia, SC: University of South Carolina Press.

Isocrates. (1929). *Panathenaicus* (G. Norlin, Trans.). Loeb Classical Library, vol. 2. London: William Heinemann.

Jago, J. D. (1975). "Hal"—Old word, new task: Reflections on the words "health" and "medical." *Social Science & Medicine, 9*(1), 1–6.

Middleton, M., Hess A., Endres D., & Senda-Cook S. (Eds.). (2015). *Participatory critical rhetoric: Theoretical and methodological foundations for studying rhetoric in situ*. Lanham, MD: Lexington Books.

Mitchell, G. R., & McTigue, K. M. (2012). Translation through argumentation in medical research and physician-citizenship. *Journal of Medical Humanities, 33,* 83–107.

Pezzullo, P. C. (2001). Performing critical interruptions: Stories, rhetorical invention, and the environmental justice movement. *Western Journal of Communication, 65,* 1–25.

President's Committee on Health Education. (1973). *Report on the President's Committee on Health Education*. New York, NY: Department of Health, Education, and Welfare.

Rabinow, P., & Rose, N. (2006). Biopower today. *BioSocieties, 1,* 195–217.

Rimal, R. N., Ratzan, S. C., Arnston, C., & Freimuth, V. S. (1997). Reconceptualizing the "patient": Health care promotion as increasing citizens' decision-making competencies. *Health Communication, 9*(1), 61–74.

Rose, N., & Novas, C. (2005). Biological citizenship. In A. Ong & S. Collier (Eds.), *Global assemblages: Technology, politics and ethics as anthropological problems* (pp. 439–463). Malden, MA: Blackwell.

Scott, J. B., Segal, J. Z., & Keränen, L. B. (2013). The rhetorics of health and medicine: Inventional possibilities for scholarship and engaged practice. *Poroi, 9, 1,* 17. https://doi.org/10.13008/2151-2957.1157

Spoel, P. (2014). Health citizenship. In T. L. Thompson (Ed.), *Encyclopedia of health communication* (pp. 565–567). Thousand Oaks, CA: Sage. https://doi.org/10.4135/9781483346427.n218

Spoel, P., & James, S. (2006). Negotiating public and professional interests: A rhetorical analysis of the debate concerning the regulation of midwifery in Ontario, Canada. *Journal of Medical Humanities, 27,* 167–186.

Zoller, H. M. (2005). Health activism: Communication theory and action for social change. *Communication Theory, 15*(4), 341–364.

Zoller, H. M., & Dutta, M. J. (2009). *Emerging perspectives in health communication: Meaning, culture, and power*. New York, NY: Routledge.

Perspectives on the Rhetoric of Health and Medicine As/Is Past, Present, and Future

CYNTHIA RYAN, BARBARA HEIFFERON,
AND T. KENNY FOUNTAIN

WHEN THE THREE of us entered the emerging field of medical rhetoric (some of us several decades ago), we joined peers invested in questions about how knowledge is made and conveyed in health and medical realms. In our pursuit, we turned to theoretical frameworks from traditional fields to situate our ideas in existing scholarly conversations and borrowed methodologies from a host of disciplinary perspectives to examine institutional and cultural messages about health, illness, well-being, and the material and social body. Simply put, like many researchers seeking a home for their ideas and interests, we turned to established disciplines for guidance at the same time that we sought to construct new ways of forging a space that would best serve our needs.

As we reflected on the rich essays in this collection, essays that we feel truly widen the scope and perspectives of the rhetoric of health and medicine (RHM), we were struck by how far scholars have come in understanding the discipline **as** a theoretical construct while defining the boundaries that indicate what RHM **is** in relation to specific health and medical artifacts, spaces, and practices. In this final commentary on the ideas and approaches in this volume, we offer our take on the field as told through the voices presented herein.

WIDENING RHM PERSPECTIVES:
THE WORK OF THIS COLLECTION

This collection illustrates the dialectic nature of RHM to both deconstruct and reconstruct, to critique and to create. The authors presented here critique cultural norms embedded in Western biomedicine to reveal disparities and discrimination in how health care is delivered, and to whom. If and when the patient's voice is lost or misunderstood, these RHM researchers suggest ways to recover them. Using different theoretical lenses and methodologies, all participate in what Segal, in the foreword to this collection, describes as "polydisciplinary" work. RHM is a rigorous and generous field with a proven record of valuing inclusivity. Not only do RHM scholars seek to recover voices of disenfranchised cultural groups; they also welcome researchers using many different tools across a spectrum that spans the humanities to the social sciences, from academic to professional health-care contexts. Indeed, RHM has constructed a bridge across difference in multiple ways to continue its openness and forward-looking research in the face of rapidly changing medicine, health, social media and culture. This collection, then, shows the ideological face of RHM as it is: a means to disrupt and reconstruct various purposes and identities in order not only to argue against the neoliberal agenda but also to reconstruct and recover a more humanistic culture.

Importantly, this new research in RHM engages productively with the historical theories and practices of rhetoric—specifically with what Mailloux (2006), drawing from Burke, has called "the double nature of rhetoric" (p. 38). In the first and likely most common understanding, rhetoric is a speech, text, or discourse that exerts a persuasive force on audiences, a force that is crucial to and that arguably co-constitutes the act of meaning-making. In the second and hermeneutic sense, rhetoric is a capacity for analyzing or interpreting rhetorical texts and discourses. RHM, then, sheds light, in Segal's (2005) words, on "the persuasive element in [medical and health] discourse" and other texts, by analyzing how those very elements operate (p. 5). In their articulation of "rehumanizing rhetoric," Winderman and Landau, in chapter 3, describe it beautifully as the ability to make human the dehumanized rhetoric of some medical texts. Nearly all the chapters in this collection engage in this double capacity in some way, specifically through (1) the analysis of texts, objects, and discourses that persuade about or constitutively produce what counts as health and medicine; and (2) the identification of meaning-making practices and modes of critique that invite researchers and nonresearchers alike to more meaningfully interact with the ideas, discourses, and actors involved in health and medicine.

Using a variety of research methods and theoretical conceptions, chapters across all sections in this anthology—Interdisciplinary Perspectives, Representations and Online Health, and Health Citizenship and Advocacy—demonstrate the useful fluidity of rhetorical concepts and formations involved in looking at multivariate forms of health and medical discourse. Scholars turn to older rhetorical concepts—such as topoi, metonymy, personification, pathos—in ways that build from, yet are not constrained by, the ancient tradition. These chapters demonstrate the generative space made possible at the intersection of health and medicine and rhetoric. In the process of making this space visible, they demonstrate the centrality of some of the key concepts that RHM shares—deliberation, communication, representation, and identification.

Because this collection also represents, in this push/pull, deconstruct/reconstruct movement, the dialectical nature of RHM, we see the essays presented here as a further development of what McComiskey (2015) termed "three-dimensional rhetorics," which seek to address multiple audiences of not necessarily oppositional views. As the scholars in this collection attest, RHM often plays the role of advocacy and negotiation, mediating between various views—and, in McComiskey's words, the various "values and interests of *different* . . . orientations competing for public attention," creating "new orientations in the process" (p. 4). Viewing the work of RHM through this three-dimensional, dialectical perspective reveals the value of projects like this collection to forge common ground with stakeholders disparately placed.

As the work in this collection demonstrates, RHM's contribution to the study of health, illness, and medicine involves more of what we indeed find in humanities disciplines—that is, a rehumanizing of the subject. In chapter 1, Derkatch and Spoel suggest that what the multivalent and overlapping approaches that make up health humanities have in common is the true "'humanizing' potential of humanities instruction within the health professions as a means of expanding practitioners' capacities for empathy and care, and for understanding patients' unique 'lifeworlds'" (p. 14). They not only pose "health humanities over [just] medical humanities," in that "'health' situates [the body] within a broader frame of living by encompassing all the factors that affect health" (p. 14); they also contend that RHM stands as an exemplar of health humanities. Thus, Derkatch and Spoel invite rhetoricians of health and medicine to take "a broader consideration of the intersections between health and human life" (p. 14).

As evidenced by nearly every chapter here, rhetoricians do indeed seek to improve the *practice* of medicine through the inclusion of humanities and an attention to rhetoric itself. Whether or not improving medical practices is the central goal of our work, we suggest that this potential effect might be viewed as an advancement over mere critique; after all, critique reveals the need for changing current medical practices, yet the creation of new ideas, perspectives, and practices builds something productive and constructive from the terrain that critique opens up. The collection does indeed widen our perspectives on what critique can be and the types of creation it can foster, as RHM here is often staged as advocacy and recovery of voices previously unrecognized. Many of the essays here demonstrate that critique and creation can work hand-in-hand to uncover and address inequalities.

In chapter 5, Friz and Overholt deconstruct an interface for a reductive technology that quantifies women's pregnancies and sexual behaviors, clearly a site where the fulsome voices of women have been severely limited. Other authors in this collection also address how sexist and racially discriminatory medical practices shape the health, well-being, and even life expectancy of women and people of color. In chapter 8, Maher, for example, looks at the role of sudden infant death syndrome (SIDS) in babies' health, to position RHM as and is a form of social justice, one that reveals the causes and effects of racial disparities and intervenes to change them. Hickman, in chapter 9, analyzes the practices and texts of one community health worker (or CHW) in order to spotlight the strategies the CHW uses to educate and advocate for the Latinx community. In the process, Hickman outlines the rhetorical economies of public health that shape the work of all public health actors. Finally, Winderman and Landau's methodology and aims, instead of providing a deconstruction of what happened to Henrietta Lacks's cancer cells, are intended to recuperate the role of emotion to rehumanize patients through rhetorical and material techniques of personification and affiliation, offering a compelling model of how to humanize medicine and health.

LOOKING FORWARD: WHERE MIGHT WE GO FROM HERE?

But where might this widening perspective take our polydisciplinary field? By way of conclusion, we would like to offer a few suggestions, if not predictions. After all, this collection offers important indications of a number of growing trends in RHM. As evidenced in this collection, in the work of Singer and Jack (chapter 6), Kessler (chapter 4), and Friz and Overholt (chapter 5), we predict a more dedicated effort in RHM to investigate the ways that new and emerging media, such as social media, facilitate our conceptions of health, illness, and medicine. There is a growing need for scholars of RHM to examine the tools and technologies of the networked, digital media—apps, devices, and platforms—that we use to monitor our health and connect with others. These pervasive multimodal texts merge the verbal, visual, aural, kinesthetic, haptic, and locative in ways that will continue to influence how we communicate, deliberate, and conceptualize our evolving forms of health citizenship.

Scholars of RHM who come from academic disciplines that study such multimodal texts are well suited to make a significant contribution. But to do this work, we must look at not only the verbal message but the visual one as well. If there is one missed opportunity in this book, it is the absence of a deep engagement with visual rhetorical scholarship in RHM. Perhaps because we perceive visual representations as unavoidable (almost irreducible) to health and medical discourse, scholars in this volume have looked past the images to the practices they make possible, in the process overlooking, no doubt inadvertently, an opportunity to deconstruct and reconstruct the visuals that shape health and medicine.

As many of these chapters demonstrate, scholars in RHM are committed to questions and concepts at the foundation of rhetorical studies. By returning to such formations as genre (Derkatch & Spoel, chapter 1), topoi (Holladay & Price, chapter 2), rhetorical identification (Singer & Jack, chapter 6), and rhetorical agency (Kuehl, Drury, & Anderson, chapter 7), scholarship in RHM will continue to demonstrate the conceptual and explanatory power of rhetorical concepts. However, as the researchers here demonstrate, RHM often puts the rhetorical tradition in productive conversation with new philosophical and political lenses. The field's increasing interest in, for example, philosophy and feminist thought brings to scholarly investigations complex understandings of ontology (Kessler, chapter 4), biopolitics (Friz & Overholt, chapter 5), embodiment (Singer & Jack, chapter 6), and ethics (Maher, chapter 8). From this intersection, we are certain to build new rhetorical concepts specific to our field, evidenced here by Singer and Jack's "chronicity" and Kessler's "rhetorical enactments." In these two chapters, which analyze the ways that chronic illness and autoimmunity are represented and conceptualized in online spaces, Singer and Jack and Kessler, respectively, show how digital and new media spaces are themselves reconceiving rhetorical theories in exciting ways to which RHM researchers must attend. By engaging with research in disability studies, feminism, gender and queer studies, and race and ethnicity studies, RHM will provide a more methodologically, theoretically, and politically sophisticated analysis of the ways that gender, sex, gender expression, and race and ethnicity—bodies and identities—shape medicine, health, and illness. Holladay and Price, in chapter 2, persuasively demonstrate the utility of integrating key disability studies concepts into the research on RHM in order to strengthen not only our scholarship but also the social and material consequences of that scholarship.

As many of the scholars here might agree, questions of social justice (Winderman & Landau, chapter 3; Maher, chapter 8) and health citizenship (Derkatch & Spoel, chapter 1; Friz & Overholt, chapter 5; Hickman, chapter 9; Kuehl, Drury, & Anderson, chapter 7) are and will continue to be a motivating force of the work we do. We are inspired by the social justice research in this collection, for instance Kuehl, Drury, and Anderson's contribution, which proposes the concept of *rhetorical* health citizenship as a way of articulating rhetoric's role in health-related deliberations.

While RHM researchers will continue to collaborate with health-care workers to study and improve medical practices on the local level, we also predict that our collaborations with stakeholders will expand to include scientific researchers who increasingly recognize and value the contribution of humanities scholars not just as teachers and advocates but as academic researchers with the potential to enrich scientific and social scientific projects as well as to impact policy. Hopefully these collaborations will enrich the scientific studies done in medicine, nursing, public health, and other health-care domains by infusing them with the kinds of interpretative, historical, and qualitative methods that are so productive in RHM. However, we also recognize that RHM research might be transformed by these collaborations, particularly when we begin to adopt more quantitative methods and larger data sets. Incorporating statistical analysis into our current methods will allow us to ask new and different questions of rhetoric, health, and medicine. These multidisciplinary partnerships have to potential to shape not just the types of research we conduct but also the audiences we address. As we participate as active collaborators on multidisciplinary teams, we might see changes in the way we present and discuss our work in venues targeted for those outside the field. We already see this in the journal *Rhetoric of Health and Medicine*'s "persuasive briefs," which are targeted in part to audiences beyond RHM.

Broadly speaking, the scholars who work in RHM are interested not only in articulating the ways that knowledge is made and distributed in health and medical contexts, but also in identifying and assessing the outcomes that arise from this examination. The inclusive nature of RHM demonstrated by the authors in the collection offers scholars a wide range of disciplines and methodologies with and within which to work in approaching key questions in the field. As a result, we enjoy the advantage of asking more compelling and complex questions regarding both health and medical issues situated in a wide continuum of contexts. As a theoretical construct and a coherent, albeit inclusive, set of methodological practices, RHM *is* a mode of critique, analysis, and interpretation that compels us to interrogate the ways that communication—in all its multivariate, multimodal, and material forms—makes health and medicine possible. Once we understand the possibilities that languages, discourses, texts, objects, and bodies both afford and deny, then we can engage with RHM *as* a mode of creation, generation, and poiesis. This as/is capacity of RHM offers new opportunities—both conceptual and practical opportunities—for reimagining how we experience health and medicine.

REFERENCES

Mailloux, S. (2006) *Disciplinary identities: Rhetorical paths of English, speech, and composition.* New York, NY: Modern Language Association.

McComiskey, B. (2015) *Dialectical rhetoric.* Logan, UT: Utah State University Press.

Segal, J. (2005). *Health and the rhetoric of medicine.* Carbondale, IL: Southern Illinois University Press.

CONTRIBUTORS

JENN ANDERSON is Associate Professor in the School of Communication and Journalism at South Dakota State University. They serve as the Coordinator for the M.A. in Communication & Media Studies program. They also founded and coordinate the undergraduate Health Communication Minor. Dr. Anderson has published over 30 peer-reviewed articles in journals such as *American Behavioral Scientist, Health Communication, Journal of Applied Communication Research, Translational Behavioral Medicine,* and *Qualitative Health Research.*

COLLEEN DERKATCH is Associate Professor of Rhetoric in the Department of English and the Graduate Program in Communication and Culture at Ryerson University in Toronto, Canada, and the author of *Bounding Biomedicine: Evidence and Rhetoric in the New Science of Alternative Medicine* (University of Chicago Press, 2016). Her research focuses on rhetorics of natural health and wellness, local food and food security, and intersections between biomedicine and other approaches to health and health care.

SARA A. MEHLTRETTER DRURY is Chair and Associate Professor of Rhetoric and Director of the Wabash Democracy and Public Discourse initiative at Wabash College. Her research analyzes the quality and character of public discourse in the US, with specific interests in democratic deliberation, political rhetoric, and religious rhetoric. Drury has collaborated on projects across Indiana, Illinois, Kentucky, Delaware, and South Dakota, focusing on topics such as community planning, poverty, race and justice, and public health.

T. KENNY FOUNTAIN is Associate Professor of English and Director of Writing Across the Curriculum at the University of Virginia. His interests include the rhetoric of science and medicine, visual rhetoric, political rhetoric, and the history of rhetoric—specifically ancient and medieval. He is the author of *Rhetoric in the Flesh: Trained Vision, Technical Expertise, and the Gross Anatomy Lab* (Routledge, 2014).

AMANDA FRIZ is Assistant Professor in the Department of Communication at the University of Washington. Her work braids together the rhetoric of health and medicine and science and technology studies, focusing on medical scientific constructions of women's sexual health, anatomy, and sexual desire. When not teaching or researching, she can be found in the Wasatch Mountains camping or skiing.

S. SCOTT GRAHAM is Assistant Professor in the Department of Rhetoric & Writing at the University of Texas at Austin. He works at the intersection of computational rhetorics and science, technology, and medicine studies. His first book, *The Politics of Pain Medicine* (University of Chicago Press, 2015), offers a praxiographic exploration of interdisciplinary pain medicine and related public policy. He is currently using computational methods to study conflicts of interest in biomedical publishing.

BARBARA SHERMAN HEIFFERON is Professor Emerita at Louisiana State University. Her sixth book is an analysis of the resistance to the first American smallpox inoculation in 1721. Other works address writing studies and medical rhetoric more generally and include *Writing in the Health Professions*; *The Rhetoric of Healthcare: Essays toward a New Disciplinary Inquiry,* with Stuart Brown; and numerous articles. Her interest in medicine derives from her first career as a cardiopulmonary technologist.

AMY HICKMAN is Lecturer in Health Promotion, at the School of Public Health, University of Queensland, Australia. She completed her doctorate at the University of Arizona in Rhetoric, Composition and the Teaching of English. Her current research interests include the rhetorics of health and medicine, feminist research methodologies, critical public health, health communication, and community health literacies.

DREW HOLLADAY is Assistant Professor of English at the University of Maryland, Baltimore County. His research combines the rhetoric of health and medicine with disability studies to examine writing about medicine, the brain, and mental health. His writing is published in *Technical Communication Quarterly* and *JAC* as well as the edited collection *Literatures of Madness*. He also co-edited the collection *Writing for Engagement: Responsive Practice for Social Action.*

JORDYNN JACK is Professor of English and Comparative Literature at the University of North Carolina, Chapel Hill, where she teaches courses in rhetoric of science, women's rhetorics, rhetorical theory, and health humanities. She is the author of three books, *Science on the Home Front: American Women Scientists in World War II* (University of Illinois Press, 2009); *Autism and Gender: From Refrigerator Mothers to Computer Geeks* (University of Illinois Press, 2014); and *Ravelling the Brain: Toward a Transdisciplinary Neurorhetoric* (The Ohio State University Press, 2019).

JENELL JOHNSON is Mellon-Morgridge Professor of the Humanities and Associate Professor of Communication Arts at the University of Wisconsin–Madison. She is the author of *American Lobotomy: A Rhetorical History* (University of Michigan Press, 2014), editor of *Graphic Reproduction* (Pennsylvania State University Press, 2018), and co-editor of *Biocitizenship* (New York University Press, 2018) and *The Neuroscientific Turn* (University of Michigan Press, 2012).

LISA KERÄNEN is Associate Professor and Chair of the Department of Communication at the University of Colorado Denver. Her research and teaching span biopolitics, bioethics, and viral discourses. She is the author of the award-winning *Scientific Characters: Rhetoric, Politics and Trust in Breast Cancer Research* (University of Alabama Press, 2010), co-editor of *Imagining China: Rhetorics of Nationalism in an Age of Globalization* (Michigan State University Press, 2017), and the author of scholarly articles about the rhetoric of health and medicine. She is a past president of the Association for the Rhetoric of Science, Technology, and Medicine.

MOLLY MARGARET KESSLER is Assistant Professor of Writing Studies at the University of Minnesota, Twin Cities. Her research areas include rhetoric of health and medicine, technical communication, and disability studies. Most recently, her research focuses on patients' lived experiences, medical technologies, digestive diseases and treatments, and the gut microbiome. Her research has been published in *Rhetoric of Health and Medicine, Journal of Health Communication, Technical Communication Quarterly,* and *Rhetoric Society Quarterly.*

REBECCA A. KUEHL is Associate Professor in the School of Communication and Journalism and Women, Gender, & Sexuality Studies program coordinator at South Dakota State University. Her research focuses on intersections among rhetorical citizenship and public deliberation, civic rhetoric and education, and women's health discourses. Her research has been funded by two Community Innovation grants from the Bush Foundation, the charitable arm of 3M.

JAMIE LANDAU is Associate Professor of Communication Arts and Director of the Center for Excellence in Learning & Teaching at Valdosta State University in Georgia. In general, her research has always explored how verbal rhetoric and mediated images influence US public policy and social change related to gender/sexuality and health/medicine. Her recent scholarship also examines public feelings, both how they are communicated and how rhetorical scholars study them.

JOHN LYNCH is Professor of Communication and a Resident Fellow at the Center for Philosophy of Science at the University of Pittsburgh. His work focusing on rhetoric of science, bioethics, and argumentation has been published within and beyond the field of communication and includes collaborative work with scholars in the sciences and the humanities. While supervising many doctoral dissertations at the University of Iowa and at the University of Pittsburgh, where he received the *Provost's Award for Excellence in Graduate Mentoring,* he served as Chair at both of those departments. He is a past President of the Association for the Rhetoric of Science, Technology, and Medicine.

JOHN LYNE Professor of Communication and a Resident Fellow at the Center for Philosophy of Science at the University of Pittsburgh. His work focusing on rhetoric of science, bioethics, and argumentation has been published within and beyond the field of communication and includes collaborative work with scholars in the sciences and the humanities. While supervising many doctoral dissertations at the University of Iowa and at the University of Pittsburgh, where he received the *Provost's Award for Excellence in Graduate Mentoring*, he served as Chair at both of those departments. He is a past President of the Association for the Rhetoric of Science, Technology, and Medicine.

JENNIFER HELENE MAHER is Associate Professor at the University of Maryland, Baltimore County, where she teaches in the English Department's Communication and Technology track and is an affiliate faculty member in the Language, Literacy, and Culture Ph.D. program. She is the author of *Software Evangelism and the Rhetoric of Morality: Coding Justice in a Digital Democracy* (Routledge, 2016), which examines rhetorics of freedom encoded in software.

LISA MELONÇON is Professor of Technical Communication at the University of South Florida. Her research in RHM focuses on innovative methodologies, place, time, and contexts. She is the co-editor of *Methodologies for the Rhetoric of Health and Medicine* (Routledge, 2018) and the editor of *Rhetorical Accessability* (Baywood, 2012). With J. Blake Scott, she co-founded and co-edits the journal *Rhetoric of Health and Medicine*. She is currently finishing a book on early modern medicine and rhetoric.

STACEY OVERHOLT is Assistant Professor in the Department of Management at the University of Utah. Her work focuses on representations of and discourses about cancer in media, as well as the surveillant functions of health technologies. She resides in Salt Lake City with her very fuzzy Yorkie named Jules.

MARGARET PRICE is Associate Professor of English at The Ohio State University, specializing in disability studies and rhetoric/composition/literacy. Her book *Mad at School: Rhetorics of Mental Disability and Academic Life* (University of Michigan Press, 2011) won the Outstanding Book Award from the Conference on College Composition and Communication. In 2017 Price was inducted into the Susan M. Daniels Disability Mentoring Hall of Fame. Price is a co-founder of the Transformative Access Project, which centers race, disability, gender, sexuality, class, and location in exploring questions of access.

CYNTHIA RYAN is Associate Professor of English at the University of Alabama Birmingham. She studies messages about health and medicine in the media and healthcare organizations, examining the implications of these discourses on a variety of stakeholders. She teaches science writing, medical writing, and magazine writing at the University of Alabama at Birmingham and publishes in both academic journals and public outlets. Ryan runs a cancer education program alongside homeless women in Birmingham called Street Smarts™ and is committed to portraying the complexities of cancer survivorship.

J. BLAKE SCOTT is Professor of Writing & Rhetoric at the University of Central Florida, where he previously served as founding Associate Chair and Director of Degree Programs. With Lisa Melonçon, he is a founding co-editor of the journal *Rhetoric of Health & Medicine*. His work in RHM includes rhetorical-cultural studies of HIV testing and prevention policy, transnational pharmaceutical policy, the sociocultural infrastructures of electronic health records, and prescription drug microinfluencers.

JUDY Z. SEGAL is Professor in the Department of English Language and Literatures and in the Science and Technology Studies Graduate Program at the University of British Columbia. Her research on rhetorics of health and medicine appears in journal articles and book chapters across disciplines and in the monograph *Health and the Rhetoric of Medicine* (Southern Illinois University Press, 2005).

SARAH ANN SINGER is Assistant Professor of English at the University of Central Florida, where she teaches courses in the Technical Communication program. Her research interests lie at the intersection of scientific and medical rhetoric and digital media. Sarah's work appears or is forthcoming in *College English, Technical Communication Quarterly, Peitho,* and *Journal of Medical Humanities.*

PHILIPPA SPOEL is Professor of Rhetoric in the Department of English, Masters in Science Communication, and PhD in Human Studies at Laurentian University in Sudbury, Canada. Her research focuses on rhetorical criticism of health, science, and environmental communication, including midwifery communication, lay perspectives on healthy living, environmental controversies, discourses of local food and food security, and the rhetoric of "citizen science" in environmental and health research.

EMILY WINDERMAN is Assistant Professor in the Department of Communication Studies at the University of Minnesota, Twin Cities. She studies historical and contemporary discourses concerning health, emotion, and the formation of collective identity. Addressing the circulation of public emotions in contexts such as the birth control movement, pregnancy loss, and abortion politics, she examines how rhetorical action circulates emotions like anger, disgust, and grief to negotiate controversies related to public health and reproductive justice.

INDEX

9 780814 255971